The Bootstrap Gu

Medicinal

HERBS

in the

GARDEN, FIELD
& MARKETPLACE

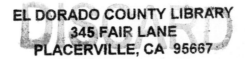

The Bootstrap Guide to

Medicinal HERBS

in the

GARDEN, FIELD & MARKETPLACE

by Lee Sturdivant & Tim Blakley

Illustrations by Peggy Sue McRae

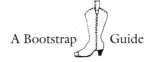

A Bootstrap Guide

Published by
SAN JUAN NATURALS
PO BOX 642
FRIDAY HARBOR, WA 98250

Book design by Jack Lanning for Words & Deeds

SAN 251-6497

ISBN 0-9621635-7-0
Library of Congress Catalog No. 98-060624

10 9 8 7 6 5 4 3 2 1

For Heather and Tal,
for always making it happen

Contents

"Small business is the understory of commerce, where new ideas and diversity arise and are processed into growth. One of the purposes of the restorative economy is to ensure that innovative commercial options have a chance to survive in the monoculture of corporate capitalism. Like any new species, the new ... small business has to find a niche, some crevice in the marketplace in which it can adapt to the dominant commercial system and then live long enough to tell the tale."

Paul Hawken, *The Ecology of Commerce*, 1993

Part I

by Lee Sturdivant

*"Between 1960 and 1986
the National Cancer Institute tested
more than 35,000 plant species—
only five to ten percent of the total plant species—
and nearly 1,400 showed anti-cancer activity."*

American Botanical Council, 1998

Acknowledgments

I write this list of people to thank with a genuine sense of humility at just how many people I have called upon and relied upon for help in getting it done. To each and every one of them I express my sincere thanks for their time and efforts. I am also grateful to those who have contacted me over the years about herbs, flowers, small business, and our Bootstrap Guides™. It is only through this continued exchange of ideas that I ever feel at all qualified to be taking on a project like this. Not so much to offer special expertise, as to help keep the world of market gardening—that happy arena for so many of us—alive and well. Working with Heather and Tim has also been a real pleasure; how lucky all medicinal herb people are to have such hard-working enthusiasts in the field—and at the word processor.

A hearty salute to artist and friend Peggy Sue McRae, for this fourth plant book she has illustrated for us. Peggy Sue has moved on to marble sculpturing; I so appreciate her taking the time to work again with us.

Special thanks to: Hal Bellerud, Tim Blakley, Charles Brun, Richo Cech, John & Louise Dustrude, Marlin Huffman, Kerwin Johnson, Alison Kutz Troutman, Jim Lawrence, Jim Macpherson, Suzette Mahr, Robyn Martin, Allison McCutcheon, John & Elaine McLeod, Heather McNeil, Mike & Lynn Monroe, Michael Pilarski, Linda Quintana, Sandy Richard, Conrad Richter, Mark Roh, Tierney Salter, Phil Schulz, Clarissa Smith, Beverly Swanson, United Plant Savers, Kelly Van Allen, Mark & Marggy Wheeler, Janet Wright, and Craig Winters.

My thanks also to my family and personal friends who put up with me during this busy time, often carrying my load in both family and community as I worked on the book. I know I owe you all. Big time.

Lee Sturdivant

A Tidal Wave of Herbs

A wave of interest in medicinal herbs has been steadily building just off the North American coastline of consciousness for several years. Constant reports of the increasing use of medicinal herbs by consumers everywhere showed the wave to be getting huge—as if poised just over the broad stream of popular culture we all call the mainstream.

I got a phone call the other day that made me realize that the medicinal herb wave has indeed already crested and cracked open; that it's now starting to flood all areas of the country.

My friend Peggy, who has been very ill, called to tell me that her medical care provider, the largest nonprofit HMO in the country, had encouraged her to switch from Prozac, the much prescribed anti-depression pill, to St. John's wort, an herbal medicine made from the flowers and stems of a small plant (*hypericum perforatum*) that is considered an invasive weed on pastures in parts of North America.

"Did you try it?" I asked, at first stunned by the idea of such a huge company making a recommendation that only a year or so ago would have seemed far beyond possible.

"You bet I did," she responded. "And I liked it. Less side effects. The trouble is, they don't pay for it. Actually, it's not that expensive."

In my drug store today, the price of Prozac pills, available only by prescription, is just over $2.50 per pill, in quantities of a hundred. At the same drug store today, tablets of St. John's wort, standardized at 300 mg. of *hypericin,* are available without a prescription, at 12¢ each. At home, the fresh flowers of St. John's wort can be rather easily combined with grain alcohol (or vodka), into what herbalists call a whole-plant herbal tincture.

It's tsunami time, I told myself. The long and fervent push from so many consumers for a more "natural" form of medicine has finally met up with the search for cost savings by the health care industry. Get ready, North America, it's time to take your herbal medicine, ready or not.

The good news (I think) is that we really are ready for such a change. Three-fourths of the people in the world have never stopped using medicinal herbs the way Americans stopped using them in the 1920s and '30s. The drug store shelves in Europe have long carried herbal preparations right alongside the other over-the-counter (OTC) medications. Many North Americans have been demanding that same herbal choice here for many years, and now that choice is actually coming on stream, with almost flash flood force.

Estimates are that over a third of the U.S. population now uses herbal remedies; that alternative remedy sales are the fastest growing segment in over-the-counter drug sales; and that by the end of this century, 88% of the North American population will be using what is commonly called *alternative care*. Will it still be called alternative, I wonder?

This book is about the small business opportunities in that burgeoning world of medicinal herbs: about the plants, products, people, and ideas involved in that world. We'll explore the ways for you to successfully grow, gather, and supply the herbs; to learn to make and sell the products; to educate yourself about plant medicine, and to become a part of this suddenly more popular health care phenomenon.

There are two of us writing this fourth Bootstrap Guide. I've been doing the interviews with all the growers, practitioners, and product makers; gathering the resource materials, and learning about the potential openings for newcomers in the medicinal herb markets of North America; an overview of an evolving and fast changing scene.

Tim Blakley brings everything back into sharp focus by sharing his long years of field work in growing, harvesting, and preparing herbs for medicine makers. His specific, crop by crop, detailed, A to Z growing chapter may be the first thing you'll want to turn to, if you are an experienced grower and now considering medicinal herb growing. Together, we aim to help you learn just how this small business sector is operating in the country, and how you can participate—at least at the start-up level.

First, a few words about the geography. Two years ago, when I began work on this book, I made a couple of fast trips across the country in search of medicinal herb growers. Although there were lots of herb users, and even a few medicinal herb practitioners in many places, in only a few parts of the U.S. and Canada were there any serious efforts then being made to grow medicinal herbs for all the new markets.

What was barely starting in other areas, was already quite obvious where I live. In my area, the Pacific northwest, the herbal renaissance had been happening for quite a few years; I've been writing and selling books about that renaissance for over ten years myself. I decided to center my own interviewing and research for this medicinal herb book primarily in the northwest, where the small medicinal herb business examples are so varied and plentiful. That would also let me demonstrate how the important herbal networks—so vital to the herb renaissance—operate in my area. Those herb webs or networks are now forming everywhere, and can become a big help in your own small business efforts.

If you live in the Rocky Mountains, the southwest, the Ozarks, the Appalachian area, or some parts of New England, you are also in a more active area of medicinal herb interest. From all those herb interest centers, with the help of several magazines and newsletters, associations, research foundations, universities and, most especially, from a remarkable group of modern American and Canadian professional herbalists, the ideas and knowledge about the medicinal uses of these plants will continue to spread across the country in the coming years.

Tim Blakley has worked as a commercial herb grower in several parts of the country including Iowa, Ohio, Oregon, and California. His work has been completely hands-on: propagating, growing, harvesting, drying, and preparing the plants for product making by a couple of the most reputable whole-plant medicine companies in the country.

Tim has also taught about herbs for years, but it's his growing efforts that bring something special to this book. The library shelves are filling up now with wonderful books about how to use medicinal herbs; ours is the first one to show you how to actually grow and then market these useful botanicals.

Our emphasis will be on the plants themselves, on organic growing, on local and regional networks, and on the importance of learning to grow and collect herbal medicines well—whether or not you ever intend to make a business in herbs. This kind of medicinal herb know-how is like knowing how to grow your own food well. It gives you a more confident stance in a commercial world that tugs at us every day to do less and less for ourselves; to become ever more dependent on product corporations for everything about our lives—from ready-made biscuits to simple headache cures. Learning about medicinal plants and herbal medicines can also tie us firmly to the earth—where we all belong—and to all people with whom we share this tiny garden of life, so filled with the remarkable plants we are now rediscovering.

Finally, learning about these plants can start you on a small business adventure full of opportunities and pitfalls. I think again of the herb business scene these days as one of huge waves crashing over the countryside. Some of the biggest companies in the world are right now trying to gain domination and ride this new consumer interest for enormous profits. We aren't going to show you how to win in some giant corporate herb medicine wave riding championship. Rather, we're going to try to direct you to a different area of the beach entirely. If you want to surf these waves and not get wiped out, we think you've got to start small and learn big. We also think we can show you how to have a successful start—and a fun ride.

A Word About Prices & Chaos

There are prices all through this book because we know our readers want very much to know what kind of money can be earned in this relatively new world of medicinal herbs. But please keep in mind that the prices you read are simply those we are finding in the marketplace at the time the book is being written. They should be seen as very tentative; very dependent on where the market is when you begin to participate. Tim and I have each found very different prices in the marketplace for identical herbs. Not too reassuring to readers, I know. Medicinal herb prices are completely unstable and very volatile; they will probably continue to be that way for some time to come.

In fact, much of the medicinal herb world is full of chaos and instability right now as it undergoes such rapid expansion, and as a part of it moves into the mass market. Very stable markets seldom offer openings for newcomers, so bear with the crazy parts; those may be the best places for market entry.

The governments in both the U.S. and Canada are also not yet finished with their regulatory concerns about medicinal herbs. This may well be a book Tim and I will have to revise fairly often, as almost every chapter had breaking news about its subject as it was being written. If you feel like you're being invited to learn about surfboard riding during an El Niño, you're wrong. It really is a tsunami.

CHAPTER ONE

Meet the Growers

Dirt First

You will meet some successful medicinal herb and medicinal mushroom growers on these next pages, and get some idea of the commitment and cost necessary to make a start in growing these plants commercially.

Actually, almost every succeeding chapter of the book will also include sections on growing, because that is the main emphasis we want to keep in the book, and because most people who become involved in medicinal herbs find that the source of the plants turns out to be of primary importance in obtaining quality herbal medicines. Growers, wildcrafters, herbal practitioners, product makers, and sellers—all must be concerned with the quality of the plants, which are the basis of their businesses.

Business opportunities with medicinal herbs truly are plentiful, whether you decide to grow herbs to sell fresh or dried directly to a medicine making company; to grow for a broker—who sells them to others; to grow botanicals to sell as nursery plants, seeds, or roots; to grow or find good plants from which to make and sell your own medicinal herb products; to become a practicing medicinal herbalist—using what you grow for that purpose; or combining several of these as many of the people in this book do. Whatever path you take, the quality of the herbs you use will help determine your success. All of this "medicinal herb stuff" one hears so much hype about these days is based on the reactions in our bodies to the chemicals in those plants. The best grown, best treated and prepared herbs will give the best results. Period.

At the end of the book, you will find many suggestions for looking further into the subject of growing and marketing medicinal herbs—in both the U.S. and Canada. That resource section may well be the most useful part for you. It's getting to be a very big world out there on the subject of medicinal herbs. Tim and I certainly don't have all the answers or all the directions; we do hope to help you find your way into and through some of that world.

Growing Medicinal Herb Blossoms

❦ *Pacific Botanicals*

First comes some inside knowledge and advice from well established, medicinal herb growers who supply many of the small to medium sized herb product companies in the U.S. Meet Mark and Marggy Wheeler of Pacific Botanicals.

Their 110-acre certified organic farm is in the Applegate Valley of southwest Oregon, where they started growing medicinal herbs commercially nearly 20 years ago. When they first moved to the area, the Wheelers intended to grow organic peaches, but they had been growing some medicinal herbs for their own health all during the '70s.

Unknown to the Wheelers, Herb Pharm, one of the earliest and best known of the herbal tincture companies, was also starting out in the same area at the same time. The Wheelers did grow peaches, but Herb Pharm bought some of their medicinal herbs and, as there weren't many places in those days to purchase organically grown medicinal herbs, the Herb Pharm needs soon led the Wheelers to plant more and more herbs.

Today, Pacific Botanicals grows more than 30 medicinal herbs for many companies. They also act as brokers for other organic growers and wildcrafters around the country, always encouraging new growers with helpful advice. They also do some importing of organically grown herbs.

Every year they experiment with growing new plants, always trying to look ahead and guess what will be in demand a few years down the road. This year the Wheelers are trying out stevia and psyllium. These plant trials keep them very attentive to the medicinal herb market.

The Wheelers also stress how important their plant trials are for figuring out their true costs. "You have to figure out what you are going to charge to make a living growing these herbs. And, if you just go out and start growing them and then decide to charge what everyone else is charging, you might lose a lot of money. Keep close track," Mark suggests, "of all your plant and seed costs, plus the time they take to get planted and taken care of, and then add in the land and water costs, plus the harvest costs. Then take your harvest plant weight and decide how much to charge, based on all those figures."

One other decision that complicates herb pricing is whether you will be selling the herb fresh or dried. About half of what the Wheelers grow is sent out fresh. That means the herbs have to be picked, cleaned, packed in ice, boxed and labeled—all by two o'clock in the afternoon to be ready for the FedEx and UPS pickups that carry the boxes to the airports. This intensive harvest and packaging allows the herbs to be delivered, on ice, to their customers' labs within 20 hours of picking. It's also expensive.

The herb company making the purchase determines whether they want the product fresh or dried, and that usually depends on what they are using it for. It's the possible loss of medicinal chemicals in plants that makes most reputable herb companies willing to spend the money for expensive air freight deliveries on herbs intended for fresh herb tinctures.

One herb the Wheelers only sell fresh is corn silk: *zea mays*, often used for urinary tract problems. "This is one of those herbs," says Mark, "that we can only sell fresh. We can do okay with it by selling it for 10 or 12 dollars a pound (the price depends on the amount purchased.) Most of the corn silk on the market comes from corn canneries; it's all brown and ghastly looking, and sells for only one dollar a pound. There's no way we could compete with that."

Instead, they grow a regular sweet corn, Golden Jubilee, that gives a lovely, lightly colored yellow silk when it's picked quite young. They pick the ears early in the morning, quickly remove the silk, then send it packed on ice to arrive in perfect condition the next day at the labs.

Not all herbal product companies or herb practitioners demand such a high quality product to work with, of course, but enough of them do to have made Pacific Botanicals one of the more successful organic herb farms in the country. They now have 10 people working in the fields, and seven people just to handle all the shipping and marketing. If you are serious about eventually becoming a large grower of medicinals, Pacific Botanicals is the kind of company you would want to try to emulate. Their success comes from lots of hard work, plus their ability to always push the ideas of high quality, freshness, and organic growing. Those three ideas would also be any newcomer's keys to opening up the doors to marketing in the medicinal herb world.

The Wheelers suggest that new medicinal herb growers might consider herb blossoms as their first crops, because they are usually easier and faster than many medicinal herb crops, and are a good way to break into the medicinals market. Blossoms are very labor intensive, but they are a relatively easy way through the door to the medicinal herb product world, as most product companies need a constant supply. They are also good plants for beginners to use trying out their own herb teas, salves, and tinctures.

Starting out by supplying a good crop of blossoms could more than likely lead a grower into the more complicated growing of higher priced crops, say the Wheelers. Much of the small but growing world of high quality, organically grown medicinal crops that this book is talking about is being built up on trust and reputation. It can take some time for growers to find just the right crop for their own area, and then the right buyer for what they are able to do well. On top of that, it can also take quite a while for growers to learn details about the medicinal herb market itself. In the meantime, say the Wheelers, consider blossom growing as a first crop, as you are learning about the other medicinal herbs.

What follows are their best recommendations on a few blossom crops, including specific hints for growing and harvesting. The prices listed were those at the time of writing, but you can send for bulk herb company catalogs anytime to determine current prices.

Calendula Blossoms

Calendula blossoms have long been used in the treatment of wounds, sores, and other skin problems. This is probably one of the easiest herbs to grow, say the Wheelers. They stress the importance of getting only calendula *officinalis* seeds—not some of the fancier garden varieties that offer lots of color shadings. The plant's sticky resins are what's wanted by the product companies, and these are most readily available from the non-hybridized seed crops. Those resins are also most available in the blossoms picked on hot, sunny summer days.

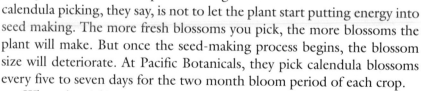

The Wheelers direct-seed calendula in April and then again in July, and can start picking blossoms 80 days after planting. They suggest thinning the crop to a 10 or 12 inch spacing, always selecting for the tallest plants—to make picking easier. Mark reminds tired out pickers to bend down on one knee every once in a while to take the strain off a bending back—and also to sit a while on the edge of your picking bucket.

They pick by hand, using their fingers like a rake, picking five or six blossoms as they rake through the stem. The important thing with calendula picking, they say, is not to let the plant start putting energy into seed making. The more fresh blossoms you pick, the more blossoms the plant will make. But once the seed-making process begins, the blossom size will deteriorate. At Pacific Botanicals, they pick calendula blossoms every five to seven days for the two month bloom period of each crop.

When the picking is good, say the Wheelers, you can pick 10 pounds per hour. It takes five pounds to get one pound of dried calendula blossoms. So if someone is picking less than five pounds per hour, adds Marggy, it is just not worth it, commercially.

This year, the Wheelers are charging $17 to $19 per pound for dried calendula blossoms, and between $5 and $7.50 per pound for the fresh. Prices depend on quantities, of course, and all their products are certified organic.

One tricky bit they have learned is that the calendula blossoms don't fully open until 11 o'clock in the morning, even though their fresh blossom harvests have to be packed and sent out by 2 pm. For fresh orders, the Wheelers start the picking at 10 o'clock and find that the blossoms actually continue to open as they are packed.

Red Clover Blossoms

Long used for both herbal teas and medicines, red clover (*Trifolium pratense*) seems to enjoy constant popularity in the botanical blossom markets. The Wheelers are paid $12 a pound for the fresh blossoms, $35 per pound for the dried. Actually, a wildcrafter near me gets as high as $50 dollars a pound for dried wild clover blossoms picked from very uninhabited island locations. Not bad for what appears to be a weed in many locations. But, like all blossom crops, red clover is very labor intensive and after picking a few pounds of blossoms, you may well think that even the higher price is not enough.

For the Wheelers, red clover acts as both a cash crop that doesn't need weeding, and as a cover crop to fertilize their soil. They drill in oats on top of their clover field, and the oats act as a nurse crop to the clover. In June they can harvest the oats and mow the field, after which the clover blooms. The clover will come back and blossom for three or four years without having to be replanted.

Their clover pickers go into the field as early as five in the morning and pick the blossoms while they are still wet. This is just the opposite of what is done to pick most blossoms, but the clover color and quality will fade fast, say the Wheelers, if you wait until the heat of the day to pick.

Pick blossoms, they recommend, that have as much red as possible on them, that are at least one quarter open, and that have less than one quarter of brown on them. The $50 dollar a pound blossoms, they note, never have even one dot of brown on them—which would mean incredibly selective picking. Hold the blossoms gently, they suggest, snapping off the blossom with a thumb nail. They pick their clover field every other day, but wait four or five days to go back over the same spot.

It takes just over five pounds of fresh clover blossoms to equal one pound of dried product. The Wheelers produce about 500 pounds a year of the dried flowers, selling them for $35 a pound.

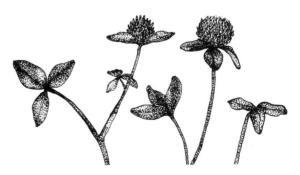

Mullein Blossoms

Here is a crop, *Verbascum thapsus*, long used for coughs and throat infections, and also to make a popular ear infection treatment. Most herb product companies probably purchase mullein (pronounced like sullen) blossoms from wildcrafters. The Wheelers have found a variety that is considered

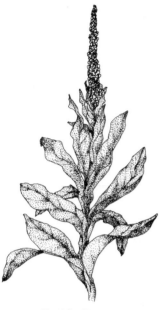 even more desirable by many herb practitioners and medicine company labs and, happily, that is much easier to pick than are the wild blossoms.

Verbascum thapsus is the mullein species they grow. It is a very, very tall biennial that produces high quality flowers in great abundance. The blossoms have excellent bioactivity, besides being easier to pick. Marggy found the variety while browsing in a European seed catalog years ago, and decided to try it.

Mullein, whether wild or grown, is a very fuzzy crop to pick, and is also attractive to bumblebees. Be careful, say the Wheelers "because, as you pick off the blossoms, the bees go to the plants ahead of you and, by the time you reach the end of the row, those same bees can be damned mad—and mean."

Pacific Botanicals sells the *olympicum* species of fresh mullein flowers for $17.50 a pound. These blossoms don't dry well, so they sell only the fresh.

The Wheelers recommend harvesting mullein flowers when the stalk is about 50% open, but say also that it's important to take the blossoms before they start going to seed. "It forms little hard seed heads along the stalk," says Marggy, "and you can end up crushing good flowers just trying to strip around those hard seed heads."

Because flowers are so fragile, they also suggest that all blossoms should be moved quickly from picking buckets to either an ice pack for shipping, or at least poured out on clean sheets. Otherwise, they can quickly turn to compost in the buckets.

Echinacea Blossoms

This is an herb that has recently been in great demand in the marketplace, a demand the Wheelers are growing a little uncertain about these days as more growers come on line. There are several species of echinacea plants used worldwide in echinacea preparations. The Wheelers have nearly always recommended growing the *purpurea* species, but they are now seeing a stronger demand for the *angustifolia* and *pallida* species.

As you will read in the next section on the McLeods of British Columbia, the *angustifolia* species is the native plant that has been collected in the plains areas of the U.S. and Canada for many years. Until recently it was believed to be too difficult to grow in cultivation. Now that the wild species is disappearing from too much careless wildcrafting, some growers are finding they can grow this narrow leafed species with relative ease. The third species, *pallida*, is the one grown and used most often in Europe. But all species, it seems, are strong stimulants for our immune systems, and all are used now in the herbal product marketplace.

In the U.S., echinacea root has long been the most popular source for herbal medicines, while in Europe, flowers, stems, leaves, and seeds have been the most used. For new growers, the Wheelers suggest growing the blossoms to sell, which can be harvested the first and second year, while the root itself must grow for at least three years to be large enough to market.

"The zingy flavor of echinacea, which apparently comes from the chemically active echinacosides, seems to move around the plant during its growth," says Marggy. "When the center cone is high, your tongue will tingle with the plant chemicals if you taste the blossom. A little later, it is the seeds that have more zing, while in the spring, the tingle comes from the leaves and stems."

They pick their blossoms in early morning, put them immediately on ice and ship them right out. These days, some labs are making first one extract out of the blossoms, then one from later seeds, and then one from the root. They then blend them all together and sell them as a whole plant extract.

At this writing, Pacific Botanicals offers echinacea blossoms only in July for six dollars a pound. From October through March, they offer the fresh root at nearly $10 a pound, and the dried root all year round at $24 a pound. In all they offer echinacea in a dozen forms.

German Chamomile

This herb (*Matricaria recutita*) is probably the fastest growing crop of all the blossoms the Wheelers recommend for newcomers. You can begin picking these flowers in as little as 70 days. Mark and Marggy only grow this herb to sell as fresh because they cannot compete with the imported dried chamomile (which they import and sell) from organic growers in France. Pacific Botanicals sells their fresh chamomile flowers for

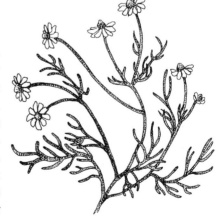

$11.50 per pound, and the imported dried flowers sell for about $17 per pound.

Many growers seed chamomile directly into the field, but the Wheelers start theirs in the greenhouse in early January. That way they can get a hundred per cent stand of flowers. Then they transplant into 26" rows—using the same row width as they do for everything on the farm so their equipment works with all. They plant out the chamomile transplants on 4" settings when the roots are white. Don't plant them too close, says Marggy, or you will have to thin the chamomile—a dreaded job on the farm, she adds.

Chamomile should be grown in the cooler seasons as it will bolt and flower too quickly in the hot summer sun. Long used primarily as a soothing tea ingredient in the U.S., it is a very important plant medicine in Europe. The demand for it is both constant and growing, and its use in America can be expected to grow, too.

🌿 🌿 🌿

Mark was also willing to answer a few other specific questions about his agricultural practices and medicinal herb selling in general.

Q. What kind of fertilizers do you use and recommend for these crops?

A. I fertilize the soil and not the crop, per se. That is, I use soil tests and indicator plants to dictate what kind of fertilizers and green manure crops I should use. I obtain the large majority of fertilizer from cover crops. I also use some compost and lime. It all depends on your soil.

Q. Do you have any recommendations on drying processes for new growers?

A. So much depends on what your climate is like and what seasons you will need to dry in. Moving air is most important. Ideas can be gleaned from other farmers in your area on how they dry their crops.

Q. Any recommendations on selling?

A. Try growing lots of different plants and keep good records of time and costs, so you know what you need to get paid. Have at least a little experience and then send a sample of the crop you want to sell. Be sure and send along a copy of your organic certificate.

Q. What are some of the most common mistakes new growers make?

A. 1. Not doing grow-out trials before going into production.
2. Lack of a good weed control program.

3. Lack of a good fertility-rotation program.

4. Lack of capital.

Mark has a final, more long term crop suggestion that I'd like to pass along. Think about the many herbal medicines, he says, that we are already getting from certain trees around the world. It may be that putting in a medicinal tree orchard would be something newcomers would want to consider. It is not something I had read much about, but Mark's comment certainly makes sense for those with the time, land, and an interest in trees.

Importantly, there must also be a willingness to do the research on how to turn these trees and their parts into viable and profitable medicinal crops. Mark was willing to share a list he is thinking about adding to his property, and I have added a few more that I've read about in other places. Actually, Tim Blakley covers a few of these in his section. I think it's very much worth looking into. I'm not absolutely certain on the exact species on these; but this list should get you started.

🌿 MEDICINAL HERB TREES

Black Haw	*Viburnum opulus*
Carob	*Ceratonia siliqua*
Chaste Tree	*Vitex agnus-castus*
China Berry	*Melia azedarach*
Elder, Black	*Sambucus nigra*
Eucalyptus	*E. globus*
Fringe Tree	*Chionanthus virginica*
Ginkgo	*G. biloba*
Hawthorn	*Crataegus monogyna*
Horse Chestnut	*Aesculus carnea*
Jujube	*Ziziphus jujuba*
Juniper	*Juniperus*
Lime Tree	*Tilia cordata*
Pomegranate	*Punica granatum*
Sweet Gum	*Liquidamber styraciflua*
Tea Tree	*Melaleuca alternifloria*
White Oak	*Quercus*
Willows	*Salix*

Growing Echinacea
❧ *John and Elaine McLeod*

Now a look at a family growing echinacea on Bowen Island, just north of the city of Vancouver, in British Columbia. John and Elaine McLeod bring a strong background to their medicinal herb growing effort, but what's most impressive about them is their intelligent, tenacious search for all the missing information—plus the path they are choosing in their marketing. Follow their example and you can succeed as a medicinal herb grower. Echinacea may not be such an important crop for small growers by the time you read this, but it's the McLeod MO, their method of doing things that is so important to notice.

Their little echinacea field will also be a good place to focus on a few details in one of the key secrets to success in growing medicinal herbs for profit: the McLeod determination to learn to grow the highest quality herbs possible. Theirs is the same idea pushed by the Wheelers. As more and more companies start meeting the growing demand for these herbal preparations, the question of ingredient quality will become ever more important in the market sectors where the start-up opportunities are. Watching the McLeods is a good way to see just what that can involve. Their first experiences with medicinal herbs also show an interesting, almost typical, path for these early herb growers.

John was once a wheat farmer in Manitoba, while Elaine took her degrees and worked in the field of early childhood education. They moved west to Bowen Island 16 years ago and opened a small retail plant nursery to serve the few thousand Bowen Island residents.

Meanwhile, their two daughters, Erin and Christine, had developed both food allergies and immune system disorders. It was the McLeod search for help with these complicated family health problems that brought them to their first encounter with medicinal herbs. This pattern is one that reappears throughout this book with the people involved in growing and marketing medicinal herbs. Personal and family success in using herbs seems to make converts of us all.

After making the rounds of all the regular doctors without much relief, Elaine was told about a naturopathic doctor in the area and decided to give him a try. The doctor, who had been trained at the naturopathic college in Portland, Oregon, put the girls on treatments that included echinacea, and they both begin to improve. John and Elaine then began to pay attention to medicinal herbs. They also became quite close to the naturopath and learned of the difficulty he was having getting enough high quality echinacea for his own practice. At that time the primary North American supplier of organically grown echinacea was sold out for at least the following two years.

That situation instigated the McLeod search for information about the plant along with the idea of growing some on the land they owned surrounding their small nursery. They first visited and gathered a little information from the Canadian government agriculture research stations in British Columbia. Then John went back to Manitoba where, because of increased freight rates, farmers were looking for niche crops instead of the usual wheat, oats, and barley. The government there, he found, was taking an active interest in herb crops and he was able to gather a little more information. Later, on a trip to the Far West Garden Show in Portland, John visited the library at the naturopathic college there ("I took rolls of dimes along") and copied everything he could find on the research done on medicinal uses of echinacea.

It is this determined and patient searching that is bringing John and Elaine past the frustration most new, would-be medicinal herb growers feel at the lack of information available on crops they know are wanted and needed in the marketplace. There are not yet a lot of textbooks for growers available on these crops; your county agriculture agents and provincial agriculture ministers are scrambling themselves to find out helpful information, right alongside the new growers.

Echinacea has become the best known and most often used herbal remedy in the U.S. and Canada. In Europe, it has long been sold as an approved over-the-counter (OTC) medicine, commonly prescribed by most doctors in Germany for prevention and early treatment of colds and sore throats.

Echinacea is a native American plant that was heavily used by Native Americans in their treatment for sore throats, toothaches, infections, and even snakebites. In the late 1800s it was touted to American pharmacists by a patent medicine maker named H. F. C. Meyer who had been selling it in his "blood purifier." Meyer was such an enthusiast for echinacea (and his own patent medicine) that he sent samples of it to well known pharmacists and physicians in Cincinnati, raving to them about the "proven" uses of echinacea. Meyer even offered to come to Cincinnati bringing "a full-sized rattlesnake, possessed of its natural fangs...." He would let the snake bite him in front of the doctors, he wrote, to make his point.

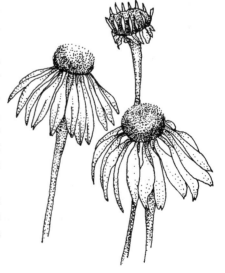

Two other men—John King, an "eclectic physician" (meaning one who used plant medicines in his practice) and John Uri Lloyd, a pharmacist (who later became head of the American Pharmaceutical Association)—eventually became convinced of the medicinal value of echinacea and began making products with it themselves.

Echinacea was then recommended by a group of doctors in America known as the "eclectics" (who included herb medicines in their cures) and it soon became a very popular medicine among all doctors—both "eclectics" and "regulars," as the other doctors were called. All found it quite successful in their practices. But echinacea has never been approved as an OTC medicine by the Food and Drug Administration (FDA).

Echinacea remained popular in the United States until the eclectics and herbal medicines both came under attack by organized medicine in the 1920s and '30s. The discovery and wide use of first sulfa drugs and then antibiotics also contributed to the downfall of plant medicines in the U.S. But in Europe, echinacea and many other herbal preparations remained popular and continue to be sold on the shelves today right along with all other OTC medicines.

The renaissance of herbal medicine in this country has now brought this plant back into popularity with millions of American and Canadian consumers, and the irony is that we must look now to Europe for all the modern research on this native American plant's properties—although some clinical studies of echinacea have recently started in America.

Hundreds of scientific research papers in Europe have shown that echinacea does boost the immune system, and is an excellent treatment for many common conditions. The government drug agencies in both the U.S. and Canada are now trying to deal with the increased popularity of this and many other herbal remedies, but in the meantime, people like John and Elaine McLeod just got busy in their fields to meet the increasing demand for high quality, organically grown herb crops.

Which brings us again to the few McLeod acres surrounding their little nursery on Bowen Island, in B.C. At the time of our visit, the first planting was only months old and already starting to show a few of the distinctive tall-stemmed purple flowers with the dark conical centers and the drooping rays, so typical of echinacea purpurea, pronounced ek-kin-AY-sha pur-PUR-ee-ah.

The Bowen land had been fallow for five years and the McLeods have applied for organic certification under the Canadian system. It is a south slope that is covered with glacial till down to about three feet. John calls it a very mineralized soil with little organic material.

They had the seed started for them in organic plugs by a greenhouse grower in the Vancouver area who does nothing but plugs, which are tiny plant pots used by commercial growers everywhere. These miniature starts can sell for 10¢ to a dollar each—depending on the number needed. Their 24,000 growing echinacea plugs were delivered during a spring storm and the clock started ticking to get these plants into the ground as soon as possible. The McLeods ended up having to hold and care for the plugs for two weeks waiting for a break in the weather to plant.

They used their John Deere to help form raised beds and then set the plants in by hand on 14" centers with 26" between the rows. With four or five people working, they could set out 2500 plants a day. Each little plug was dipped in water and rolled in bone meal before being set in the ground.

The plants went in before the irrigation system, so that meant hand watering for the next few weeks. That first planting of only a quarter acre added up to nearly two miles of rows to tend.

"We practically lived out there night and day hand watering," said Elaine. "The sprinklers would have simply missed too much. So we took hours and hours to drag hoses very carefully over the field." But that early hand watering, they believe, made the big difference in giving the plants a great start and keeping their plant losses to almost zero—only one hundred of the 24,000 plants needed replacement.

Their water is from a surface pond with a pump and T-tape system, delivering about one half gallon per 100 feet. Some of the rows have black plastic for weed control; one has been top dressed with chicken manure; one control bed has had no fertilizer, and several are being fed a locally made and tested compost material. Living on a ferry-serviced island can often mean extra expenses; bringing loads of fertilizer across from the mainland would add too much to the cost of the crop. These test plots were very important in their plans to add more echinacea plantings to the rest of their land.

At our visit, the McLeods were realizing that they were going to need a small rototiller to cut down on the hand weeding between the rows. John estimated his basic farm equipment to be worth about 80 or 90 thousand dollars, but figures he can probably do 10 acres of echinacea, or other medicinal herbs, without much more investment. They both also realized that the other expenses involved in putting in even this small field have been far greater than they first imagined. The fact sheets put out by the B.C. Agriculture Dept. seriously underestimated the costs, says John. And the plugs costs them several thousand additional dollars, but seemed necessary because their own greenhouse space was committed to their nursery plant needs.

John and/or Elaine have walked the fields nearly every day since first planting. It's like getting to know someone, they say, learning all their habits, and learning how the plants react to the patches of different soil types they found in preparing the field. Every two weeks they have counted the leaves on each plant, measured the plant height and then recorded everything in journals. In the evenings they read everything they can get their hands on about the plant itself, attend herb conferences whenever they can, keep in touch with agriculture offices in both B.C. and Manitoba, and consider their choices for marketing as the plants develop.

In Germany, they have learned, the root has not been used for medicine at all—only the leaves, flowers, and seeds. Elaine has wondered if that would be the most practical thing to do: harvest only the top parts.

And wouldn't they be better off, they've also wondered, learning to actually make the tinctures themselves, and then marketing them in the area? Their naturopath encourages this and that suggestion has set them off on that new path to learn about tincture making.

This determination to learn everything they possibly can is what sets the McLeods (and other very successful medicinal herb growers) apart from those who would try their hand at medicinal herbs (or anything else) and come up short. Grow culinary herbs, flowers, or market vegetables, and you can no doubt find lots of information in your local library or book store to answer all your questions. You can also find a ready outlet at your Saturday market, your local grocer, or restaurants. But grow medicinal herbs and you need to plow new ground in more ways than one.

"When we started this idea only a year and a half ago," said John, "no one had a clue around here what echinacea was all about. Now we keep running into locals who know all about it. Last week, a 10 year old rode by on his bike, stopped to ask what this plant was, and when I told him it was a medicinal herb called echinacea, he said, 'Oh yes, I know about that,' and off he went."

The McLeod daughters, meanwhile, are gaining back their health, with one of them being given echinacea, thuja, and baptisia—a strong combination of herb plants used in Germany and sold under the registered name of Esberitox N.

There are several species of echinacea, the *E. purpurea* species being the most commonly used for medicine in the U. S. The native plant, first used by the Native Americans, was actually *E. angustifolia*, a shorter plant with much narrower leaves than *E. purpurea*. The McLeods were told that *E. angustifolia* didn't like rain, so they only planted a tiny test plot of it. At our visit that plot had done so well that Elaine said she thought they might be willing to try it now. Others around the country are also finding that *angustifolia* is not impossible to grow, so more of that cultivated species will be appearing.

Echinacea pallida (for pale) is the third species that is used medicinally. Until recently it has been considered not quite as good medicinally as the other two varieties, but that, too, may be changing with new test results. Actually, the *pallida* species has long been grown in Europe and sold as *angustifolia*, because of an early mistake in seed identification. It is this kind of identity error that has driven the FDA and other herbal medicine critics so crazy in the past. Medicinal herb growers are starting to realize that paying closer attention to where the seeds come from, to even having their seeds scientifically identified in a botanical laboratory, may be required.

In all, there are actually nine different species of echinacea growing around the world, but only these three, *purpurea*, *angustifolia*, and *pallida*, are so far considered useful for medicinal purposes. Most medicinal herb people have been turning more towards the use of the *purpurea* species of echinacea because it is considered fairly easy to grow, and because of the recent decimation of the wild *angustifolia* plantings all across America.

Just as with wild ginseng and goldenseal, echinacea has now become known for its increased value in the market place and the get-rich-quick screwballs are out there in parks and along roadsides, pulling up the wild plants by the roots and throwing everything into the backs of their pickup trucks before tearing off down the road looking for someone to buy their *valuable crop*.

The parts of the plants that could be used for fresh tinctures are easily spoiled by this kind of careless treatment; the parts that are used dried for medicine making should be harvested at certain times, dried at certain temperatures, and treated like what they are: material for use as medicine.

People like John and Elaine McLeod are making the work for future medicinal herb growers a whole lot easier by their thorough, careful approach and their willingness to share their learning with the rest of us. When I last checked in with them, they had added lots more crop, were trying several other herbs, and were well into the process of learning how to make herbal extracts. That puts them even further along the route to becoming successful medicinal herb growers and marketers.

Growing Ginseng

🌿 *Jim Lawrence*

Next comes a story of sexual rejuvenation and very big payoffs; lots of hype and occasional cheating; large cash outlays; endless problems; real skill and effort; and a big dose of long term patience. And I mustn't leave out an almost daily threat of sudden and total failure. Whew! Sounds like I must be preparing you for a typical Hollywood movie script. Instead, here comes (tah dah!) ginseng root.

Larry King never made ginseng real to me. My local farmer, Jim Lawrence, has. Years ago, King, now a well known CNN television celebrity interviewer, used to pump up a verbal head of steam for a ginseng product every night between his interviews on early talk radio. That product went from sales of $1 million per year to about $40 million per year—the first time in history that so many Americans took up with ginseng.

One thing to keep in mind here is that ginseng is really not an American-style medicine. It's what herbalists (especially Asians and Europeans) sometimes call an "adaptogen"—something taken over a long, long period of time to stay healthy. Not something you take temporarily to deal with an illness or sudden health problem. And not the quick-fix that Americans seem to prefer.

Since the Larry King ads, Consumers Union, publisher of Consumer Reports, has done extensive tests on ginseng products sold in America, and concluded that many of them have so little actual ginseng in them as to be considered virtually worthless. Many ginseng products, in other tests, have also been found to be adulterated with ingredients not even mentioned on the label. But the hoopla continues.

There is also some hullabaloo building around the case for ginseng growers in America: that you can earn REAL money on a small plot of land growing this one plant. My local farmer, Jim Lawrence, along with a lot of other small farmers, has been listening. Cautious, suspicious about the hype, but listening. And eventually willing to make a try at this herbal brass ring.

The big retail market for ginseng has never been with Americans, but with Asians, who have apparently used this plant and its close relatives since before their written history began. Its reputation in Asia to enhance a long, healthy, and sexually active life still fuels the trade in ginseng. Until very recently, the North American trade in cultivated ginseng has rather quietly taken place between a few ginseng growers in the midwestern U.S. and Canada, and a very few Asian brokers in Hong Kong.

A series of recent events is causing the market for growing, buying, and selling ginseng to open up a little. It is these events that have brought Jim Lawrence into the ginseng picture, along with three other new growers—just on my own tiny island. I can only imagine how many others are out there trying hard to become a part of this new, slightly changed and possibly more hopeful scene in the old ginseng movie.

For the first time, midwest ginseng growers now have competition from growers in Western Canada and in the states of Washington and

Oregon. In contrast to the heretofore tightly held agricultural information on the crop in the midwest, both western groups are remarkably open and helpful to new growers.

Throughout Canada, government agriculture offices and university agriculture departments are now promoting ginseng as a viable crop to consider for production in many parts of their country, and are putting out lots of information on it. A small group in both public and private agriculture circles in Washington state is equally eager to share what they know.

The so-called New World Economy has so shaken established agriculture and marketing systems that every area of North America (and the world?) is suddenly scrambling to come up with new possibilities to keep their local economy alive. Ginseng, and medicinal herbs in general, are becoming a big part of that scramble.

The recent change-over in Hong Kong (from long British colonial to mainland China rule) has occurred during the writing of this book, causing major price concerns and possibly another one of the scene changes in the ginseng market.

There has also been an enormous influx of Asians to North America during the 10 or 15 year run-up to the Hong Kong change-over. Recent estimates place the Asian population in such centers as Vancouver, British Columbia, as high as 25%. This is creating an entirely new (virtually local) market for ginseng—something the farmers of the far west are certainly taking into consideration.

And now there is talk of American tobacco farmers in the southeast looking into ginseng production as a viable replacement crop. Ginseng seems to be one of those crops long believed possible to grow in only a few areas—until it is tried and grown successfully in other places.

The Chinese like the kind of ginseng grown in the U.S. and Canada. There are several species of ginseng, but the species that interests us here is known as American ginseng: *Panax quinquefolium, quinque* meaning five, *folium* meaning leaves. Each mature stem has one leaf with five leaflets.

American ginseng is considered a yin, or cooling herb in Traditional Chinese Medicine. Asian ginseng (*Panax ginseng*) is considered a yang, or heating herb. The third commonly used ginseng, by the way, is Siberian ginseng (*Eleutherococcus senticosus*), which belongs to the same botanical family as the other ginsengs, but to another genus altogether. There is also a recently discovered ginseng species found in Vietnam: *Panax vietnamensis.*

Asians consider American ginseng to be almost as good as their original native-grown ginseng which, as a result of over-harvesting, disappeared from China many, many years ago. Herbalist Steven Foster says that there are still "about six pounds of wild-harvested Asian ginseng dug in northeast China each year, and a single root may sell on the Hong Kong market for $20,000 or more." Wildcrafted ginseng in America, I have read, can bring up to $600 per pound, with less and less found every year.

In Canada, there are fairly new, extensive ginseng growing operations in British Columbia. Chai-Na-Ta, a publicly traded Canadian company with headquarters near Vancouver, B.C., now grows over 1500 acres of ginseng. Another company, Imperial, has also put in large plantings of ginseng in the B.C. interior.

In Ontario, where ginseng has long been grown, nearly 5,000 acres of ginseng production were recently reported, an annual 70 million dollar industry. Ginseng has a special and long history in Canada where Jesuit priests, in the 1700s, were the first to recognize the plant as the same one being used so widely in China. It was first cultivated under artificial shade in Ontario in the 1800s.

In Washington and Oregon, two men seem to be most responsible for the recent interest in growing ginseng, although there are many reports of the plant having been grown earlier in many areas of the far west—especially where Chinese forced labor had been brought in to work on the building of railroads.

A former midwest ginseng grower, Don Hoogesteger, moved to southwest Washington state a few years ago to set up a ginseng growing operation. He began reaching out to teach other growers in the area and, by chance, his operation was near the offices of Dr. Charles Brun, a horticulturist and county extension agent who thought he recognized good potential prospects for Washington farmers. Brun has now become somewhat of an expert himself on all of the existing ginseng operations in the Pacific northwest region.

Dr. Brun goes to many agricultural conferences speaking out on ginseng possibilities; telling what he has learned of this fabled crop. First I'll relate some of what Brun tells those who want to consider ginseng growing, and then I'll take you to visit Jim Lawrence, one of our local growers.

Brun views ginseng growing as an "alternative to Wall St. investing." It's ideal, he says, "for someone about fifty years old, who is willing to work hard now to make sure she or he can retire a bit early and stop driving the freeways to work." Plant a quarter acre of ginseng a year, says Brun, and in five years you'll start having a very decent payback. Dried ginseng root, he says, can yield up to $55 per pound.

It needs to be said right up front that Brun is not talking here about organically grown ginseng, which is worth considerably more money, but which Brun thinks may just be too difficult to grow. We will be discussing organically grown ginseng when we get to the Lawrence farm.

The investment in getting into ginseng is not small—up to $16,000 per acre, says Brun—although he strongly suggests that new growers start out with a quarter acre at a time. That quarter acre cost would probably be about $5,000.

The ideal soil is believed to be a silty loam on a south slope of not more than a 10% grade. The crop needs a good 18" of very good drainage, and many farmers have had to put in drain tiles to keep the water tables low in their fields.

"Run your rows north and south," Brun advises, take down any big trees around the field and "clean up all the trash." He also stresses the importance of getting all the weeds out ahead of time and that "you should consider using a cover crop first."

Ginseng requires 80% shade for growing, and even one day of full summer sun can ruin your crop. In parts of the midwest, ginseng grows naturally under high canopy shade trees, and commercial growers in those places also plant under those same tall trees. In most other areas, the shade is created by expensive post and shade cloth installations.

Rent a post pounder rather than an augur, advises Brun, to put in your posts, as the augur can cause your posts to sink in too far. The shade cloth expense is high: up to $8,000 per acre (21¢ a sq. ft.) but it lasts for years if carefully cared for. And it must be put in properly with special extra wires holding all the posts together so they cannot be pulled out by the wind. The shade cloth gets pulled aside for winter and tied up like dropped sails on a sailboat boom.

The plants get mulched with sawdust—not straw, because of slugs. And remember, says Brun, that fir mulch works better than alder mulch—which can bring endless mushrooms to the fields in the northwest.

Ginseng grows only from stratified seed, and can take 18 months or more to prepare seed to germinate. He suggests new growers start with purchased seed from someone like Hoogesteger to be able to start harvesting their own seed after the second year of growing. Stratification, to break the internal dormancy, is done by placing seed in washed sand and sealing it up for 18 months—away from cats and mice. Stratified seed costs are about $35 per pound, and an acre takes about 100 lb. of seeds.

Far west growers, says Brun, can take advantage of mild winter climates to dig up young ginseng roots and slant-clip the bottom one third off the root to give it the shape desired by buyers. This winter transplanting cannot be done in the climates of Wisconsin, Ontario, or inland B.C.

Many of Brun's recommendations are given a slightly different emphasis when made by others for growers in different parts of America and

Canada. The reference section at the end of this book will lead you to much of the current information available on ginseng growing in the U.S. and Canada.

The main things to realize are: that the plant is susceptible to many diseases, bugs and critters; that drought, moisture, heat, and even air pollution can affect it; that ginseng requires 80% shade, expensive seed, careful harvesting, drying, and packaging and that marketing may take special efforts.

The ginseng market is still primarily in Hong Kong (through brokers who buy from individual growers in the U.S. and Canada) and can be quite volatile. As I write this paragraph, I have just learned that the Canadian Corporation, Chai-Na-Ta, has decided to defer selling their ginseng crop for the rest of this year as prices are at historic lows. Apparently the takeover by China is having a very big effect indeed. There are also recent reports that the Chinese are becoming quite adept at growing American ginseng under shade themselves, and plan to be self-sufficient in that crop by early in the next century. But that they are growing ever more interested in woods grown ginseng, which may prove of real value to those trying to grow ginseng in the southeast. Talk about a volatile market!

And one more thing. American ginseng is listed as an endangered species under the Convention on International Trade in Endangered Species (CITES). This does not mean that international trade is limited in ginseng, but that the international trade must be documented. Before importing or exporting American ginseng, a permit must be obtained from the exporting country.

If all these costs, chores, uncertainties, and admonitions haven't scared you away from considering ginseng as an herb crop, it's time to meet my friend Jim Lawrence, and find out the real life problems of growing this ancient plant. And the real allure of it.

A long time artist and commercial fisherman, Jim has owned his 22-acre Thirsty Goose Farm for 25 years. Fishing these days in the northwest is too often reduced to only a small window that opens to allow an occasional fishing day—or even just a few hours. And what's left of the fishing season is now always accompanied by the rankling din of blame-saying and finger pointing around the issue of just who and what have caused the near disappearance of our once fabulous salmon resource.

For our small island economy, fishing was one of the few things to help keep young families here. Jim and his wife, Lisa, are raising two daughters: Mara is 10, Natalia is 14. Jim's and Lisa's parents live here, along with other members of their families. Picking up and moving away is something they are trying hard not to have to contemplate.

And the Lawrence family remaining here is something the rest of us islanders have a stake in. A diverse population is essential; so is a diverse economy. Our collective nightmare is having these islands become nothing but a monoculture playground for only the retired, or only the very wealthy. I listen to Jim's dreams about the possibilities of the ginseng crop and I find myself buying into it, too. Maybe, just maybe…

"I've wanted so desperately," says Jim, "to find a crop that can be grown on this island that will earn a family as much as $30,000 a year an acre. That's a real alternative to all the land development and speculation that's going on here. We could keep our open spaces and our own way of life, and not be reduced to just tee-shirt tourism and rich man's real estate."

The Lawrence family grows their own food, plus an almost year-round supply of organically grown mixed salad greens for our food markets, lots of summer basil and tomatoes for everyone, and a fine organic crop of U-Pick strawberries. Most recently they are making an expensive, determined effort on the ginseng. A very different crop indeed.

Jim started with a third of an acre. He looked into the shade cloth installation recommended by Brun and tried to figure out a cheaper way to go. Jim spent many days at the south end of our island, where all the driftwood washes in, retrieving and then splitting enough logs to make his own posts—168 of them. For shade cloth he has so far had to spend $5,000 for his nearly three year ginseng effort—although it should last for at least 20 years. And he's had to buy expensive, stratified seed, of course.

Another expensive factor is simply that ginseng is a root crop and takes a long time to grow. Jim says he knows of crops that have taken as long as seven years to mature. Whatever lives and grows in the soil itself can feed on and attack ginseng roots during those years. The parts that grow above ground are especially inviting to certain bugs, creatures, and fungi: rhizoctonia disease, alternaria leaf blight, to name a couple, and lots of root rot. Ginseng is the devil of plants for such problems.

Jim Lawrence admits to being, like a lot of us, a selective listener. "It's like getting married," he said. "Who wants to hear about all the possible problems." He was told and read about all the potential problems with ginseng, but what he heard was the information bits that made this crop sound so perfect for our island.

He heard that deer don't eat ginseng. That's a big plus for the San Juan Islands; we love our expanding population of handsome deer; they love most everything we grow.

He heard that farmers in the west are harvesting up to 3,000 lb. of root per acre—while in Wisconsin, they can only get an average yield of 2,000 lb.

"Look," he said, "you and I are sitting here at the first of March and I'm expecting that those ginseng greens could pop back up any day now. I know I'll have to have this shade cloth back across the top by Easter. And

I also know that Wisconsin will still have two feet of snow on the ground when I do."

The other big plus he heard about was that ginseng grown in most other places requires sprinkler systems because of heat in the summer. Sprinklers mean moisture, which means fungus. Our island pattern is for a dry, fairly cool summer. We usually get about 20 to 22 inches of rain— about half that of the Seattle area. Most years we get little of our rain in the summer.

He also heard ("but wasn't really listening") that ginseng requires a special site for growing. In the wild, ginseng prefers moist but well drained soil. Drainage is very critical.

Jim's best soil has always been where he puts his strawberries. So that's where he put the ginseng. Wrong. That patch is as rich as a river bottom, he says, and as low lying. The ginseng showed signs of disease and rot the very first year of growth. He had to dig them all up—90,000 tiny young roots—and move them to a higher piece of ground near the woods.

And the one problem he hadn't thought about at all began to do him in early, too. Slugs. "We've had 'em by the train load," and how they adored the tender green shoots of ginseng. A third of Jim's crop simply disappeared. He then did what many of us might decide to do with that kind of investment in that kind of dream crop. He bought and spread slug bait in the woods near his ginseng field, thus giving up his organic status on that one piece of his land.

Next, the fungus problems appeared and Jim bought some foliar spray to try to battle them off.

"This whole thing has been so hard," says Jim, shaking his head, "that it's really hard for me to admit just how hard it has been."

Jim's anxiety to protect his investment, to move ahead on his dream to grow a well paying crop, actually cost him dearly: organically grown and dried roots can bring quite a bit more per pound than regular ginseng. And though Jim easily admitted and believes that medicine crops should absolutely be organically grown crops, he was also aware that most of the ginseng shipped to the Orient is not organically grown; that most ginseng growers in the U.S. and Canada use chemicals rather freely on their crops, because of the common problems. Jim's advisors also told him he was trying to walk on water to grow this crop organically. And the plant losses just kept coming.

"I'd get together with the other ginseng growers here and we'd all have these looks of terror on our faces. Sometimes I'd be shaking—like I'd run over the neighbor's dog or something. When the first field flooded I spent all day out there trying to dig a ditch. You can dig forever on flat land and the water won't go away. I felt so crazy that I just kept digging. Those ginseng gods just laughed at me."

Since then, Jim has calmed down a bit, met a couple of other organic growers and has reconsidered his actions. He's decided not to give up on the organic part. He won't be able to sell his first batch as organically grown, and he is now taking another very different tack in his overall plan.

"I was just too concerned with the money and investment," he says. "I really needed to spend a whole lot more time and effort learning to know and grow this plant. I've added in smaller amounts the last two years. In fact, this year, I only added in a very few new rows."

Jim's original field is now in transition back to organic. He knows his crop will be in the ground for several more years, and he's prepared to wait it out, take his losses and know that he'll end up with a lot of knowledge—although maybe not a lot of money for quite a while.

Meanwhile, he's considering ways to sell the crop in Washington, and forgetting about the big brass ring in Hong Kong—which may prove rather tinny after all. He's learning much more about the medicinal aspects of ginseng, about its growing use in the area. He's talking with people about ginseng products, how they are made and used around the world, and realizing his best market might be right here in the Pacific northwest. After all, he asks, "wouldn't you rather take a ginseng tonic or capsule grown right here, where you know the grower, know how it's been grown, and know exactly what's in it?"

"Better believe I would," I answer.

Medicinal Herb Starts

❦ *Alison Kutz Troutman*

Even with all the new interest in medicinal herbs, I was still surprised this last year or two to see so many unusual medicinal herb starts show up in northwest plant nurseries, mixed right in with the regular culinary and ornamental herbs. I had naively tried to sell medicinal herbs years ago when I first began selling herbs. They mostly just sat there. Something has obviously changed. This year I could buy a little start of codonopsis, or Chinese dang shen, from an ordinary plant nursery I happened to stop at one day on the mainland.

I saw by the label that the supplier was one of the main northwest potted herb suppliers, Alison Kutz Troutman, of Cascade Cuts, in Bellingham, near the Canadian border. I gave Alison a call to ask about the change. "We have developed a wonderfully diverse customer base in our region," she said. "Our customers have totally rallied behind our desire to grow the unusual. We are niche marketers—because that is what we love, and that is how we'll survive in our sophisticated marketplace."

Every year she is adding in new herbs, many of them considered very exotic just a few years ago. Alison insists, as do many herbalists, that almost all herbs are, or have been, used medicinally at one time or another. Lavender, rosemary and thyme, she reminds me, are certainly considered strong medicinals. I suddenly remembered reading recently that one of my favorite herbalists, James Duke, uses a rosemary based rinse after a hair wash, as a way to fight off old age memory problems. (I've now begun doing it myself, actually.)

Alison also sees that her job is more than raising good plants. She has to constantly educate her wholesale accounts so they can become her partners in selling a more exotic variety of herbs.

"Of course," she says, "it's easy to get too far out ahead of the trend and a bit overzealous on some of our projections. So, let's just say we have to make constant adjustments to our growing program." I can hear that tone of the real medicinal herb enthusiast, tempered by the realities of the marketplace. Push out, pull back; wait a bit and push out again.

Alison also expresses some cautionary advice to other growers, a need perhaps to be a little careful on several other issues. One is putting out anything that could be toxic if overused. She grew and sold foxglove for years, but has now stopped supplying it because of what she sees as fear and confusion in the marketplace. "There is a real leeriness out there on the part of retail stores that I have to stay aware of," she says.

Monkshood, she reminds me, is far more dangerous, if ingested, than is foxglove, but aconite is sold in almost all plant nurseries. Of course it's sold as a perennial, not as an herb—a term that usually signals safe eating to many people. The herb category makes Alison cautious and careful.

She's also careful not to pick up on things too quickly. Kava kava, the Polynesian plant, looks to be a trendy plant coming along soon, but Alison is in no hurry to learn to grow it until she's convinced it's perfectly safe. There are so many herbs being used around the world that being cautious on a few of them still leaves her plenty to play around with.

Cascade Cuts does about 90% of its own propagation in house, and she constantly seeks out new varieties of herbs from around the world—which has her producing things like Vietnamese and Japanese corianders. She takes great pleasure in procuring and promoting Chinese and Ayurvedic herbs; which puts herbs like gotu kola and fo ti right out there for ordinary gardeners like myself. Even a few years ago I would have sworn that those herbs would never sell anywhere in this country. Now I watch each year to see what new herbs come along for me to try in my garden. And there are many people like me all over the country, trying to learn about these herbs, how to use them, how to grow them. Companies like Cascade Cuts are making it lots easier, and keeping our gardens ever more interesting.

I am suggesting that there is probably going to be a much better business opportunity now in these medicinal plants for the garden than ever before. I wrote about how to start a little herb nursery business in *Profits From Your Backyard Herb Garden*. Now I am seeing that anyone with an herb nursery business should allow more time and space for medicinal herbs. These plants are starting to sell very well.

Chinese Medicinal Herbs

North America is a much more ethnically diverse region these days than it ever has been before. Yet it lags far behind the rest of the world in its use and appreciation of medicinal plants. If we stop and think that three quarters of the world's population have never stopped using plant medicines, that most people around the world actually use plants from their own areas as their medicines, we can begin to realize just how enormous the potential for botanical medicines might be. Even though the medicinal herb market may have taken off with such an explosion lately, we are probably just at the opening salvos.

Chinese medicines are the exotic world botanicals we seem to want to learn a lot about first. You'll see in the section of this book about herbalists that the study of Traditional Chinese Medicine, including acupuncture, is drawing more and more converts because it is one of the few paths towards a recognized license to practice herbal medicine in America.

As more and more herb practitioners choose that path, their own needs for traditional Chinese herbs will increase. Many of the plants used in TCM are now imported. You don't have to read all that much about modern Asia these days before learning that pollution there is becoming a problem of such huge dimensions that it won't be long before many North Americans will be questioning the value of getting any medicinal herbs or herb products from that part of the world. Organically grown Chinese and Ayurvedic herbs should be in far greater demand as time goes by. Maybe very soon.

For those of you considering medicinal herb growing, following is a list of a few well known Traditional Chinese Medicine herbs that can be grown in North America. Some of them are covered in Tim's section. There are also seed and plant sources listed in the reference section at the end of the book, as well as recommended books to read about the subject. If you have someone in your area practicing TCM, you will want to give them a call to talk about their plant uses and needs. I'll be mentioning this again in the selling chapters.

TRADITIONAL CHINESE HERBS TO GROW

Achyranthes	*A. bidentata*	niu xi
Angelica	*A. sinensis; A. dahurica*	dang gui
Asian ginseng	*Panax ginseng*	ren shen
Astragalus	*A. membranaceus*	huang qi
Codonopsis	*C. pilosula*	dang shen
Eucominia	*E. ulmoides*	du zhong
Fo Ti	*Polygonum multiforum*	he shou wu
Ginger	*Zingiber officinale*	sheng jian
Licorice	*Glycyrrhiza uralensis*	gan cao
Red Sage	*Salvia miltiorrhiza*	dan shen
Rhubarb	*Rheum palmatum; R. officinale*	da huang
Siberian ginseng	*Eleutherococcus senticosus*	ci wu jia

CHAPTER TWO

Growing & Marketing Medicinal Mushrooms

"Why wait until we get cancer? We want to eat these (medicinal mushrooms) and add these healthful cancer protectors in our diet all along the way. To me, this is like the best type of health insurance that I can have."

Christopher Hobbs, herbalist, author, and founder of the
American School of Herbalism

The Other Magic Mushrooms

Why medicinal mushrooms in a book on growing and marketing medicinal herbs? They're in here because I think medicinal mushrooms are a special crop that could be considered by anyone looking at growing plants to meet the coming demands in the marketplace for more natural medicines.

Medicinal herbs are getting much of the press coverage these days, but I think medicinal mushrooms are going to also be in great demand as the studies now being done on them become much more known.

"The most fascinating aspect of the medicinal mushrooms is ... enhancing the function and activity of the body's immune system," says Andrew Weil, M.D., faculty member of the University of Arizona College of Medicine, and author of the best selling books, *Spontaneous Healing* and *8 Weeks to Optimum Health*.

"Shiitake mushrooms contain lentinen that boosts immunity and inhibits growth of tumors," writes Jean Carper, former senior health correspondent for CNN television news and author of *Food—Your Miracle Medicine* .

With reputable experts like these promoting the health values of medicinal mushrooms, it seemed entirely appropriate to add a section to this book on the commercial production of organically grown mushrooms— especially of one delicious gourmet mushroom considered world-wide an excellent cancer fighter: the Shiitake.

An immune-stimulating polysaccharide called lentinen, which is known to attack tumors, is one of the key active ingredients in Shiitake. Polysaccharides are large complex molecules of many smaller sugar molecules. They apparently resemble bacteria molecules, and can "fool" our bodies into producing an immune response. This response sets off an increase in killer T-cell activity, plus other antibiotic and antiviral processes that can be very helpful in fighting disease.

These are the same polysaccharides, by the way, that appear in herbs like echinacea and astragalus. Scientific studies are going on worldwide about these herbs, the polysaccharides *and* the Shiitake—along with other medicinal mushrooms, including the Maitake and Reishi.

Mushrooms, as you no doubt know, are the fruiting bodies of an underground tree-like system of tiny cottony roots called mycelia. Mushrooms feed on organic matter in the soil, release spores after they fruit above ground and then, when conditions of temperature and moisture are just right, the growth cycle begins again.

You probably also know that mushrooms are members of the fungi kingdom, and that penicillin was obtained from a fungus in 1928. There are about 100,000 fungi species; about 38,000 of them are mushrooms—and only a very few of those have been named and studied.

The Shiitake mushroom (*Letinus edodes*) is the second most common commercially produced mushroom in the world because of having both medicinal and food value. Most of the market has long been in Asia, but

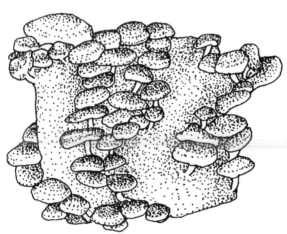

Americans are now consuming more and more Shiitake every year.

In Japan, thousands of small scale Shiitake growers use log culture to provide the majority of mushrooms sold to markets there. This model has also been adopted by Europeans and North Americans with some success.

Log culture is a simple and natural growing method, although quite labor intensive and slow in comparison to the newer methods of growing on sterilized sawdust. I have not been to a log culture operation, but there are excellent books about it which make fascinating reading. With both methods, there are strong associations to assist new growers. The reference section on mushrooms should be helpful.

Shiitake are usually quite expensive in the retail market (a big plus for growers) and are considered a grand gourmet treat by cooks and diners everywhere. The flavor is far superior to that of the common market mushrooms.

Shiitake are available dried in many super markets, and are now available more and more often as fresh. It is the fresh production that interested me—especially organically grown mushrooms.

I knew that the regular button (*Agaricus*) mushrooms that are found in every market around the country are grown in animal manure of one type or another, and with lots of chemical sprays used along the way. According to Christopher Hobbs, "many commercially cultivated mushrooms are among the most heavily sprayed items in the vegetable section."

What would it take, I wondered, to produce organically grown mushrooms?

Snow Peak Mushroom Co.

🍄 *Jim Macpherson*

Jim Macpherson of the Snow Peak Mushroom Co. was listed as just such a mushroom producer in a directory of Northwest Organic Growers. He agreed to let Tal and me come for a visit to his farm in Lebanon, Oregon—peaceful farm country in the middle of the state about 25 miles east of Highway 5. We arrived at the farm having no idea what to expect; we left his place a few hours later converted to enthusiasm for this unusual crop.

I have visited and talked with other growers since then, have read several books on mushroom growing, and think this can be a very strong crop for the future. It must be noted that, like other well paying crops, commercial mushroom growing is not cheap to take up seriously; it is not especially easy, and it is certainly not fast. It really has no get-rich-quick attributes about it.

Macpherson began his mushroom growing efforts about 10 years ago after his brother gave him a magazine article to read about Shiitake growing. Jim first tried growing Shiitake on oak logs but soon switched to making his own substrate medium for growing blocks. His entire operation is contained in several large, pale green Quonset style buildings.

In the first production step, Jim, or one of his few employees, loads about two yards of hardwood sawdust into a ribbon mixer, then adds measured amounts of water, wheat bran, and millet to create a nutritious mix in which to grow Shiitake.

Jim has the mixer rigged to a "bagging machine" for building his substrate growing blocks. Five pounds of the mix is carried up from the mixer by a continuous belt, tips over the top and then falls into an open plastic bag. An employee picks up the bag and gives it a sharp tap—squaring it up into an instant mushroom growing block.

The bag top is folded over and closed with a clothes pin. A little air vent in the center of the bag allows some air exchange, but will prevent the entry of contaminants. The filled plastic bags are placed on a cart to eventually be pushed into a long, cylindrical autoclave sterilizer at the other side of the building.

When 800 of these little five pound blocks have been filled, Jim closes up the sterilizer, sets the temperature at 250°, and lets it all cook for seven hours.

Eight hundred substrate blocks, then, is his daily production capacity. After 14 weeks, those 800 five pound blocks can produce about one thousand pounds of fresh Shiitake mushrooms. But Jim does not just sell the fruit—he also sells the blocks to other commercial mushroom producers.

The sterilized blocks must be inoculated with mushroom spawn before the Shiitake life cycle can begin. This is done in the spawn room which is fitted with a HEPA (High Efficiency Particulate Air) filter to remove any airborne bacteria along with any different fungi spores. The fairly recent development of this air filter is one of the things that has so changed the gourmet and medicinal mushroom farming scene in America.

The spawn room smells of rubbing alcohol; everyone wears sterilized gowns, aprons, and gloves. This is a serious and expensive part of the business. Jim buys his mushroom spores from a lab in Corvallis, Oregon. In the wild, mushrooms produce spores which are often genetically different from the parent mycelium. For this reason, growers purchase pure strains of mushroom spawn from specialty labs.

After inoculation, each bag of substrate is dated and moved into another one of the large buildings where the blocks are stored on shelves and held for a fourteen week stay at exactly 70°, in order for the mycelia to grow. All the buildings are completely light, humidity, and temperature controlled. This fine-tuned management of the environment for these growing blocks is the primary job of the commercial organic mushroom grower.

"This can be done anywhere," says Jim, "but it is obviously easier and cheaper to do in a place where there is a fairly mild climate with some humidity."

At the end of this incubation stage, the bags look different. The color has changed, the bags seem more solid, some even have bulges on the side—all signs of thickly grown mycelia. The blocks are then removed from their plastic bags and moved into a different environment: a cooler, much more humid (RH 90%) building where they are set on rebar shelves and induced by this fake, fall-like environment to bear their fruit.

It's a strange sight, really. The blocks are now dark brown, like oversized loaves of pumpernickel bread. Water is dripping everywhere. It's dark and dank—looking for all the world like a huge, long abandoned storeroom behind a German bread bakery. From the side and top of each loaf, the small exotic shapes of Shiitake can be seen. Two employees come through each day snapping off the ripened fruit, then boxing it for market.

I notice that one of the women is wearing an air filter mask—a result, she tells me, of a slight allergy caused by constant exposure to the mushroom spore. That is not uncommon, says Jim, who keeps in touch with other growers across the country through grower associations.

Jim sells his fruit to only one or two wholesale produce brokers on the west coast; his substrate blocks to mushroom growers everywhere. He is one of the largest Shiitake growers on the west coast; the largest grower, he tells us, is in Pennsylvania.

Individual Shiitake substrate or natural wood logs are available these days, I notice, in all the garden magazines. For $25 or so, you can have one shipped to your home with full instructions on how to grow it. Jim gave us one, which our young niece, Stephanie, promptly turned into her science project at school. "It just grew one big, huuuuge mushroom," she later related, holding her hands out in a foot wide circle, "but I was afraid to eat it."

Shiitake growers get about $5 per pound for the fresh mushrooms at produce wholesalers, $6 or $7 per pound from chefs. The blocks produce from one to one and a half pounds per block in the six to nine months of their productive life. Jim sells them, in quantity, to other growers at $2 to $2.25 per block. At any given time, Jim and his employees are looking after about 60,000 blocks that are incubating and 20,000 of them that are fruiting.

His operation is obviously very, very successful. And, just as obviously, very expensive to set up and operate. Know of any small operators, we asked?

Fungus Among Us

◖ *The Monroes*

Enter Lynn and Michael Monroe, who also took a trip to Jim Macpherson's Shiitake farm in Oregon, became Shiitake enthusiasts, and are now small, full-time commercial growers in Snohomish, Washington. Fungus Among Us is the name of their company.

Actually, Lynn and her brother first started growing mushrooms as a home hobby. She later heard about Macpherson, and then she and her husband, Mike, visited the Lebanon farm when they wanted to look into serious mushroom growing.

The Monroes lived in Seattle at that time, where they had extra space in a garage they thought they could spare. They decided to turn that into a little mushroom room, starting out with 100 blocks that they purchased from Jim. They've been seriously "into mushrooms" ever since.

The first things the Monroes wanted to talk about were the pitfalls. "The two main things people need to realize about this business," said Mike, "are that it isn't cheap to get into, and that you have to do it every day."

"Mushrooms don't stop growing on weekends," added Lynn.

Lynn and Mike are friendly, delightful young people with total enthusiasm for what they are doing, but it's now well tempered by the investment and hard work they have had to put in.

They just "played around" with the Seattle garage operation, building a tiny room in a part of the garage out of rigid foam ("that pink stuff") and installing fans.

They laugh and talk simultaneously, remembering the experiment.

"Whatever you do, don't ever put a mushroom operation inside your house."

"What a mess."

"Humidity City."

"Rot it out."

"Needs 85% to 90% humidity."

"No room in a home can stand that for very long."

And all the time showing me through their present mushroom operation that keeps them both occupied nearly full-time. Their mushroom buildings were once a small barn and a large greenhouse, with the concrete pad for another building being spread that day as we walk and talk.

The Monroes say they had to put in 12 and 14 hour days at first, just to get this new place going. Now they can have shorter work days, but they have to be there every day because of all the cooling and humidity systems that may need repair, because of all the care needed to keep contaminants out of the system. Contamination can come in through the growing medium, on tools, through the air, and even on the bodies of people coming into the room. This kind of mushroom growing doesn't seem to be a good crop choice for careless people.

Mike and Lynn have been working with students at the Seattle Institute of Culinary Arts, inviting the would-be chefs to come out, see how the mushrooms are grown, and learn to do more cooking with fresh gourmet mushrooms.

The medicinal aspects of the mushrooms are of special interest to the Monroes and they are already learning to grow other exotics—like the Oyster, the Maitake, and the Lion's Mane. All of these mushrooms have studies done about them in Japan and China that show they are worthwhile candidates for possible anti-cancer drugs. The new building at the Monroe farm will house a special section for doing more work with these different varieties. When the medicinal aspects of the mushrooms become more well known in America, the Monroes will be ready.

Meanwhile, Lynn has managed to place their mushrooms in the nicest supermarkets of the Seattle region, the organic sections of Puget Sound Consumer Co-op stores, and many of the fanciest restaurants.

At this time they can incubate 5,000 blocks at a time, and believe they will be going to a maximum of 15,000 blocks eventually. They sell individual growing blocks through a mail order seed company, but not yet to other growers.

Diversity is one of their primary concerns, and to this end they have already produced a mushroom cookbook, learned how to dry the mushrooms successfully, created mushroom growing and cooking gift baskets, and have put all this on their Internet site—where they now get electronic orders and feedback from interested people around the world.

The Monroes credit Macpherson and *Shiitake Growing Handbook* author John Donahue for their own success. They keep a file on everything they can find about medicinal mushroom research worldwide, and are very confident that the demand for their product can only increase.

Most of the present Monroe customers don't yet have any idea about the special medicinal values of the Shiitake or the other exotic mushrooms the young couple are learning how to grow. The gourmet part of the market is carrying their business along quite profitably as they wait for the medicinal research information from around the world to catch up with these North American customers. A well-paying business waiting for the next exciting steps to happen.

San Juan Mushrooms
🍄 *Fungi Phil*

There's one more person to introduce on the subject of mushroom growing: meet Phil Schulz, recently known on our little island as Fungi Phil. Our island supermarket carried a splendid shelf of unusual mushrooms last year—"locally grown" the sign said—to my delight. I purchased and prepared the mushrooms, but when it came time to do the interviews for this section, I found that Fungi Phil's shelf of market mushrooms had disappeared. He had not left the island—just the world of growing for awhile.

Phil grew up in the northwest and some of his earliest memories are of walking through the mushroom barns his family had when he was a little boy. They grew Agaricus, the common button mushroom, and Phil began growing those a few years ago based on his own memories of how they were grown by his family. He used the manure-laden straw available from our county fairgrounds each year after everyone brings their animals to the fair for a week of showing and judging.

Phil also started reading about mushrooms, took a workshop or two, and learned of the much higher value of exotic mushroom crops—especially those that are organically grown. He decided to give the exotics and organic cultivation a try.

Phil's regular work is in electronics. He was unmarried at the time, and started his new mushrooming venture after regular work hours, in a closet in his house. He soon found that each type of mushroom could require a different temperature, a different humidity, and even a different growing medium. I could hear in his voice just how crazy his life must have become as he got deeper and deeper into the mushroom world while still keeping his regular job going.

"I started selling oyster mushrooms, then oyster and Shiitake both. I used decomposing straw for growing oyster mushrooms, and that attracted pests that were too much for the Shiitakes in the same growing house."

Phil spent $30,000 for a large greenhouse, but then couldn't afford an autoclave in which to sterilize the soil. Instead, he used pressure cookers (48 quarts of soil at a time) and the time it took to accomplish that nearly drove him crazy.

"There were just so many details," he remembers, "so much to keep track of, so much attention that must be paid. My greenhouse would hold 1,000 Shiitake blocks, but I could never grow that many because of the additional space needed for incubation."

He kept both the incubating and the growing blocks together in the same greenhouse, and when he filled that up he'd stash the blocks all over his house.

"I just got carried away," he said, "making my own blocks and then trying to create appropriate environments to put them in all over the house. In cupboards, even under the beds. It got to be a mess. I'd come home from work at night and have to deal with whatever had happened during the day," he said, and soon even more started happening.

"Mushroom growing was hard work," he says now, "and I didn't ever make enough money at it to quit my day job. I got pretty tired of fighting molds and pests." A final blow came last winter when a hundred year snowstorm put down his (and many another islander's) greenhouse.

"When it came time to slow down and get married," he said, " I was ready." Now he is rethinking the whole idea. Phil still wants to be involved in growing a crop—but he doesn't want to get back into such a frantic fight to stay ahead of so many potential problems.

"Maybe something without so much expense," he says, asking if I know anything about growing ginseng or goldenseal. Oh, brother, I think; why can't Phil be happy growing red clover, or maybe echinacea? He just keeps choosing the tough stuff. But, of course, it's the tough stuff that can bring in a very good income over a long period, IF IF IF. And statistics do show that people who fail at attempts like this often come back with another try and succeed quite well—having learned from their own and others' mistakes.

The exotic mushroom idea is a good one because Americans are only now beginning to discover the health benefits of these delicious mushrooms. In Japan, I have read, Shiitake growing leveled off in the '60s until the whole country discovered their medical aspects. Now, because the Japanese government has approved the use of Shiitake (and the chemicals derived from them) as anti-cancer treatments, Shiitake farming has continued to grow at a steady rate. As more and more research is done on these truly magic mushrooms, we can surely expect some of that same increase in interest in this country.

The retail and wholesale prices right now seem very high—but what will happen as new growers get into the market every year? Learning to market mushrooms will be the key for newcomers—and every bit as important as learning to grow them.

Creating a market in your own area will actually be the ingredient for success in gourmet/medicinal mushrooms **or** in medicinal herbs. You must learn to grow well, of course, but the marketing will be just as important. With mushrooms (just as with fresh herbs) you will quickly learn that freshness, quality, and good service are the keys that open the doors to sales. **These are truly going to be the determining factors for small growers.** The same ideas we will cover in the section about marketing medicinal herbs are the ideas needed to sell exotic and medicinal mushrooms: concentrate first on your own area; push the ideas of high quality, fresh and organically grown. And then be certain you are able to deliver what you promise.

With gourmet mushrooms, you will probably also need to become an educator, as so few people now purchase and use exotic mushrooms. In my first book on herbs, I encouraged new growers to put on little culinary herb tasting demonstrations at their market accounts or at their farmers' markets, to teach people about the taste value in fresh-cut culinary herbs. I think the same ideas can apply for gourmet/medicinal mushrooms in the '90s and well beyond.

At our Saturday Market this year, my friend Sam Pope is selling packages of his Kulu Farm ostrich meat. He sets up a grill, gives everyone little tastes of cooked ostrich sausages, hamburgers or steaks, and we all go home with packages of meat—even though my family seldom eats red meat! Such is the power of a tasting demonstration. Of course, Sam also hands out printed information on the ostrich meat showing how much leaner it is than other red meats—plus recipes, too. That's just what a person can do with exotic mushrooms at a supermarket or a farmers' market. Demonstrate their delicious flavor and give out lots of consumer information. You'll need to learn the medical information yourself; you can start with the reference section at the end of this book. As the medicinal aspects of the mushrooms become ever more publicly known, the popularity (and your sales) can only increase.

Medicinal tincture companies are starting now to produce and sell Shiitake (and other exotic mushroom) extracts. The best tincture companies will want to use mushrooms that are organically grown. Now I find that little packages of dried exotic mushrooms from Asia are offered in many Asian, gourmet, and health food stores. I've yet to see a package of them marked as organically grown. I feel certain that combination of organically grown exotics can offer new growers real clout in the marketplace as the anticancer properties of Shiitake become better known.

CHAPTER THREE

Wildcrafting Medicinal Herbs

"If it should turn out that we have mishandled our own lives as several civilizations before us have done, it seems a pity that we should involve the violet and the tree frog in our departure."

Loren Eiseley, The Star Thrower, *1978*

Michael Pilarski

Maybe I can just skip the subject of wildcrafting in this book, I told myself. I had covered it somewhat in *Herbs For Sale*, and since that time had become ever more skittish about the whole subject. It's hard to pick up a single herb newsletter, magazine, or herb book that doesn't shine another light on the crazies out there, removing the remaining wild stands of echinacea, goldenseal, and ginseng and somehow finding buyers. I get a phone call or an e-mail from one of them every now and then.

"I just scored some fresh echinacea. Even got the roots. Where can I sell them for the best price?"

In hell, I want to answer. Instead, I go through the drill about the disappearance from the wild of our native species; how important it is to not take whole plants helter skelter—blah, blah, blah—feeling all the while that the whole conversation (or correspondence) is hopeless and that there's really no way of convincing idiots to behave sanely. Over time, I have managed to convince myself that there are big bus loads of idiots out there grabbing everything and that maybe wildcrafting itself ought to be banned.

Michael Pilarski has now convinced me that I may have gotten a wee bit twisted on the subject, a little like one of those other paranoid types we all know who watches a few too many crime stories on local television news channels. Pretty soon "everyone's a criminal and we've got to crack down ever harder." (All the while the crime statistics are going down but the television coverage gets ever more bizarro.)

Anyway, I'm choosing to present the important subject of herb wildcrafting through the far more experienced eyes and ideas of a man who has spent the last 20 or more years of his life thinking about and acting on the ideas of species protection and conservation. He certainly makes a lot more sense on the subject than I ever did.

Michael Pilarski is the founder of Friends of the Trees, a long time environmental organization in the west that has overseen the giving away and planting of over 170,000 trees and shrubs. Forestry restoration is his specialty, along with worldwide networking on permaculture and sustainable agriculture. He also wildcrafts medicinal herbs himself.

Michael has published a thick volume on restoration forestry, along with a complete guide to growing kiwi fruit in northern climates. He has started apprentice programs for organic farms; he collects and maintains seeds of over a hundred wild species growing in the northwest. Nowadays he also puts together specific country or region reports for people traveling overseas to work: the contacts, resources, and detailed information to make their third world travel more successful. He teaches classes in ethnobotany and, most importantly for this chapter, in wildcrafting medicinal herbs.

Pilarski has probably spent more time wandering the mountains and foothills of eastern and western Washington state than anyone else I've met. And for twenty years he has made and used medicine from the plants around him. I'd probably be hard pressed to find many who have learned and thought more about wildcrafting than he has.

"Most people automatically assume," says Michael, "that as soon as we are taking something from the wild we are depleting the resource. Not true. We can do sustainable wildcrafting; we can even do wildcrafting as restoration. After all, burdock, St. John's wort, tansy are all plants people often want removed from their land," he reminds me.

I can immediately think of others. On our island, the few remaining cattle raisers are often complaining about too much hawthorn on their land. And how about all the land in the southern states that is full of kudzu vines? All of these plants, I know, are used medicinally. All are invasive and prolific beyond imagining in some areas of the country.

So it's really not the taking of the plants so much as it is the question of exactly which plants, from which areas, and how to take them in a more responsible manner. Ethical wildcrafting, then, is the real subject, and that is Pilarski's world.

Ever think of weeding as wildcrafting? Pilarski does. "I get my supply of horsetail from an organic farmer who has horsetail as a weed in his row crops. I carefully go through and remove the horsetail; the farmer and I are both satisfied." Horsetail (*Equisetum arvense*) is used as an astringent and diuretic.

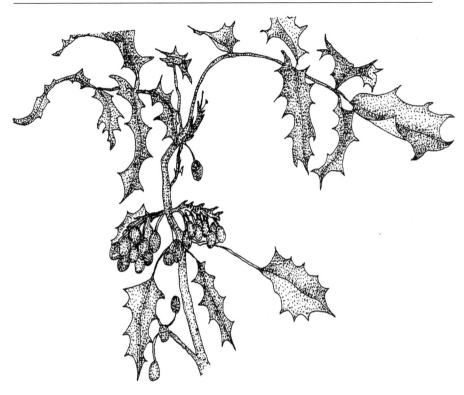

Pilarski has overheard herbalists on the east coast worrying about too much wildcrafting of Oregon grape (*Mahonia aquifolium*) on the west coast. It is used as a substitute for goldenseal, whose natural stands are disappearing rapidly.

"You may be able to take too much from one stand of Oregon grape," says Michael, "but even that might be hard to do as the roots break off as you harvest, leaving rhizomes in the ground to continue growing. There really is Oregon grape everywhere, throughout much of the northwest, and in amounts that are truly abundant.

"Most people think of our continent as untouched when Europeans first arrived. That's not so. It was a landscape modified by the Native American people who met all their needs from the land gathering and changing the environment as they went. But they apparently did it in a sustainable way. That's what we have to strive for. And it will mean taking different things in different amounts, and it will have to vary from region to region."

Pilarski uses devil's club (*Oplopanax horridum*) as an example of his overall view and method of wildcrafting. One of the lesser known ginseng relatives, devil's club was a primary medicine of the north coast native peoples and Michael believes it will soon take its place as an important medicinal herb in the American marketplace.

"If you live in Northern California and hear that I'm wildcrafting this herb you would be shocked, as it's becoming quite rare there. But, as you go further north, the stand sizes begin to increase. And once you get to Alaska, it is incredibly prolific.

"I primarily want recumbent stems when I collect devil's club, as it is the bark that is important for medicine. So I take the stems, prune the tips, and shove the stem tips back in the ground at the base of the plant, to replant them. If conditions are right, some of these tips will take root and start new plants.

"This particular plant also likes partial sunlight and, as the shade deepens, the plant will become shaded out. It has an advancing edge and a retreating edge. I need to harvest from the area it is dying out in; so I take from the retreating edge. That way I know I'm doing very little damage, besides replanting as I go."

Sometimes Michael will bring home the growing tips of devil's club and give these to organic farmers who are wanting to get into growing medicinal plants. "Eventually, we need to learn to grow all our medicinal herbs, " he says, "but wildcrafting is still going to be an important part of herbal medicines. We must learn to do both things better."

When deciding to wildcraft a medicinal plant, here are the kinds of things Pilarski feels must be known and considered about each plant before taking it:

- Is it a non-native, invasive, widespread, abundant, weedy plant? Wildcrafting in these cases can be a profitable alternative to using herbicides for weed control. Examples in Washington state: St. John's wort, burdock.
- Is it a non-native abundant plant species generally not considered noxious? In many cases, stands of these species can be harvested in a way which doesn't reduce the resource and so enables long-term yields. Examples in Washington state: dandelion, mullein.
- With native plants, are they widespread and abundant everywhere, or simply widespread and only locally abundant? With these, more care must be used, smaller quantities taken. Examples here would be: Oregon grape, elder.
- Are they native plants that are rare, threatened, and endangered locally, but not throughout their range? Much more caution now must be used, and much more known of the plants and their environments. Michael's examples here are Pacific bayberry and sweet gale.
- Native plants which may be abundant locally but are threatened in most other parts of the range should not have any harvesting,

says Pilarski. "Let's not take the best stands that are left!" Small amounts of seed and propagation materials can be judiciously harvested, but only to bring into cultivation.

- Native plant species which are officially classified as rare, endangered, or threatened are illegal to harvest. All parts are protected. But this list is far too short, says Pilarski, and many more species must be added.

Wildcrafters, says Michael, must know the status of each species throughout its range. If they take the time to really educate themselves about these special plants they can play a part in the future of medicinal plants in their own region.

They can then successfully bring native botanicals into cultivation, they can get contracts to harvest in an area before clear cutting or road building, and they can help divert non-native medicinal plants scheduled for destruction in a restoration area. And yes, they can earn money from selling medicinal plants to medicinal product makers. Almost all herb medicine makers use some supplies of wildcrafted plants.

What really comes through in talking with Michael Pilarski are the 20 years of learning that have gone into his education as a wildcrafter. And what scares both of us is the free swinging, greedy mentality that can start people along the wildcrafting path in search of the bucks, but without any of the learning.

There's another aspect to the uglier side of wildcrafting that worries Michael more and more. "Many cultures around the world are totally without concerns about sustainability," he notes. "And many immigrants from those cultures have come into the country to seek work—and are very hard working people. People we don't want to keep out of the country, but who have a very different sensibility than many of us do. All too often, they see our forests and our plant-covered lands as chock full of resources that are up for grabs. Simply there for the taking. Without any limits."

He is talking specifically now about the floral trade and its endless need for salal and sword fern; about the wild mushroom market and the now fiercely competitive search for those high value crops. All this picking has been taking place in our forests with, so far, almost no oversight from the forestry people. Most of the pickers are immigrants.

"The forestry bureaucracy needs to be more involved in this and more educated, too," says Michael, and he is working to stay involved with them in order to help draw up some sustainability guidelines for the industry and the forest service.

"Last year," he recalls, "I went in to get a permit from a forest section I'd never worked in before, and the ranger on duty said that I was the first person in his 15 years of working there to come in and seek a permit to pick. 'I know there are lots of pickers out there,' he said, 'but they never come in for permits.'"

If you intend to wildcraft in your area, be aware that the regulations regarding picking on state land, U.S. Forest Service land, and private lands can be very different. The whole issue of wildcrafting is in a state of flux around the country right now as everyone is starting to take a look at the issue anew.

In the future, says Pilarski, "we will have to see more guidelines and regulations on harvesting medicinal herbs on public lands." Which also means that the question of learning to grow native plants will become ever more important as time goes by.

The U.S. Forest Service is presently putting together new plans for its Special Forest Products Division for different regions of the country. This is the federal department that is concerned with collecting from the wild. In several places in the country, it is seeking herbalist information in order to work together on better protection of the forests.

United Plant Savers

"At the same time as 80% of the world's population depends on traditional medicine systems, chiefly herbal medicine, the accelerating need for phytomedicines, pharmaceutical drugs, and other industrial applications has caused over-exploitation of medicinal plants, resulting in genetic erosion and threat of extinction of many source plants harvested in the wild."

Conclusion from the First World Congress on Medicinal & Aromatic Plants for Human Welfare, Netherlands, 1992

🌾 🌾 🌾

It's not just the forestry people who are getting involved in these questions about wild medicinal plants. Herbal people all around the country are awakening to many of these problems and one of America's leading herbalists, Rosemary Gladstar, has recently stepped forward to help found a new, nonprofit organization, United Plant Savers (the herbalist's UpS). Dedicated to saving endangered and threatened medicinal plants, this organization for herbalists and people who love plants hopes to help ensure the future of our rich diversity of medicinal plants.

UpS offers wonderful inducements for their new members: conferences and workshops around the country; free seeds and roots of endangered species; slide shows of "at risk" medicinal herbs for their members to share in local communities. I am now awaiting the arrival of a dozen free goldenseal roots that UpS is shipping to all their interested members across the country. What better way to see if this precious and disappearing plant can be shown to grow in many areas of the country.

Most importantly, UpS offers a united effort, based on up-to-date information, to prevent the great botanical medicine reserves of North America from being depleted by careless greed and ignorance. "Native medicinal plants are under siege," says Dr. Richard Liebmann, Executive Director of UpS. "In the United States alone, over 2400 acres of native habitat is lost every day."

United Plant Savers' goals include identifying and compiling information on threatened medicinal plants in each state and/or bioregion. This is the information they hope to get out to the herbal community around the country, along with lists of resources for obtaining seeds, roots, and plants for replanting and restoration. This is just the kind of national group that can make a big difference in the future of medicinal plant wildcrafting. I hope readers of this book will consider supporting them in their efforts by becoming members. See the resource section for their address.

Here are the UpS basic guidelines for *Wildcrafting with Integrity:*

- Always wildcraft with thoughts of beauty. Put beauty into your work. Ask yourself how much more beautiful will this plant community be when I am finished gathering.

- Think first about the plant community and how many plants it can manage without, not how many plants you need in order to make products or profits.

- Treat the native plant complexes like the fine perennial gardens that they are.

- Do not upset in any manner undisturbed native soil— it is rare and precious.

- Take only as many plants as you can reasonably use; strive for zero waste.

- Replant the areas you are harvesting from. Scatter seeds, replace crowns and plant roots. Leave plenty of mature and seed-reproducing plants to reproduce.

- Start a replanting project in your area to help re-establish endangered and threatened species.

- Know the endangered plant species in your bioregion.

In the fall of 1997, UpS sent out the following draft copy of an indigenous medicinal plant list for their members to comment on. These plants are the ones UpS feels are already truly endangered.

⚜ UpS AT RISK PLANT LIST

American Ginseng	*Panax quinquefolium*
Black Cohosh	*Cimicifuga racemosa*
Bloodroot	*Sanguinaria canadensis*
Blue Cohosh	*Caulophyllum thalictroides*
Echinacea	*Echinacea spp.*
Goldenseal	*Hydrastis canadensis*
Helonias Root	*Chamaelirium luteum*
Kava Kava (Hawaii only)	*Piper methusticium*
Lady's Slipper Orchid	*Cypripedium spp.*
Lomatium	*Lomatium dissectum*
Osha	*Ligusticum porteri, L. spp.*
Partridge Berry	*Mitchella repens*
Peyote	*Lophophora williamsii*
Slippery Elm	*Ulmus rubra*
Sundew	*Drosera spp.*
Trillium, Beth Root	*Trillium spp.*
True Unicorn	*Aletris farinosa*
Venus Fly Trap	*Dionaea muscipula*
Wild Yam	*Dioscorea villosa, D. spp.*

The following UpS list is of plants the UpS feels may be at risk, but need further research. Some plants are "abundant in one bioregion and quite rare in another." But they are plants that need watching in many areas of the country. UpS also invites suggestions from their members for additional plants for these listings.

These are also plants that need to be organically cultivated, if at all possible. That has to be one of the real answers to our over-harvesting and loss of habitat problems. If you are wondering which medicinal plants to grow, which ones might be wanted in the future, these lists are certainly good places to start in your thinking. If you can provide organically grown supplies of these plants, you should easily find good markets for them.

Michael Pilarski and I also both agree that all of the companies who purchase medicinal herbs grown in the wild need to take a stronger interest in just where those plants are coming from and how they have been harvested.

In the Rocky Mountains, an excellent effort at cooperation between sustainable pickers and growers along with ethical medicine companies is already taking place.

🌿 UpS PLANTS TO WATCH LIST

Arnica	*Arnica spp.*
Butterfly Weed	*Asclepias tuberosa*
Calamus	*Acorus calamus*
Chaparro	*Casatela emoryi*
Elephant Tree	*Bursera microphylla*
Eyebright	*Euphrasia spp.*
Gentian	*Gentiana spp.*
Goldthread	*Coptis spp.*
Lobelia	*Lobelia spp.*
Maidenhair Fern	*Adiantum pendatum*
Mayapple	*Podophyllum peltatum*
Oregon Grape	*Mahonia spp.*
Pink Root	*Spigelia marilaandica*
Pipsissewa	*Chimaphila umbellata*
Spikenard	*Aralia racemosa, A. californica*
Stone Root	*Collinsonia canadensis*
Stream Orchid	*Epipactis gigantea*
Turkey Corn	*Dicentra canadensis*
Virginia Snakeroot	*Aristolochia serpentaria*
White Sage	*Salvia apiana*
Yerba Mansa	*Anemopsis californica*
Yerba Santa	*Eriodictyon californica*

The Rocky Mountain Herbalist Coalition in Boulder, Colorado, began compiling a list a few years ago of those growers and wild herb harvesters willing to follow strict ethical standards in plant collecting and growing. The directory of these companies is offered to anyone with an interest. The address is in the resource section.

A small but important group of wildcrafters and growers from around the country are listed in the directory. So are wildcrafting ethics and guidelines, a wildcrafter's criteria sheet, a voucher specimen information sheet, and a list of botanists around the country to contact for botanical verifications. Each company in the directory also provides a representative list of a few plants they harvest, along with a current price per pound.

There's also the question of our own responsibility as herbal medicine consumers: where do the medicinal plants we are consuming come from? Sustainable wild harvesting has to become much more than a trendy phrase if any real progress is to be made on this important issue.

If you want to take up wildcrafting and sell what you collect to herb companies, you will find ways to contact these companies in another part of this book. You will also find helpful wildcrafting resources in the resource section. It's obvious from looking at any catalog from a company selling bulk medicinal herbs that much of the product from many of them is still wildcrafted. The effort at learning to bring those plants home and cultivate them commercially is quite new—especially this organized nationwide effort.

There will be a long time need for wild harvested plants. For some people this can offer a decent income. The important thing is to make certain that any wildcrafting we do becomes a part of the solution to the need for ethically harvested wild medicine plants—and not a part of the continuing problem of their disappearance.

Consider joining UpS and using their resources to help spread the word in your community about the wild medicinal plants of your area. When you're in the northwest area, give Michael Pilarski a call. Take his wildcrafting classes, have him teach or speak in your area, and set yourself on a path towards wildcrafting enlightenment. You might also thank him, as I do, for sharing his resources and knowledge.

CHAPTER FOUR

Selling What You Grow or Collect

"The medicinal herb world needs dynamic people with curiosity who will work hard to achieve their goals. People who want to enter into this field should not expect to get information served on the plate. They need to be prepared to experiment to some extent themselves. Those who do not have that inquisitive mind and that are not ready to experiment themselves, I don't think this is for them. They better go in to some more conventional and well established field."

Dr. Branka Barl, Saskatchewan Herb Research Centre,
Univ. of Saskatchewan, Saskatoon, Saskatchewan,
Burnaby, B. C. Feb. '98

Herb Marketing 101

For years, herbal medicine enthusiasts have been out banging the drums to get everyone's attention focused on the great potential to be found in these remarkable plants. They have been succeeding. Herbalists for years have also been fighting to stop efforts from the Congress and the FDA to limit the availability and use of these herbal products. They have also been succeeding at that.

As a result, it is estimated that up to 60 million Americans now spend an annual average of $54 each year on medicinal herb products. That adds up to a North American market worth more than three billion dollars a year. In that same year, it is estimated that the German population alone spent $3.5 billion for medicinal herb products. The American herb market is still quite young; the German market is more mature.

According to Peggy Brevoort, CEO of East Earth Herb, Inc., and former president of the American Herbal Products Association, the **top selling** U.S. herbal products for the year 1997 were those made from ginkgo, ginseng, garlic, St. John's wort, echinacea, and saw palmetto. The products from herbs showing the **greatest increase in sales** during that same time were St. John's wort, green tea, kava kava, elderberry, grape seed, saw palmetto and nettles.

It's not so much the size of these markets that is causing so much interest these days, as it is the rate of growth in the markets. Medicinal herb sales have been growing from 15% to 20% per year in both the U.S. and Canada for several years. But the real growth in herbal product sales, and the market news that is actually driving the current tsunami of medicinal herbs in North America, is the fact that there has been a very recent 80% increase in the use of herbal products in the U.S. **mass market**: drug stores, discount houses, super markets, etc.

Previously, the sales of herbal products had primarily been through the more than 10,000 to 15,000 health and natural food stores in North America. Until recently, much of this sales activity has been with products made by small to medium-sized herbal product companies; often the same companies who have been leaders in the political and regulatory efforts to keep herbal products available in the marketplace. Some of these companies have had great business success the last few years as more and more Americans have taken up the use of herbal preparations.

There are several things driving this continued increase in herbal medicines: the constant increase in health care costs, discontent with many aspects of the present health care system, and a very large and aging baby boomer population that has discovered both the health and cost effectiveness of herbal preparations. There are almost daily reports now on the results of new studies on botanical medicines and the major newspapers and television news stations have recognized the increased audience and reader interest in all things herbal. The use of herbal medicines, incidentally, is also increasing all round the world, including Asia and Europe.

All this increasing interest is reflected throughout the North American market and is pushing the herb product market further and further into the mainstream, creating both new markets for herbal products and new manufacturers of those products. Along with such mainstream success has now come the avid interest and involvement of corporate, worldwide business interests that have awakened to the fabulous profit potential in America's new found love affair with all things herbal—especially medicinally herbal. These large business interests are already all over the medicinal herb market and, of course, aren't worried about making or leaving small business opportunities for you or me. This market change is creating a new mass market for herbal products. It is quite different from the one centered in the natural food store market that has been there for some time now. I think it's important to understand this changing and dual market if you want to start a small business based on medicinal herbs.

There are many small business opportunities in the natural food market sector; there are not going to be so many chances in the mass market area. We are all used to taking over-the-counter medicines in manufactured forms that are made to be shipped around the world and to keep safely on the drug store (or health food shop) shelves for years. Those are the kinds of herb medicines that the large drug corporations are now rushing to put out for North American consumers. Should you be wanting to consider providing herb plant material right away for such large company products, you are mostly dreaming. You might as well consider supplying next year's salt and pepper needs for Campbell's Soups. Never gonna happen.

Sometimes I feel sure we are headed towards an herb medicine system that is simply a replica of our allopathic, or regular, single strong chemical drug system: single herb constituents extracted from plants, over-processed by megacorps, and shoved into little silver bullets to be swallowed and aimed at one isolated health problem. That's the system we've all been trained to. It's the system I hope many of us can continue to resist.

Yes, there absolutely and definitely is a place for small and new growers in today's medicinal herb market. The place to sell medicinal herbs is the same place we all need to be as far as our own herbal medicine purchases are concerned. Small and beginning growers need to concentrate on local or regionally owned and operated, small to medium-sized herb medicine companies; those that deliver high quality medicines made from carefully and organically grown, or carefully wildcrafted, **whole plants**. These are the companies looking for growers to supply their needs. These are the companies you'll need to learn to find and learn to grow for.

If you concentrate on this part of the market you will get a good start. And all the things you need to learn for this market you would also need to know should your efforts ever lead you into a much larger operation. Growing, harvesting, drying, cleaning; getting the crops to your customers in the best possible condition. Learn to meet these demands in the smaller, high quality and organic herb market and you will prepare yourself for the future—no matter how large you intend to become.

The resource section contains the results of a random survey I did of a few such herbal medicine and medicinal tea companies across the country. I found these names in one of the herb business directories. Some of them I know, others I don't. I suggest you familiarize yourself with these surveys, note the similar patterns in their replies to my questions, and ask yourself how you can learn to meet the needs expressed in these surveys. Spend a little time going over these survey responses; they are quite revealing. These companies are springing up everywhere. Many will be able to buy and use your well grown herbs.

First of all, talk to your local practicing herbalist or naturopathic doctor, if you have one in your area. (If you don't, chances are you will have before long.) Where are they getting their herbal medicines? Often these practitioners will be wanting to make at least part of their own medicines and will be interested in finding fresh, locally grown product.

Following that, I suggest you look in your regional phone books, and go into your local and regional food co-ops, herb shops and health food stores. Look at the labels on the herb medicines, especially those made with organically grown whole plants, especially those produced in your own region. Start a list of those companies you will want to contact.

What I'm really talking about here is an on-going working relationship with a medicine company or herbal practitioner. If you look at one of the herb resource directories I list in resources, you can find many, many herb businesses around North America—and the world. You can also make a trip to your local library and look in the Thomas Register for a listing of herb businesses. But first of all, I would concentrate on the businesses in your own area.

Attending herb conferences is also an excellent way to meet and talk with herb medicine makers, as they are often the speakers at these conferences. The conferences give a brief overall picture of the part of the medicinal herb world that this book is about. It's the part that's full of opportunity for new and small growers. A listing of coming herb conferences can always be found in the magazines featured in the resource section.

Okay, you say, I can do all that, but how would I know what to charge for my herbs? You can send for catalogs from existing bulk herb suppliers. Start out by looking at their prices. Then consult other herb company brochures; or look some up on the Internet. Tim Blakley also gives current prices in his listing of herbs in this book. These prices change all the time, of course, as I mentioned in the introduction to this book.

A main point to remember about pricing is that this is a very volatile, fluctuating market you are going into; any price published today could be up or down tomorrow. And quality, quality, quality, will, and should be, the determining factor in the prices you can receive. If a company isn't seriously selling quality in their products, you really can't afford to be dealing with them.

If you grow for a small tincture, herbal product or tea maker, you can easily get the going market price for your herbs. If you can save your customer freight costs, if they can see your garden and your methods; if they can learn to trust your product, then your prices should probably never be any less than what these larger, more well known companies are charging—assuming you do a great job at growing, harvesting and/or drying. Sometimes your prices can be even higher.

Many people read about the burgeoning medicinal herb world and decide they want to "grow the expensive stuff and earn a lot of money fast—before other people get into it." I get e-mails and phone calls from such people all the time: "I've got five acres, just tell me what to grow. Something that brings a great price. And doesn't take a lot of work."

I'm sure you know the type. If you read the surveys, you'll see that the need for growers is real—but it's definitely not a get-rich-quick scheme.

Pacific Botanical's owner, Mark Wheeler, whom you probably just read about in the grower chapters, contacted me recently to suggest that I not "overdo" this book's enthusiasm on echinacea growing. There are so many echinacea growers these days, he said, and the price in the market is fluctuating so much, that he's just not sure about its future. "We may be seeing supply catch up with demand this year."

On that same day, an ad in the classified section of one of the herb newsletters I get had a notice from Marlin Huffman, of Plantation Botanicals in Florida, wanting to buy 10,000 pounds of echinacea root. Whoa, I thought. Are these two guys really in the same business? The answer turns out to be: yes and no.

When I spoke to Marlin Huffman on the phone about my question, he was kind enough to lay out his view of the current picture on the echinacea market in America, along with a few other insights that new growers should add to their thinking about the medicinal herb market.

I wrote about Marlin Huffman and his operations in a previous book, *Herbs For Sale.* He's one of my all time favorite herb people: forthcoming, funny, and with a sharp, knowing eye on all things in the herbal marketplace around the world. Huffman, who started out as a wildcrafter long ago, is now a very successful part of that large corporate world herb market. But he's never forgotten how he started out, and always has a keen sense of how newcomers and small growers ought to position themselves in the herb market.

"There is money to be made by small growers in echinacea, and other herb plants," says Huffman, "but it will be by the small grower with ¼ to two or three acres of a crop who can, perhaps with family help, plant and weed by hand; collect their own seeds; grow their own starts; and never stop to ask themselves how much they are earning an hour. They just have to figure out the jobs that need to be done and get out there and do them.

"Those kinds of growers," says Huffman, "don't have to purchase $100,000 tractors, $30,000 sprayers, or pesticides and herbicides; they don't have high labor costs, high irrigation costs, and their land is often already paid for."

They can cater to the organic market, he says, "where that term still has some meaning," and keep their expenses low and their profits at a very decent level. "I can't really compete with such a grower," he says. "And they can deal in a market that I can't deal in. Just as they can't deal in mine."

"A metric ton of dried echinacea root right now," says Marlin, "is worth about $58,000. Small organic growers can probably get $50,000 to $52,000 for the same ton. With their low costs, that should be quite profitable."

Most large product companies won't deal with someone whose biggest growing effort would be only 2,000 pounds, says Huffman. "Larger companies often need about 60 tons of an herb like echinacea. They really don't want to hear from single ton growers. That takes too much expense and time." And no one can predict the future market price in a crop like echinacea as more and more growers from around the world hear about its growing popularity and start growing the crop. For some farmers, he says, echinacea is already becoming a commodity crop, and that kind of competition will always drive the prices down.

Huffman grew and harvested over 60 tons of echinacea this year on farms in South Dakota, Texas and Kansas—and purchased another 70 tons from other growers. His little ad, he said, only reflected that he needed still more to meet his market sales. But these suddenly ultra-popular herbs, he says, are not where new and smaller growers should be concentrating their efforts.

"If you had a warehouse full of dried, well grown St. John's wort today, you could probably come close to naming your price," says Marlin Huffman, who happened to still have at least a small warehouse full when we spoke recently. "But those price changes are known around the world very fast now," he says, "and huge growers in South America are planting as we speak. This herb can well become a commodity for those of us who can learn to grow it well and cheaply. Today's big price cannot last very long."

He operates in quite a different world from that of Marggy and Mark Wheeler of Pacific Botanicals. Or almost any one else I mention in this book. Huffman can react to media stories like the one this last year on the *20/20* television program about St. John's wort. I have been told that just that program alone drove the sales of St. John's wort up more than 1,000 per cent with accompanying large price increases. By the time new growers can learn how to grow the herb well and in quantity, the price can be down—way down—driven there by very big growers.

Marlin's comments about the state of organic growing and marketing in the U. S. are also particularly revealing. In the bigger corporate world of medicinal herbs, says Huffman, the term organic has no meaning. "I wish it did, I'd like for it to, but it doesn't. There is such chaos in the marketplace around that term and so little policing, that it can too often become a fraud."

A few years ago, he recalls, "I sold some organic saw palmetto to a buyer who put my organic certification number on his product label. He left it on there for three or four years, without ever buying from me again. I know all the organic growers of that crop, so I called them all to see if the man had purchased from them. He had not. So here he is, selling many, many tons of that crop, using my certification number to help sell it to unsuspecting buyers, and I finally had to threaten to sue him just to get him to stop. And he can get away with it very easily because the term organic has become almost meaningless," says Huffman,

"I have bought organic echinacea from places like Trout Lake Farm," (the largest organic herb grower in the U. S.) he says, "but organic now means so little in the larger world picture, that I don't even price those goods up any higher. Even when I've had to pay more for them because they are grown that way. It just doesn't mean anything at that market level. My echinacea goes to a European extractor who turns around and puts the processed extract back in the American market. He doesn't care at all if it's organically grown."

It's interesting to note here that growing for the organic market is seen by even one of the larger medicinal herb growers as the almost exclusive territory of smaller growers. If you step out of growing for the organic market, you step into the limbo I think of as mainstream oblivion, and your competitors increase a hundredfold, especially in size.

That limbo-land is the world of the super-processed constituents being used for the herbal products coming into the mass market—though they can now be found in the natural foods market, too. I think of them as the instant coffee products of the herb medicine market: tiny little globules of a few plant chemical constituents that are then sold as "standardized" medicines to those who are reassured that a "standardized" product must be both healthy and safe. More about this later, but it's just another reminder to stay on the organic and the "whole plant" side of the herbal medicine world. That's where your opportunities are.

If you are reading herb newsletters and magazines, attending herb conferences, and staying in touch with at least some parts of the medicinal herb world, you will also start hearing about the newest studies being done around the world on herbs. Soon you'll find yourself predicting what will be gaining in popularity, and learning to grow it. At that point you can, of course, take advantage of price increases in the market that come as different herbs gain in popularity. There are several thousand potential medicinal herbs out there, and there is finally money being put into research on these plants. According to many experienced and educated herb experts: we ain't seen nothin' yet. The medicinal herb market will continue to grow and grow.

Meanwhile, get reading on these surveys and start your own market research for what you intend to grow. Soon you may hear about a new (to you) medicinal herb; then read or hear about it again, perhaps in a different context, and then again, and you'll begin wondering about that herb. Is that an herb that may become more popular, more used? Should I learn to grow a little of it before it becomes very popular?

Here's an example of how that might work. I did some wondering recently about the herb osha (*Ligusticum porteri, L. spp.*), when someone asked me why Tim wasn't covering that herb in this book. I started a little book research, found that osha is related to one of my favorite culinary herbs: lovage, that it grows and is collected mostly in the Rockies; that it has a scary resemblance to and shares the same habitat with water hemlock; that it is considered a great flu medicine by some herbalists, not very worthy by others; that it has previously been considered impossible to germinate and domesticate; that this year both Richter's and Horizon Herbs are offering seeds with hopeful instructions; that it is listed for sale in several catalogs at between $24 and $48 per pound, dried, etc.

To continue this search, I would next see if it is offered for sale retail in my health food store, or herb shop—and in what form. I would notice if it is listed as an ingredient in herbal teas, etc. I would do a little search on the Internet about it; see what herb enthusiasts on there are saying about it. I would ask my herb friends about their experiences with it, and would just keep it in the front of my mind as I continue poking into this and that corner about medicinal herbs. I would probably start a little file on it if it began to look like something I really want to know a lot more about. Let your own curiosity about medicinal herbs and their future lead you down the path, one or two plants at a time. Put in only a few plants, or a few rows to begin with. Learn how it grows, harvests and dries. Then just keep on learning.

After you start growing medicinals, be sure and get yourself listed in the organic grower guides put out in your state and region. Consider an Internet web site to let people know what you are growing; start building an herb network through your own area and keep educating yourself in every way that you possibly can.

Perhaps some people can grow a crop of one single medicinal herb and, without knowing anything about it (or very much else), end up selling it for a decent price, as though it were onions or broccoli. But medicine crops are not treated the same as food crops in the marketplace, and I don't think successful growers can act as though they are.

These ancient plants are now part of a relatively new marketplace, and a new market often means room for newcomers. It can also mean operating without all the information you might need, and taking a few more risks than you might if you stayed on the broccoli wagon. The time you spend working on this marketing aspect is going to be just as valuable (or more so) as the time spent in the garden, field or hillside.

Take some time now to look at the company surveys. They begin on page 287.

CHAPTER FIVE

Meet the Medicinal Herbalists

"A factor that may have a profound influence on herbal medicine in the next century will be the economic advantage of keeping persons well rather than treating them after they become ill. In ancient China, people paid their physicians as long as they remained healthy and ceased to pay them when they became ill."

Dr. Varro E.Tyler, Lilly Distinguished Professor of Pharmacognosy, Purdue University, Herbs for Health, *March, 1996*

The Herbal Network

This is a chapter for those with a curiosity about, and an interest in, the actual one on one practice of medical herbalism, especially for those wondering what it takes to become an herbal practitioner. Few states do any legal licensing for such a vocation, and just the idea of offering any kind of health advice or care without a license is often enough to scare most people right off the subject. But there are herbal practitioners everywhere now, and it's time to take a look at who they are and what they really do.

Of all the new business possibilities in the medicinal herb renaissance, this one may prove to be one of the most popular, because there has been such a change in the ways we now seek out better health and well being. Not that many years ago, we didn't have a massage therapist, a hypnotherapist, a fitness trainer, or a biofeedback specialist in our community. Now we have several of each on the islands. People with a very good knowledge of plant based medicines and preventives are also among the new professionals many people are willing to consult with about their health. Professional herbalists usually charge from $40 to $75 per hour.

My selections here are very much based on my own prejudices, and a few words on those might be appropriate. I often use herbs in my own everyday health care, and I sometimes seek advice from herbalists. I read a lot of books on herbalism, and I consider myself very sympathetic to medicinal herb possibilities.

But I start to get a little squeamish with medicinal herb advice based on astrological signs. Or pendulum swings over herbal preparations. Or solely on writings from early centuries in Europe. Or the so-called Doctrine of Signatures—which was also big a couple of centuries ago but seems a tat incongruous these days.

I'm consciously choosing to direct readers down an herb path based more on reason and modern botanical medicine studies, as those are what make herbalism meaningful to me. A truly well educated, plant-based herbalist is someone whose advice I would always seek. They have taken the time and trouble to learn how the chemical compounds in plants may react in our bodies. They respect the history of the people's medicine enough to have learned previous herb uses and beliefs, but they also respect what modern labs are proving And they also know some plants can be dangerous. Because something is "natural" doesn't mean it's harmless—by any means.

Just as modern medicine has its share of quacks and quackery, so does herbalism—or any other system where some people will pay money to others to tell them what to do to feel better. Medicinal herbalists are far less regulated than most health practitioners and that makes room for lots of quackos and whackos. But our disappointment with parts of the more regular "cattle call" medicine has become so deep that many people everywhere want to try other approaches: Ayurvedic, homeopathic, holistic, traditional Chinese, to name just a few. We are, after all, a consumer society above all. So we look around and make our choices and remember always: *caveat emptor*, let the buyer beware.

The herb practitioners I will show you in this book are those who stress their own education and knowledge of the plants above everything else. I believe they are bringing us a genuine alternative to the medicine chest of very strong single chemicals we have all been visiting so freely for the last half century.

🌿 🌿 🌿

Before we meet these herbalists, I would first call your attention again to the importance of the herb webs, or networks, that are being woven in different regions of the country. At the center of each web are people who have been involved in herbs since at least about the 1970s, and who are always teaching or writing about the plants and the medicines made from them. Their outreach has been, and still is, quite remarkable. Those with new herbal interests are lucky to have the knowledge of these early herb people to draw on. They continue to build a strong and impressive network over which American herbalism is growing—very, very well. Medicinal herbalism is definitely not a fad. It will be with us for a long time to come.

A few of those early herbalists have now built up successful herb product companies; yet many remain very active as teachers. Herb people attend conferences endlessly. They are always getting together, exchanging information, spreading the word about the world of herbs. If you want to take a strong step along the medicinal herb path, attend one of the herb conferences that's probably being planned for your part of the country soon. It can tie you in, almost instantly, to the herb web of your region. The dates for these conferences are always given in the herb newsletters and magazines listed in this book's reference section. As I've said before, medicinal herbalism is very strong in a few areas of the country, and not yet so in many others. But I have no doubt that it will soon be reflected, although perhaps a little differently, in every part of the country.

It's time to meet some herbalists from my area. See if you can find a part of yourself in any or all of them, and see if you can also recognize the pattern of herb web building that is taking place in your area now. Much of the North American medicinal herb renaissance has been spread across the land in the most bottom up, grass roots fashion—which I think you can easily see at work in the following interviews.

🌿 *Janet Wright*

Janet Wright is one of my favorite would-be herbalists, always giving of her time and knowledge with grace and generosity. Janet is a full time schoolteacher in my town, so her interests in medicinal herbs are strictly for fun and knowledge at this point. Even so, Janet is very much at the center of our island network of herb people; I love being a part of the herb web she has built here.

For 15 years, Janet and her husband Dick, also a schoolteacher, have traveled to the Grand Teton mountains during the summers, where they camp out and spend as many weeks as possible learning all the birds and wild flowers, the trees and plants of that area. The Wrights are the kind of amateur naturalists you always want along when taking long walks; between them they know an incredible amount about what's overhead and underfoot.

More than a dozen years ago, Janet saw a notice of an herb walk being offered at the park where they were camping, and decided to attend. The walk was led by Rocky Mountain herbalist Clarissa Smith (more about her later) and, with that one "life changing" walk, Janet stepped fully into the world of wild medicinal plants. She came home inspired—and loaded with ideas and book titles to poke into.

All Janet's spare time the following year went towards reading about wild plants as medicine. She returned to the mountains the next summer, and many summers thereafter, to look up Clarissa Smith, and to attend any classes she might be offering in the area.

"I was totally taken with all of it," says Janet, "but quite hesitant to share it with anyone at home or at work. Herbs weren't all that popular then. People around me still thought they were weird."

Janet didn't just learn to identify plants with Clarissa, but also how to dig them properly, bring them in from the wild, dry or process them, and finally, to make simple medicines. She and Dick began trying the medicines to solve everyday health problems. It was a revelation to them both. "They worked," she laughs, remembering that time. "It was such fun."

Only then did she start to mention her interest in herbal medicine to others. Not surprisingly, she was soon asked by her colleagues for solutions to their problems:

"I keep getting colds, Janet, got any ideas?"

"I have been having the worst digestion problems. Can any of that weird stuff help?"

"I'm getting this crazy insomnia; wake up in the middle of the night and can't get back to sleep. Just hate taking sleeping pills. Would herbs be worth a try?"

So much had happened in the world of health care during those years when Janet was spending her summers learning about herbs in the Rocky Mountains, that now she could suddenly look around and find that everyone was interested in new and different approaches to taking care of themselves.

In 1993, the New England Journal of Medicine printed the results of a poll showing that more than 34% of Americans were already using some form of alternative medicine —and had spent nearly $14 billion doing just that during the year 1990 alone. Both of those figures have increased considerably since that time. And both of these often quoted figures have acted as somewhat of a wake-up call to many parts of the health care and pharmaceutical industries.

Herbs, which had virtually disappeared from the medicine chests of this country 50 or more years before, were now seen by many as new ways to treat old health problems. Herbs were less expensive, had fewer side effects, were more "natural," and had a long history of safety and efficacy all around the world. Herbs often stood in sharp contrast to the never ending supply of new and expensive doctor-prescribed medication: medicines at an ever greater cost, and often with more and more dangerous side effects.

The new popularity of medicinal herbs, combined with her own growing knowledge of the subject, brought Janet Wright into a more active role with herbs in our community. She invited Clarissa Smith (who, in the meantime, had moved to Seattle) to come to the islands and teach a few all-day classes to those with developing herb interests.

Janet also helped form a small local herb group, where interested

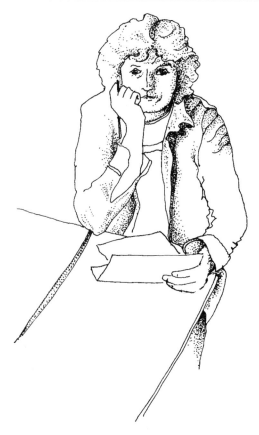

islanders gather once a month to share all they know and have learned about one single herb and, over time, have helped each other become better family herbalists. That's really what Janet sees as her primary role: to learn enough to be of real medical help to her family and friends.

Over the years, she has learned to grow some of the plants that she finds the most useful in her medicine making—plants that will grow on her relatively shady land: arnica, hops, black currants, motherwort, self heal, uva ursi, echinacea, rattlesnake plantain, mints, and violets. Other herbs she orders from Frontier Herbs in Iowa, and still others she picks from wild stands on the island: Oregon grape, St. John's wort, and nettles—lots of wild nettles. In the spring, Janet prepares and serves her friends a full flavored lasagna made with layers of fresh green nettles.

I would wish every community a Janet Wright or two. Her kitchen has a counter top full of jars filled with herbs "cooking in their menstruums." She makes and keeps a constant supply of herbalist Susan Weed's *Old Sour Puss Mineral Mix* on hand: a medicinal herb vinegar of common medicinal "weeds" (yellow dock, dandelion, plantain, nettle, raspberry, mugwort, comfrey, and red clover) combined with clean egg shells and left to sit in cider vinegar for six weeks. "Best and easiest source of calcium," says Janet.

"Who knows," she worries aloud, "what the FDA could eventually decide about some herbal medicines. I just feel it's important to learn all I can, to grow all I can for our own use, and to teach anyone who's interested in all I've learned."

Does she ever charge people for the advice or medicines she gives them, I wonder?

"Not really," she answers. "If I have some direct costs for something I make, I will pass that cost along. But really, I'm an elementary school-teacher. That's my serious work in life. I'm just having a good time with the herbs, and learning a lot. Maybe some day, after I retire, I can see that I may become more serious about the commercial aspects. And, if our retirement money ends up a little short, I guess I would think seriously about getting into that for some extra money. Right now I'm way too busy with my job, and just having too much fun with the herbs to even think about that more commercial part of it."

🌿 *Sandy Richard*

For a slightly different look into the more commercial aspects of an herbal practice, Sandy Richard is a good example of what it can take to get very serious about earning your living in the world of medicinal herbs.

With a B.A. in history from Rutgers University, followed by an M.A. in history from the University of Washington, Sandy thought she was headed for a U.S. State Department career—until she made a few trips to the San Juan Islands.

The incredible beauty of these islands can and does make all-consuming claims on people. But the islands offer very few career paths—or even decent job prospects for newcomers. It is not unusual here for our postal clerks to have advanced degrees, or for our house painters to be part-time research scientists. To make a permanent home on the islands often requires a lot of sacrifice—just to earn a living. To stay here and also be able to do meaningful work can take genuine resourcefulness. I never cease to be amazed at Sandy's tenacious determination and capacity for both hard work and creative versatility.

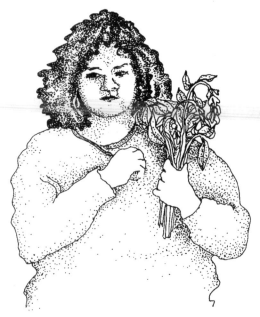

Sandy first did a few years of clerking at our local post office while she thought seriously about herself and other island work possibilities. Many who decide to stay on the islands often settle for work that can be seen as well below their own skills and capacity—willing to trade off the fuller life that can come from challenging work for a beautiful and peaceful environment.

During that time, she also decided to build a home for herself here and, in typical Sandy Richard style, chose to be her own contractor. That required late nights reading and learning about construction, to be ready to deal with the workmen who showed up early in the morning. Then she'd go off to her regular job, working on the house in the evenings and on weekends. The house, by the way, is long finished and quite handsome—filled with ethnic art Sandy finds on her budget trips to the earth's far corners.

A bout with Graves disease—an auto-immune thyroid disease—got Sandy thinking about alternative therapies. "I didn't dislike western medicine," she said, but like a lot of us, she had begun to question the system based so often on treating a disease as if it were somehow separate from the rest of the body, and the body somehow separate from the mind.

Sandy heard about a massage school in California that taught a speeded up course—one she could take in the few weeks she could get off from the post office.

"Something about it seemed right for me, and I just decided to go for it. I wouldn't give up my job, but I felt I just had to go and learn something different. And alternative health was pulling at me."

A few weeks later Sandy returned to the island, purchased a massage table—which she set up in her living room—and began working on her friends. Sandy has powerful upper body strength, and she was very soon known as a great massage therapist—one who could relieve the tightest muscle and tension knots anyone brought her.

Sandy worked at massage only in the evenings and on weekends, but her reputation spread quickly and before too long she found that her massage income nearly matched her post office income. She simply quit the post office.

She also recognized her own deeper interest in her clients' overall well being—not just in the relief of their daily stress, or help with a momentary back or neck pain. Sandy is a very good listener, and she began to tune into a pattern she heard from her clients: almost all were feeling short-changed with their visits to their own doctors.

Time with an M.D. had begun to seem measured in half minutes to most patients, and that up-tight scheduling left little time to talk about underlying problems.

"Once I had a client who went to the doctor and was prescribed Valium when she was simply grieving the death of her husband," said Sandy, amazed that such natural and deep feelings should be seen by a doctor as needing medication to repress. "I often felt that just the time I spent listening to someone was more healing than the massage itself."

Massage therapy led Sandy to discover at least one area that much of the alternative health care world now operates in quite successfully: helping people find their own mechanisms for healing. It takes time, patience, and a sympathetic ear, but it is proving to be one of the most powerful of all health care treatments.

That was eight years ago and now Sandy is taking another big leap, going still further into the alternative health care world to earn her living.

A few years ago, Sandy attended a day-long herbal walk on Shaw Island, and met Clarissa Smith, Janet Wright's herbal mentor from the Rocky Mountains. Sandy had been using Wyoming Wildcrafter's arnica salve in her massage practice for years; Clarissa had started the company. Sandy had had a culinary herb garden for years—now she was to begin learning abut medicinal herbs in earnest.

She attended all the classes Clarissa taught on the islands, went to a three-day international medicinal herb conference given on the east coast, and was soon drawn further and further into the world of healing plants. She read everything she could get her hands on about medicinal herbs and, just as she did with massage, tried out her home remedies on her friends. She made her own arnica salve and St. John's wort massage oil, and then began making a few tinctures.

There were some economic factors working on Sandy, too. She saw insurance companies opening up a little to alternative health care, but usually only for physical therapists, not very often for massage therapists. Physical therapists often do just what massage therapists do, but patients have a hard time getting their doctors to recommend massage therapy.

And every time Sandy left the island to travel for a month or two, she'd come back to find that another massage therapist had set up here. The island is growing all the time; people need jobs here, and massage is fairly easy to learn and get into. "Besides," says Sandy, holding up her short, powerful hands, "I also began to realize that I do such deep work with massage that my joints could easily get into trouble. I've been at this work for eight years already."

Sandy says that she always felt a bit "shortchanged" in her science education. "Actually, I had some very poor teachers. So I finally decided to go back to college and take some basic science classes, plus anatomy and physiology. I loved it. I've always loved learning. I'm a born student. "

In the meantime, Clarissa Smith was attending a Chinese medicine school in Seattle, learning both acupuncture and Chinese herbalism. After looking at several other school choices, Sandy also soon made the decision to invest her time, money and future in becoming a licensed acupuncturist.

Acupuncture is one of the few alternative health care practices, around the area of medicinal herbs, that carries a national U.S. license to practice. It's a license given only after an extensive two-day national exam held twice yearly—once in the west, and once on the east coast. The test is expensive ($800 as of this writing) plus air fare, etc. Some states will even require additional testing or education before granting a license to practice. But getting that credential, after a successful completion of years of course work, gives any would-be herbalist a very firm, legal platform from which to practice.

The National Institutes of Health (NIH) has recently given acupuncture treatments a big boost of approval following a review by health care experts who found "clear evidence" that acupuncture is effective for a limited range of conditions, and may well be effective as an "adjunct or alternative" to more conventional treatment for many other conditions. Acupuncture is moving rather quickly now towards being a part of mainstream medical care. The FDA also regulates the use of acupuncture needles, just as they do other medicinal devices.

Acupuncture is based on a system of hundreds of points on the body, identified by Chinese practitioners, as connecting "lines of energy" or meridians, for the treatment of many diseases and health problems.

Sandy's choice of studying Traditional Chinese Medicine (TCM) means she must also learn a health care system based on this flow of energy through the body. TCM aims, through very careful diagnosis, to find the root cause of an illness, and then, through treatment, to bring the whole body into an energy balance—without excess or deficiency. The effects of acupuncture, herbal medicines, and even certain foods on the patient are used to direct the body's energy system into better balance. This yin/yang system approach means that TCM students often speak of body processes, diseases, symptoms, and cures in terms of hot and dry, cold and wet—excess cold or heat. Of too much (or too little) fire or water.

Sandy is now busy supporting herself and this decision with her massage work, as the school cost is significant. But I must report Sandy as happy—although even seeing her out and about on the island these days is quite rare.

"For four days a week at home, I get up in the morning, do massage work all day and then study until I fall asleep at night. Then I leave the island and go stay in Seattle for three days where I attend classes from 1 PM to 9:30 PM.

"From 1 to 5 PM we are in clinic with an experienced practitioner. The practitioner does all the laying on of hands and needles, but we listen to the patient's interview, take pulses, look at tongues, try and figure out what's wrong, even discuss possible treatments." It is this clinical training that Sandy finds the most fascinating.

In the evening classes, she studies herbs, all the acupuncture points, how to diagnose using the TCM system, and also the Chinese language.

What will she do when she finishes school three years down the road? Practice herbalism, acupuncture, and no doubt continue with her massage therapy. All probably right here on San Juan island. There is an acupuncturist who now comes to the island weekly to practice, but Sandy knows there will be far less competition in this field than she was beginning to see in massage. She has finally found a field where she can spend a lifetime in learning and still find lots more to learn; Sandy is and always has been a student above everything else. The harder the learning, the better she seems to like it.

Meanwhile, she has planted a hundred *Echinacea purpurea* plants on the spare ground around her house, and is feeling good knowing that she'll also end up being able to make even more of her own medicine when she is finished with school. She can probably sell some of the roots, too; she'll no doubt need the money, after the cost of years more of schooling.

❦ *Clarissa Smith*

It's time to introduce the professional herbalist of this book. And through her to follow some of the recent history and possible future of modern herbalism in America.

Clarissa is an attractive young woman with a friendly smile, who always makes me think about being outdoors. When I attended the first herb walk she led on the island, her soft spoken, friendly confidence said to me:

> *Here's what I've learned about these plants. You're welcome to follow along and learn from me, but I won't be offended if you aren't interested. I'm not selling anything.*

That line between the medical plant enthusiast and the herb fixit sales-person can be a fine line, but it's an important one to me. With so much hype around *miracle cures* for everything these days, I always value time with people like Clarissa, who simply set aside all the malarkey and speak plainly about their own experiences with using the plants.

Clarissa grew up in New England surrounded by woods where she "hung out a lot." She had "no family tradition with herbs" while growing up, but some of her earliest memories are of being in the woods and know-ing that some of the plants were "good to eat."

"I'd actually tell other kids to eat certain plants. Of course I didn't know what I was talking about and I sometimes got into trouble with their parents. Luckily no one actually got hurt, but something was there for me with the plants." It's obviously still there.

She also remembers being sick a lot as a child—and that every vaccina-tion would bring a terrible reaction. At 22, Clarissa had what she calls "a turning point" when she went to a medical doctor who started "yelling at me telling me that my illness was all in my head. He made me cry and I remember walking out and thinking: *I'll never go to a doctor again.*"

About this time she picked up a book by Adelle Davis, a prominent

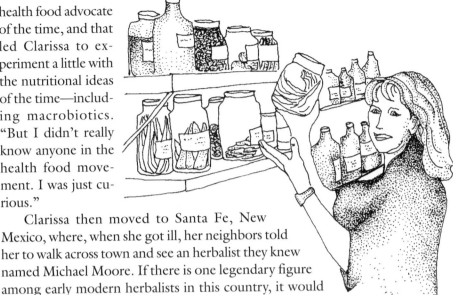

health food advocate of the time, and that led Clarissa to experiment a little with the nutritional ideas of the time—including macrobiotics. "But I didn't really know anyone in the health food movement. I was just curious."

Clarissa then moved to Santa Fe, New Mexico, where, when she got ill, her neighbors told her to walk across town and see an herbalist they knew named Michael Moore. If there is one legendary figure among early modern herbalists in this country, it would surely be Michael Moore. I have never met him, but have listened to him speak, read his books, and often visited his web site, where he so generously shares a prodigious wealth of knowledge about all things herbal.

When Clarissa visited Moore in Santa Fe many years ago, she found him "scary... a real kook. But he gave me some weird stuff to try and I got better."

She moved soon after that to Los Angeles where she took up body work, "but something about that Moore guy and his knowledge of plants stuck with me."

After a couple of years, Smith decided she wanted to go back to New Mexico and see if she could learn about plants from Moore. His first book, *Medicinal Plants of the Mountain West,* had been issued, along with Michael Tierra's book, *The Way of Herbs.* This was probably in 1979, Clarissa remembers, and those were just about the only two books she had found on the subject that was beginning to seem so important to her to learn.

She returned to Santa Fe, took a summer course with Moore and then signed on for his longer course at the Santa Fe College of Natural Medicine, where Moore taught about herbs and others taught nutrition and classes in science.

"Michael is what I treasure so much about herbalism," says Clarissa. "He is a bio-regional herbalist; one who believes it is absolutely essential to come from an earth-based, regional-based herbalism—that the connection to the land and the herbs is first. That kind of herbalism doesn't need exotic herbs. They know what to do and how to use what grows right around their own area."

New Mexico appears to be one of the primary places where modern American herbalism got reborn. In Santa Fe, all Clarissa's neighbors were Hispanic. "They all used plants, every day, and always have. The Anglo communities in the area picked up the Hispanic and Native American herb uses and built on those traditions. Michael Moore was one of the earliest (and best) of those first herb teachers."

Those next few years spent in the New Mexico school bring broad smiles and great memories to Clarissa now. "We would take crazy trips; maybe 30 people caravaning through different areas in the mountains— or on out to the coast and desert for weeks. The Anza Borrego, where we'd visit the native tribes; or to the Chiricahuas in Arizona. It was fabulous, but I definitely got the idea that where people live, people get sick in different ways. And that the plants that grow there can be of help."

Michael Moore's approach influenced Clarissa completely. "The herbs and the land are his whole life. But he brings a good mix of science and **knowing what you're talking about** as far as the plants are concerned, along with a complete awareness and appreciation of the indigenous use of that plant. He always honors that, too."

There was another aspect to Moore's teaching that Clarissa found appealing and that I notice in many of the long time herbalists I have met in preparation for this book. That is a sense of being somewhat of an outlaw, and not worrying very much about that part of it at all.

"Being an herbalist then meant you worked with people's health. There was almost no herbal product business then, so making your own plant medicine and giving it out to people was what it was all about. There was none of this sense of it being illegal to practice medicine without a license. The herbal tradition in New Mexico was still a very strong tradition and no one thought anything about it."

When Clarissa finished the school she got what she calls "a great gift" when Michael asked her to run his little store for him. He had started a small business to make herbal medicine from the local plants—just for the people in his area to use. Now he was also being asked to go out and speak around the country about medicinal herbs, and needed some help to keep the little business going.

"I said yes, of course, that I'd take the job—knowing it was my lucky break—but what an experience that turned out to be.

"I started the morning after I finished school and Michael left on a trip that same morning. For the first three weeks people would walk in and say, 'Are you the herbalist?' and when I said yes, they'd start laughing. But that didn't really last too long, as it got me up and running very fast.

"The store was like a clinic; there was no question in those days about the FDA. Besides, in New Mexico, there have always been healers everywhere. It was perfectly normal behavior. I was just thrown right into the big middle of it. People would walk in and show you awful oozy scabby sores, or be so hoarse they couldn't talk. And I'd try to figure it out. It was strictly a one person operation. You'd deal with customers all day, plus make medicines and stock the shelves. There wasn't even a cash register. I remember there was an old planked floor. I guess it was almost third world stuff.

"I learned on my feet, and when Michael would come back, we would work together, so I kept on learning. He always made you feel like an equal—would always call me his co-worker, and always ask my opinion—even on business decisions, advertising, and so forth."

A few years later, Michael sold the retail and product company to Daniel Gagnon, who still owns it. I visited that company, Herbs Etc., in 1994, and wrote about it in *Herbs For Sale*. It was fun to hear more about the early days with Moore from Clarissa. She stayed on through the transition to Gagnon and then left the company and started her own small company.

Michael Moore had always refused to make medicines for other stores and all the time Clarissa worked in the store, she was asked by health food stores to make some of the medicines for them. After leaving the Moore shop she decided to do just that. She started Dragon River Herbals, a medicinal products company, in the early '80s. A year later, she sold the company and moved to Wyoming. It seemed time for a change.

Clarissa settled in a little cabin about 20 miles outside Jackson, and then set about to learn her new landscape. "I spent the first six months outside every day, all day, with a camera and guide books. I talked to everyone: park rangers and botanists, ranchers, anyone who knew anything about the land and local plants." She had expected Wyoming to be very redneck cowboy; instead she found people to be incredibly open. It was very much an attitude of people doing their own thing.

"I think they actually liked the idea that I was doing something a little outside the law. I had started Wyoming Wildcrafters and was selling bottles of herb medicine out of the back of my pickup truck and they thought that was just fine."

Clarissa drove all over the southwest and then over into the Pacific northwest looking for herbal practitioners and stores that wanted her products. "They were totally hungry for herb products in those days."

At this point in time, Clarissa knew of two good herb medicine companies: Michael's old company and Ed Smith's Herb Pharm in Oregon. She wanted her work to be as good and as reputable as those products were.

"I took no short cuts. I did everything as carefully as I possibly could. I had maybe three lean years, but I put everything I had into making those the highest quality herbs imaginable. Within a year I got a building and, after three years of only selling wholesale, I opened a retail store in Jackson."

By this time the whole herb renaissance was coming into bloom and Clarissa and her little product company were swept up into a wave of consumer demand that no one could have possibly anticipated.

"By year three, I had five employees; year six it went to eight. The business simply went crazy. We never had a bad day. Never went below the figures of the day before. It was so new and there were so few of us producing that it was quite unreal. I never spent a nickel on ads. All I had to do was knock on doors and people would buy whatever I had.

"But almost no one knew anything in those days, so I had to spend so much time explaining things to everyone. I taught classes—anywhere they wanted to hear me. Sometimes I made only $50, sometimes $200. If anyone, anywhere wanted to know about herbs, I would go and talk. I felt so much confidence from my work with Michael Moore, and everyone was so eager to learn. It was great timing, I guess, but I worked so very, very hard." What an exciting time that must have been for those so caught up in the first flare-ups of the medicinal herb wildfires starting to sweep across the land.

After a while, slowly at first, the magic just began to drain away for Clarissa. Exhaustion, probably, as much as anything else. She was still teaching, had an active practice in her own clinic, as the product business itself simply exploded under her. Everyone advised her to quit the clinic and the teaching so as to be able to deal with the business, but her heart was just not there.

"I felt sucked into more business discussions and business decisions; there was less and less about health and the plants. Sometimes I would start daydreaming about learning Traditional Chinese Medicine and acupuncture. Yet I knew small, fast growing businesses didn't allow time off for such things." Pretty soon, she remembers, her employees were actually running much of the business part and she would just try to concentrate more and more on the teaching and the clinic.

"There were all these changes then in the herb business climate. Suddenly the whole focus was: we've got to get more plants for the herbal product business; wildcraft more for the product business. Everything turned to products only. There was never much talk of healing, of better plant growing, of sustainability, of habitat. It was very disheartening. And frankly, it just smelled of so much greed. Then, on top of all that came the whole FDA business about clamping down on herbs. I knew there were lots of shoddy products out there and lots of people coming into it that didn't know anything at all.

"In the early days of my business, I would spend the day working with employees in the lab, talking with them about the medicine, looking at herb shipments, talking with customers, experimenting with plants and new formulas. A few years later my days would start with a meeting with the insurance agent, or the accountant, followed by a trip to Denver for a meeting with other herbalists about the FDA problems. I just started hating it, mostly because I didn't know what I was doing. The more my business got away from the plants and the patients and their healing, the more unhappy I became. The demands on me to be a bigger and better business person were just not the demands I wanted on me. Wake up, I told myself, you've got to get back doing what you love. And what I love is working with people's health, with herbs, with teaching. So I simply sold out and left."

That's been several years ago, and only recently, says Clarissa, has she come to terms within herself about the herbal products business. "There are still so many wonderful people involved in the herb business—all parts of it. I just couldn't take the rapid changes, the too-fast growth."

She also realizes that herbalists coming out of classes and schools now are doing some pretty amazing things. They have better books, better teachers, more accurate knowledge than she got—and they are helping people with very serious problems. But they are also coming out knowing they have to play the game.

"We really had a luxury in those days," she says now, "in being able to be radicals and outlaws. That's just not possible now. Nowadays, no herbalist would try and deal with a very serious wound. You would just tell someone they had to go and get emergency medical help. In those early days we were taught how to take care of almost anything in emergencies.

"I guess I got thinking," she says with a wry smile, "that I was some sort of a village healer, with lines of people coming to a clinic with no supplies. And then," she laughs, "I got bummed out that there just wasn't any village after all. And it all turned into just another big business."

At this writing Clarissa has just finished up three years of studying at acupuncture school. As a licensed acupuncturist, she has joined a Traditional Chinese Medicine practice in Portland, Oregon, for more hands-on experience. She has also accepted a one day a week job in a western medical clinic across the line in Washington state.

"Imagine," she says, "an herbalist being wanted to work in a regular clinic in a logging town. Boy, have things changed.

"Herbalists these days," says Smith, "are going to be up against a world of licensed practitioners. Well educated herbalists know a lot more about herbs than either a licensed acupuncturist or a naturopathic doctor. The big difference is that the acupuncturists and the naturopaths and the chiropractors have all gotten licensing for themselves. The herbalists haven't. Lots and lots of them really do know their stuff, but they are still going to be illegal. That's why I just spent three more years in school."

She is accommodating to new realities in the world of medicinal herbs. As the herbs become more accepted, the health care people using them will have to become more and more professional and accredited.

Yet Clarissa hangs on to her dream of staying closer to the land and the plants as she becomes more and more of a professional herbalist by today's changing standards.

"What I really hope to do one of these days is to have my own practice somewhere, with some land nearby for growing. I want to learn to grow Chinese herbs, as I love using them in practice. I don't want to be part of a big business deal. I just want to practice what I know best in the best way I think it should be practiced."

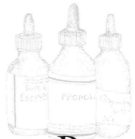

CHAPTER SIX

Meet the Product People

"If the millions working in offices and those having taxing brain work knew what these things (herbal tonics) would do for them, with no harmful after effects, the herb business would increase a hundredfold."

Jethro Kloss, Back to Eden, *1939*

Turning Plants Into Products

If you take up growing or collecting medicinal herbs, it won't be long before it will cross your mind that you might well consider processing your herbs into products yourself. Selling fresh or dried bulk herbs to another company so that they can turn them into products may well make you feel like you are missing out on the more profitable idea. Knowing the financial benefits that can come from value added products, it's time to talk herb products in more detail. If you have been following the suggestions in this book, you are already actually making some simple herb medicines and products for yourself and your family.

As the medicinal herb wave continues to sweep across the country, there are going to be more opportunities for medicinal herb product makers to try out their best ideas on the ever growing population of herb consumers. I've noticed recently that even paper products now have herbal scents added to help raise the retail price. Chamomile toilet paper, anyone?

Herbs For Sale deals with several important herbal products including medicinal herb teas; medicinal tinctures or fluid extracts; and aromatic pillows. I won't repeat what I've already covered in that other book, a copy of which you can always get through your local library; that's also the best place to look for basic small business start-up books.

Additional products that you might want to consider for medicinal herbs are salves, liniments, oils and lotions; tonics, capsules and lozenges;

bathing and soaking preparations, and medicinal herb soft drinks. To see what else is possible in the way of herbal products, just visit any health food store, any cosmetics counter, any up-to-date drug store. You will be amazed at the variety of products now being offered which are made with at least one medicinal herb.

This part of the book will not show you how to make herbal products, but the resource section will offer both direction and supply sources for those wanting to learn how to make all sorts of medicinal herb products.

It's important that you first take a realistic look at your local market-place, where most new products need to make their start. Consider taking aim at a market niche that isn't already too crowded in your area—one in which you can make and promote a high quality product that will sell repeatedly to new customers and old. This section will show you several people involved in herbal products at distinctly different levels. Reading this chapter should get your brain going in the direction of medicinal herbs turned into something that can be more valuable than what you harvest from the garden and field.

A little personal note before the commercial product talk begins: Tim Blakley and I agree that we will be quite content if our efforts in producing this book lead primarily to more and more people learning to make and use their own herbal medicine products for their families and friends. We both agree that's our more important work. Although product making is certainly legitimate, we don't claim to be experts in that field at all.

As bigger and bigger companies come on line with herb medicine products that more and more start to resemble regular medicine products (here she goes again) we want to point out that whole plant medicines are quite easy and inexpensive to make at home using the simplest equipment; are almost never dangerous to take, and best of all, can work very well for you and your family's improved health. Going commercial can be fun, interesting and profitable—but learning to successfully do your own medicines for your family should come first, and can also give you the confidence to then place products in the marketplace.

So now, let me introduce some people from my own herbal web area who are involved in making and marketing medicinal herb products. All of them, you will see, either continue to grow all or most of their own herbs, or stay as close as possible to their own growers and suppliers. They are plant people first. Of course you can make herbal products from herbs purchased from others (we offer a short list of reputable bulk herb companies in the resource section) but we promised ourselves to keep the book focused on herb plants and plant growing, so bear with us. Those are the main examples we will show.

Llama Mamma Herbal Salve
🌿 *Kelly Van Allen*

Kelly was in a very early stage of herb product development when we first met. She came to the product path in the same way so many others had come; by learning to give good herbal health care to her family. And, in this case, to her animals.

She lives with her husband and two children, ages 13 and 14, on Wind Dancer Llama & Herb Farm, 15 acres of pasture and woodland just south of Bellingham, Washington—a half hour's drive from the Canadian border. After her young children's problems with ear infections, Kelly finally visited a naturopath who cleared up their chronic ear condition with one visit. Kelly sat up and starting paying attention to herbs, first growing them and then learning to make her family's medicines.

Within a few years, she was being asked by her neighbors for herbs, and she now operates a small herb farm on the property, selling herb starts in the spring, offering classes to teach others in her area what she's learned—a perfect example of how the herbal network is spreading across the country.

The Van Allens also raise llamas and chickens, "and any other stray animal that happens to come along," so it wasn't long before Kelly was trying out a home-made salve on a skin condition she noticed on the llamas during rainy winters. Northwest llama people call it "rain rot," she says, a fungus that furry animals can get from too much rain. "With horses it's called rain scald."

After a vet prescribed an expensive salve with an antibiotic in it, Kelly wondered about trying "to make a salve from the plants that act like antibiotics." Choosing the anti-fungal, antiseptic, and antibiotic herbs like echinacea, mugwort, comfrey, and angelica, she followed herbalist James Green's method of salve making (see the resource section) and came up with small jars of:

Llama Mama Herbal Salve:
Rain Rot Salve, Good for Man or Beast.

She was selling a small (3.5 oz) jar for $3.50. "It actually works like a miracle," Kelly says with a shy blush.

At the time of our visit, Kelly was still making the salve in very small batches, and only selling it at llama shows. She had just learned that some breeders actually wanted it in much larger jars, and was putting up 8 oz. jars and wondering what to charge. A few breeders from around the country were starting to call her, as word of her product had begun to spread through the circles of llama and alpaca people.

To make the salve, Kelly first chooses the herbs growing in her garden. She says she is still varying the recipe as she feels that using the "freshest, strongest stuff" for each batch is the best way to go. She then writes down everything she's using in that particular batch, in order to have a good record; then chops up the herbs, and makes "only a small batch at a time."

Kelly first dries all her herbs before making an oil infusion of them. "There's less chance that way of getting mold into the mix. I'm able to break them up and use more surface area of the plant," she says. Mold growing on infused oils is definitely something to watch out for.

She uses only stainless or glass utensils, never aluminum, and often uses her crockpot for the cooking. Kelly puts the salve up in small glass jars, but may have to switch to plastic for the larger jars.

Importantly, she tries to keep in touch with those who purchase the salve, so she can get feedback on how each batch seems to be working on the animals. At our visit, Kelly was debating with herself about whether or not to standardize the recipe. She felt that using what seemed the very best and freshest herbs really might be the main reason her salve is so successful, yet wondered how long she should keep on varying the recipe.

Standardizing a formula is a very tricky question for many herb product makers, and can take a long time of change and experimentation. Most herbalists recognize both the changes in plants as they grow, and changes in the person, or animal, under treatment. By keeping good records and also keeping in touch with her early customers, Kelly hopes she can clarify her thinking on this and make the right decisions as she works towards a more standardized product that can hold up well in the marketplace.

She was also looking into building or working at a commercial kitchen. She has "communicated with the FDA," uses herbs she feels are "approved by them" for salves, and at the moment is feeling no pressure or worry from regulators about her product.

When beginning a little product business at this level, the regulatory agency you might think about first is the FDA—as there has been so much publicity about this agency regarding herbal remedies. I write more about these national issues in the chapter on regulations and safety, but for now I just want to encourage you not to worry very much about these FDA questions in the very first stages, as you try to work out good herbal products. The FDA is concerned with prod-

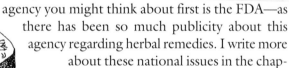

ucts that will be marketed across state lines. It is much more important at the beginning to figure out how to make a **high quality, safe-to-use product**. That should be your most important consideration in early product development.

Use herbs that you know are absolutely safe, and you should know that both from your own experience and from the experience of many other herbalists. There is so much literature available now on these plants that anything used in a product can be very thoroughly researched through your library, bookstore, herb conferences, magazines and newsletters, and on the Internet.

Most herbal product businesses begin at or near the kitchen sink, just as Kelly Van Allen's did. They begin with your own use of the product, use by your family and friends, constant product improvement with feedback from the users, and only then, after this careful experimentation, could come the possible retailing or wholesaling to others. At that point, your local rules concerning a small business are the ones that will be more important.

Small businesses like Kelly's often get their retail start with sales at local farmers' markets, at fairs or, in her case, at livestock shows. Some states are now recognizing these venues as the little business start-up engines they really are, and sometimes even making things easier for those first experiments so necessary for the start-up entrepreneur.

Meanwhile, when you decide you might have something special to sell, your town, your county, and sometimes your local health department offices are the ones to see for the rules concerning product preparation at home, the need for a local business license, any zoning restrictions that might apply, etc. These local officials will tell you if you need to contact any state offices, so make a few phone calls to your town and county to see what rules you must concern yourself with at first. Often your local chamber of commerce can offer information on exactly whom to call for small business licensing in your area.

If you like, you can also do a lot of early research from your home and library on more detailed information about FDA requirements on herbal products, just in case you are wondering about those questions for a much larger endeavor. I try and cover that in the regulations chapter and in the resource section, but they can be confusing details and I want to stress here that if you take Kelly's approach with a new product, you won't get into trouble.

One of the questions in Kelly's mind concerns insurance, and at what point you have to increase your coverage to cover the risks involved in a new business like hers. For advice on this subject, I turned to a local insurance broker, Kerwin Johnson, whose advice for start-up herb businesses seemed especially appropriate. Here are some of his thoughts on the matter.

First off, he said, you need to know your own tolerance for risk, your own comfort zone. The more local your business is, the less severe your exposures are. Ask yourself, what are the chances of anyone being hurt by what I'm doing? Chances are at the very local level most people start out at, there is seldom much risk at all. It's when you start moving out of that very local area: your local grocers, farmers' markets, and so forth, that your need for insurance grows.

Once you get to marketing through someone else—a regional show or showroom, a distributor or broker—business insurance can become mandatory. Other people that you need to help you extend your business will require that you have liability coverage. Just adding on to your homeowners insurance, says Johnson, is really not an appropriate choice for most small businesses—as once a product leaves the house, there really is no coverage for it.

The first thing you need to work out with your insurance broker, he said, is to find a classification that's fair. After that, the business and product liability policies are based solely on receipts (the amount of your sales), or on the number of employees, if you happen to be in a service business. With start-up companies, the minimum premium required to get any coverage at all can often be more than the total receipts of the small business.

One problem with working in an area like medicinal herbs, said Kerwin, is that there are probably not yet very many insurance underwriters who know much about the subject. When the press runs tabloid-type stories on herbs, those underwriters can be influenced, even if they don't mean to be. He compared it to the Internet business world where most underwriters are still trying to figure out what the real risks are. The recent scary newspapers stories about pedophiles finding their young victims through the Internet crossed my mind and made his point quite well.

Johnson says you can help to keep your insurance premium rates as low as possible by giving your insurance broker enough information to show that you know what you are doing in your field and that you know your product—in this case herbs.

Put together a package of information that shows your expertise, he suggests, and give it to your broker to take out to underwriters. Write down just what you do, what you know about what's in your product. If you have good scientific studies showing how safe your product is, give copies of those; bring in the best information you can get.

Underwriters are certainly not experts in every field, he adds, and what you want to do is to basically "sell down the price" of your coverage. Good information, says Johnson, can definitely work in your favor.

Any other bits of advice, I wondered? "Never get outside your comfort zone. Some people get beyond where they should be and that's where they get into trouble."

Kelly Van Allen is still operating the herb farm, still teaching classes—both there and at the nearby community center—and is now considering making herbal tinctures for animals, as she's certain a good herbal tincture could help other llama people with the "weak and compromised immune systems of some crias"—the name for llama newborns.

Kelly doesn't want to use alcohol for such a tincture, so she's now looking into a glycerin base instead. There are so many things to think about, she says, but doesn't want to go too fast or "get too serious about business" until her children are more grown. Shortly after our visit, Kelly was contacted by a mail order catalog in the east wanting to list her product, and she had decided to say no, as she didn't feel "quite ready yet to take things that seriously." Staying within her comfort zone, my insurance pal might note.

At last contact, Kelly had just been called by a llama organization in Florida, wanting her "to help them with medicinal herbs for their llamas." She was also considering going back to school, or "perhaps doing an apprenticeship, in order to focus more on my herbal path."

Kelly is typical of many who start out in herbal products: moving slowly, experimenting, always keeping in touch with her early customers, trying different herbs, and learning that it's the plants that make the difference in the product. It may take her several years to develop a line of herb products for animals, but her primary efforts are in slowly learning more about the product ingredients: the herbs themselves. That's the work she's doing that will lead to a good product line.

"Herbs are my habit," says Kelly. "And one of these days I would like to be able to earn enough to really support that habit. But it will have to come along quite slowly, as the family still has to come first, of course." And the herbs, I must add. The plants have to come first, too. Just as they have with Kelly Van Allen.

O-LALA Farm

🌿 *Robyn Martin*

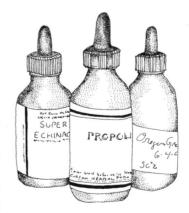

Robyn Jean Madrona Martin, her husband, Arlo Cubit Acton, and their O-LALA farm (who could resist visiting all those wonderful names?) were listed as organic medicinal herb growers and wildcrafters in one of the grower directories I collect. They live in North San Juan, the town, in the Sierra foothills; we live on San Juan, the island, in Puget Sound. Surely we were destined to meet when Tal and I drove to California for a family visit near Sacramento.

Our own area is filled with sailboat cruisers "gone to ground" on these lovely islands. I think Robyn's gorgeous area is filled with '60s escapees from the San Francisco Bay area, "gone to the hills" long ago to escape the crowds and craziness that became California.

Robyn and Arlo, who have two teenagers still living at home, were artists in San Francisco "in the old days." Now he grows organic vegetables for the local markets, while Robyn pursues a long and deep interest in medicinal herbs from their 200-acre family farm.

For the last 15 or 20 years she has scoured the hills around her area, learning about everything that grows there and collecting medicinal plants, like yerba santa and grindellia, for tincture makers in Oregon. Slowly, over time, she developed an allergy to some of the plants and her interest has turned more now to developing products she makes at home.

"I taught other people who live around here how to gather and dry herbs for those companies. Now I'm starting to concentrate on these little products," she says, bringing out first one small jar and then another to show, giving out her hints for new herb people all the while:

"Tell them to learn what's in their area. Bring the wild plants home and learn to grow them."

Robyn has 20 gallons of St John's wort oil she's prepared because "it will become very important soon." (This visit was more than a year before St. John's wort made its big appearance on the ABC program, *20/20.*)

They came to the farm in 1974 and, for almost 20 years, lived without electricity as they built two houses—one of which burned down a few years ago—and now earn most of their money at the farmers' markets nearby, and at crafts fairs in the area.

Robyn makes up imaginative names and labels for her products:

Fall Off the Wall, for "rubbing on your joints every time you fall off the wall." She puts in arnica and St. John's wort, along with several other herbs.

Hand Maid is prepared from St. John's wort, comfrey, plantain, calendula, and mallow.

Product labeling is another one of those subjects that can be intimidating in new small business product development. Many of the things I said about federal regulations can also be said about labeling. It can be confusing, and herb product labeling requirements for national (interstate) products are in the process of change right now as they are being brought into line with recent new dietary labeling laws. But don't spend a lot of time worrying about these issues to begin with.

With new products, make sure first of all that you make a safe, well tested product, and then keep the labeling simple and follow the basic rules. Show on the label how and where you (as the manufacturer) can be contacted, and list all the ingredients in the product. Show them by listing the major ingredient first, then the second most added ingredient, etc. You should also give the weight or measurement of the product, but this can vary by product and state.

One simple method is to go into a store and find a product that closely resembles the type of thing you are doing (salve, lotion, tea, tincture, etc.) and follow the example of the already established product.

One other simple rule with herbal products is not to make any serious health or cure claim on the label. Many small product companies simply stretch the product name so that it hints at what it should be used for (TranquiliTea, Sinutone, Hypericalm, etc.)

The use of so-called third party literature to explain recent findings on the herb is considered quite acceptable. You can legally give out such literature, or place it near your product: a magazine article, for instance, that shows the results of recent scientific studies on the herb you are using in your product. If you want to chase after the more complicated details, see the resource section on regulations.

Once you get involved in the subject of medicinal herb products, you will start reading and hearing fairly arcane discussions of such things as *structure and function claims,* or *cosmeceutical labels.* In the beginning, I recommend that you just keep it legal, safe, and simple.

At the time of our visit, Robyn was looking into purchasing organic grape alcohol to use in her tinctures, instead of grain alcohol. A couple of tincture companies have worked with California wine producers to develop an alcohol product made from organically grown ingredients. Others in the tincture world say that 190 proof grain alcohol is so strong and pure that seeking out the organically grown product is, in this case, unnecessary. "Grain alcohol," they argue, "just doesn't let anything else survive."

Home tincture makers, small herb business start-ups, and even some very small medicine companies use 100 proof vodka in making their first alcohol-based tinctures. Later on, when they want to increase production, they look around to find a supplier of the much stronger 190 Proof USP grain neutral spirits, usually called Everclear. This is combined with differing amounts of distilled water to make most tinctures.

Some states allow the sale of this 190 proof grain industrial alcohol over the retail counter; others require a special permit first. To find out which rules apply in your state, ask at your local liquor store. Washington state requires a special permit, given by the liquor licensing division of the Washington State Liquor Control Board. An annual $5 fee is charged to purchase five gallons or less; $10 is charged for the permit for purchases over five gallons. The present retail cost of Everclear in my state is a little over $25 per gallon.

Herb conference participants often discuss the pros and cons of basing medicine products in alcohol. Alcohol is the most common solvent used in medicinal tinctures. It gives a very long shelf life, and puts the herb chemicals quickly through the body. Dried herbs should not be used after a year of shelf storage.

The other common tincture solvent is glycerin, which is a sweet oil-based product obtainable, to begin with, from your local pharmacy, or from a pharmaceutical supply house. Glycerin is usually used in tinctures made especially for children and animals.

A typical dose from a tincture preparation is ¼ to ½ teaspoon taken several times a day. For those who worry about drinking or serving any alcohol, most tincture makers point out that even four to six doses per day of a typical medicinal tincture would still add up to considerably less than an ounce of alcohol in a 24 hour period. And there certainly are other ways to take herbs.

One other simply made product used for taking herbs internally is putting dried and ground-up or freeze-dried herbs in little capsules. Some herbs have quite bitter tastes, and some people just don't like using the tinctures. Empty capsules are available in bulk, and several companies for such products are listed in the resource section. Medicinal herb teas, of course, are an even simpler way to take herbs.

For salves and other external products, dried herbal ingredients are mixed with different types of oils—including essential or aromatic oils, and a thickening agent like beeswax.

All of these choices are the ones that new product makers will have to make. The books and guides listed in the resource section can help in your decisions. Simple methods of medicine making will often be taught in classes given by herbalists in your area. Check with your local herb farm, nursery, or health food store to find out about such class offerings.

The formulas, or recipes, for tinctures and other preparations have been freely distributed through the medicinal herb communities by people like Michael Moore, the well known herbalist from New Mexico—who has been so influential for the people in the herb network in my area. Moore has put many of his formulas on his web site and in inexpensive little booklets. See the resource section for more details. Some people also seek out older copies of the National Formulary or the U.S. Pharmacopoeia, both of which give details on the way these medicines were prepared in the past.

But, as Robyn Martin would point out, the important thing about any herb preparation is the quality of the herbs that go into it. She brings out a jar of her wild yam creme ("it keeps the whole family greasy"), one of lavender creme, and something she called *Body Block*, "a fantastic sun blocker, but no one got it."

Like most people who get involved at all in consumer products these days, Robyn is having to pay more and more attention to exterior packaging. "You can't get people to look at anything these days that doesn't have really great packaging on it." She grimaces, just as I do, hating the change, but knowing it's absolutely true. This increased over-packaging is one of the primary reasons for the rising cost of every product, and for the increased cost and continuing problems over our landfills.

Meanwhile, Robyn and I will both continue to push for the quality of the herbs inside the medicines, and acknowledge at the same time that if you want to sell very much of something in the marketplace these days, you have to make it look better and better.

The world is becoming awash in goods of all kinds, and people are making many of their purchasing decisions based more and more on how something looks. Those are the realities of the marketplace, and the further from home we put our products, the tougher the competition gets and the more important those externals become.

I take pleasure in telling about Robyn and Kelly and their new products—and take genuine pleasure in just knowing such good folks are "out there" making fine herbal tinctures and salves; keeping a little human-scale authenticity in the medicinal herb business world as it makes its big lift-off into giant global arcs and spins into that other mass market "real world."

Wonderland Teas, Herbs and Spices

❦ *Linda Quintana*

Next I'd like to detail a couple of herb product operations in the northwest that are much more developed than the previous little start-up companies, yet are totally in keeping with the **whole plant medicines** outlook of this book.

Herb stores can offer their customers a wide range of products, and they operate most successfully when run by educated and well trained herbalists. I'm convinced from my own visits to the following businesses that they have a lot to teach anyone interested in the subjects of herbs and herbal products

In the older downtown section of Bellingham, population 90,000, the tiny store called the Wonderland Tea, Herb & Spice Shop is so well established that it's regarded as part of the community health care system. I have friends who regularly stop in there for what they call little "health consultations," with its self-educated herbalist owner.

In the last few years, even a few of the local regular doctors have started sending their patients to the shop. Owner Linda Quintana's best remedies for chronic conditions like sinus problems, or repeated ear infections, are now valued by the local medical establishment. There are also so many naturopaths around Bellingham now—a University town with a fairly sophisticated population—that the miniature shop and its remarkable, self-educated owner stay busy much of the time.

The shop operates almost exclusively on the herbal products produced from the owner's Alpine Herb Farm, some 20 miles east in the Cascade foothills. Linda opens the herb farm once a week to visitors; gives plant sales a couple of times a year; and the rest of the time the rich, incredibly varied medicinal garden at the farm gives up its extensive offerings entirely for the shop product line, which is created by Linda.

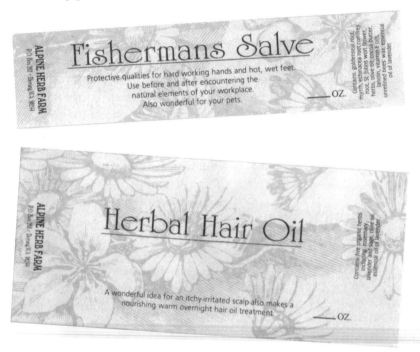

She carries only a few products made by others; she doesn't sell her harvest to other manufacturers. Her everyday efforts go into learning how to grow, dry, and then process into products the harvest of her magnificent garden. She knows these plants she grows so well, has used them for so long, that she has complete confidence in what they can do to help her customers. In a world fast filling up with container ship and train loads full of herbal products, Linda Quintana offers a tiny shop filled with the herbal bounty of her own garden. Very refreshing, and now quite successful.

The herb farm garden area has been cut out of the thick evergreen forest that runs alongside the Nooksack River, and looks exactly like what it is: a garden dedicated primarily to medicinal plants of the northwest that can help people with the typical health problems of the area—illnesses of the wet and damp world.

She understands perfectly the critical difference between providing information to her customers, and any attempt to actually diagnose, prescribe for, or treat a disease. She makes clear to her customers that they must make their own health care decisions. Herb shop owners and workers must work primarily at the education level.

Linda Quintana grew up in Alaska with a German mother and a Pennsylvania Dutch father who homesteaded on their 160 acres without benefit of electricity. They built their home from logs growing on the land, raised five children who worked daily in the food gardens at home and walked two miles every weekday morning to ride a bus one and a half hours to school.

"We were all incredibly healthy," Linda remembers. "Probably because we were outside all the time, eating highbush cranberries off the bushes, wild mushrooms, blueberries, wild burdock. We learned so early which plants were good and which to avoid: birch leaves were so sweet in the spring—but we mustn't eat the aspen."

When the family moved to Bellingham, where Linda attended high school, she remembers what a hard time she had "adjusting to the city life. I really have to have nature nearby." She certainly has it on the herb farm.

On my visit, she sits at the dining table stripping motherwort seeds from dried plants; on the stove is a big pot of soup, to which she has added medicinal plants: dandelion leaves and roots, plantain, basil, and parsley—"which are also medicinal," she reminds me.

"Medicinal herbs are foods. All herbs are foods. And we need to eat them and use them every day." That's Linda Quintana's basic herb doctrine and she has based a successful business and a very healthy life on that belief for more than 25 years.

Linda's favorite herb/food cures usually begin with teas.

Teas make you slow down, Linda says, and take extra time for yourself. "Medicinal teas can help you relax and lighten a little of the stress that may be causing so many health problems these days."

Tinctures, she thinks, can sometimes move through the body too quickly. "And I agree with herbalist Roy Upton," she continues, "in that we may be doing too many tinctures these days; just to be doing. People are always bringing me a dozen tincture bottles others have told them to take, and they can't even remember what to take them for. There's too much multi-level marketing out there," she grimaces, with the same eye roll, head shake and cynical laugh we're all feeling about the sudden over-commercialization of all things herbal.

Linda first asks her customers how they prefer to take their herbs.

"You need to take this herb regularly, so in what form will you be most likely to take it?" she asks, hoping to get them thinking about the herb, "instead of just popping another pill. I try and get them involved in their own care right way. But you have to level with them about tastes, too.

"This motherwort, for instance, isn't very tasty, so they might not like a tea made from it. Actually, a tincture might be better in this case, as motherwort doesn't really hold up that well in capsules, either. Sometimes tinctures are the best, but I always like to try and start people out with teas."

After high school, Linda volunteered a day a week to work in a tiny, 120 sq. ft. storefront in Bellingham, where a small group of local herb growers had a loosely organized co-op. She took on four other jobs to pay her way that year, but Linda's heart was in that tiny shop, where she also found and read her first herb book. "It was by John Lust and I read it through four times."

She also started growing herbs as she worked there, making endless tea combinations, herb oils and salves, and recognizing within herself that strong pull of the plants that would only grow and strengthen with the passing of time.

"One day, when the co-op leader announced that the shop idea wasn't working out very well, I spoke right up and said I'd buy it. I gave them $800 for everything, including all the stock, and then immediately took everything apart, painted it, cleaned it all up, and put it back together. Then it was all mine, and I was in heaven."

For 12 years she stayed in that tiny shop working seven days a week while slowly, slowly building up her knowledge and the little herb business at the same time. An additional spot of space finally opened up next door and she took that over—still only ending up with a shop of 600 sq. ft. That's the size of her shop today, and it's in the same location on Railroad Avenue in Bellingham, near a very popular bagel shop.

These days she works in the store a few days a week, blends her teas there, and makes the other products at the farm in a small workshop attached to the drying barn. Linda's mother also works part time in the shop, along with one or two other part time employees. But it's still very much Linda's business—and life.

Linda Quintana gains much of her herb and business confidence because she can step out of the door of her farmhouse and step right into the medicinal garden, the daily source of her continuing education and her shop product warehouse. But what about someone working in the heart of a big city? How might they go about establishing and running an herbal product business? It's time to meet Tierney Salter.

The Herbalist

🌿 *Tierney Salter*

The name of Tierney's shop in the Ravenna District in the city of Seattle, population 1,000,000, is also the professional title she's earned for herself as one of the most knowledgeable practicing herbalists in the northwest area. Tierney Salter, smiling and friendly, looks ever young and nearly glamorous. She runs a big city operation, yet her herb products are always listed by American herbalists as among the most well made in the country.

The Herbalist store is 2,000 sq. ft., open seven days a week, with 15 people working to handle the business—some of which comes in by mail responding to her mail order catalog, or to the more recently established multi-page web site. Tierney manufactures much of her product line in a nearby facility, and her herb products are available in other stores around the country.

Tierney also started out in the '70s in Michael Moore's Southwest School of Botanical Medicine, right alongside so many other now well known American herbalists.

"Michael Moore gave us his all," she says. "Learning from him was worth so much to me." Worth so much, in fact, that Tierney cleaned houses for 18 months in Santa Fe, just to stay in those classes. And afterward, she worked in a clinic in northern N.M. for six more months of training.

Salter was 24 years old when she got back to Seattle and began looking for work in "something to do with herbs. I still looked like a hippie in those days. We all had so much hair."

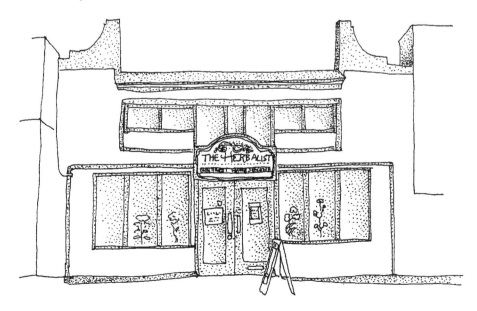

A place called the Herbal Health Center was looking for six women to help open up another center in Bellevue, a fast developing residential area across Lake Washington from Seattle. "They said that I had to know about iridology, and that I had to cut my hair, pluck my eyebrows, and put on lipstick. I'd already studied iridology with Michael Moore, and I realized that I was probably willing to change my own appearance a little, because I saw that people were being put off from using herbs just because of the way we all looked," recalls Salter.

"I figured herbs were going to be great for all of us: my parents, their friends, everybody, so if I had to look a little more straight to get them to listen to me, that was going to be okay with me. I'd been brought up in a pretty conservative household, so it wasn't all that foreign to me. And I knew I could easily let my hair grow back anytime I wanted to."

Tierney moved into the 3,000 sq. ft. office building in Bellevue, and took another few months training in iridology—which uses the inspection of the iris of the eye as an aid in determining a person's health or in diagnosing a health problem. The company sold their own line of herbs and vitamins and also taught classes with slide presentations to the employees of the banks and finance companies in the area.

She soon talked the company into letting her open up her own mini-pharmacy inside the larger store, where she could make up custom herbal tinctures for the customers, as she had learned to do from Moore. She called that tiny space The Shepherd's Purse.

"No one was doing anything like that in those days," she recalls, "and the customers were delighted."

But the business itself wasn't really her cup of tea ("Just too too much emphasis on the dress-up stuff") so Tierney spent those next two working years looking for a location for her own store, while trying to locate the best quality herbs to use in products.

"Michael had so stressed herb quality; for that is really what makes herbal medicine work. Most of the commercial herbs were just junk. Like the floor sweepings from a decent herb grower. I had to do better than that."

She eventually opened up in a 900 sq. ft. retail space adjoining a branch of the well known Puget Consumer Co-op, north of the University of Washington campus. A great deal of her focus in those early years had to be on education, she remembers, "teaching the medicinal wonder of herbs."

That early realization, of having to spend lots of time and money in educating people about herbs, is another reason for her great success. Today, Salter still teaches endlessly: in the local colleges and universities, in her shop, at herbal conferences and retreats, wherever and whenever she's asked. Every month the shop will offer varying classes such as aromatherapy, herbal soap-making, nutrition and herbs, and Traditional Chinese Herbalism.

"If you want to run a good full-line herbal product business, and you can't grow all your own plants," says Tierney, "you have to do two important things. First you have to become educated enough to know good herbs when you see them. How they look, smell and taste—all the different parts of them—whether they are dried or fresh. You simply have to work with people who know their plants. And you have to become a person who really knows the plants. Period. There is no shortcut.

"Secondly, even after you know all that, you still have to get samples, visit with suppliers, visit with growers, meet and get to know the people you are dealing with. Try and keep your sources as close to home as possible, just so that you can do that. Of course," she smiles, "I've never minded having to visit places like the South Pacific to meet growers and suppliers of kava.

"I would just keep stressing to any newcomers in this business that main idea of herb quality. Quality of herbs equals quality products, which gives a person quality results. Your customers can't trust your products unless you can trust your herb suppliers."

I know one of Tierney's primary herb suppliers: Ryan Drum, a humorous, over-educated botanist/herbalist, who lives on an isolated non-ferry-served island near my own island and harvests his herbs from some of the most unpolluted land remaining in the country. I think he probably charges more than anyone I know for what he grows and harvests; but his products are always in demand.

"Michael Moore used to bring herbs to the conferences in the old days," recalls Tierney, "and I can remember racing Ed Smith of the Herb Pharm Company, to Michael's van, just to try and have first choice of those herbs."

Those old days are full of both good and bad memories for Tierney. "First there was all that public skepticism about what we were doing. Any practicing herbalist was on the fringe. Period. The perception was so different than it is now. And then this big black cloud moved over all of us when the FDA said that since these herbs have drug-like qualities, we must turn them all into drugs. I, and many others, had worked very, very hard up to that point on something we really believed in, and it suddenly looked like it would all be taken away from us."

In 1992, Tierney Salter and a health food product consultant named Craig Winters, along with several others, decided to try to get all the Pacific northwest health food merchants organized to try to stop the FDA attempts.

"We actually organized ourselves," she remembers, "based simply on where we were sitting in the room at the first meeting: you be chairman, you be vice chairman, and so forth." They formed Citizens For Health, which began to meet regularly and to map out a plan that soon took off in health stores all around the country.

"We put black ribbons over the products that would be affected, got customers to sit down and write to the White House and to Congress. It was a crazy, busy time." Their campaign actually succeeded very well with the enactment of the Dietary Supplement Health and Education Act, which I tell more about in the chapter concerning regulation. But that battle set up a very fearful time for herb product makers and retailers.

"We trained our employees to be able to get across to customers their own beliefs in the power of herbal medicines without being seen as prescribing or practicing medicine without a license. To tell people what you would do if you were in their position. To tell what others have done, what traditional use this herb has had, and so forth."

And then one day the FDA agents actually showed up at Tierney's store, and gave her a real scare. "I was at home when an employee called to say they were in the store 'in full suits and briefcases.' I dropped everything and went over there, my knees knocking, and never even noticing that I had just gotten dressed for a Christmas party. I had on a big black hat with a red ribbon on it, with sparkles all over everything. I must have looked pretty strange for a business owner. Or maybe they thought I fit their expectations of a crazy herbalist in that outfit."

As it turned out, the agents were not there to bust Tierney or her store for any illegal activities. An herb product containing the desert plant chaparral, or creosote bush, had been implicated in several recent cases of liver damage, and the agents were asking Tierney to cooperate in a nationwide attempt to remove the herb from store shelves. She, and most other herb retailers, agreed readily to the removals, although the case against the plant was never really proved.

The Herbalist store moved a few years ago just half a block down the street to a larger facility. They feature their own products, but carry many, many products made by other companies. They have a wide array of books, and even have an herbal tonic bar, one of the newest big-city-style medicinal herb offerings.

I've also visited Tierney's manufacturing site, a few miles from the store. Lee Pereira runs the facility using Tierney's formulas. The herbs for tinctures are first identified and checked for quality, a record made for each batch of herbs received, and then they are weighed to determine the amount of solvent (*menstruum*) needed.

Lee uses a very large 40-quart chopper/processor for the first steps, adding the menstruum (usually alcohol and distilled water) according to

Tierney's formulas. This mixture then sits in barrels (*macerates*) for the next two weeks before having all the juice squeezed out of it with a hydraulic press that puts 2400 pounds of pressure on the mixture. That process leaves behind a semi-dry pile of depleted herbal matter, called the *marc*, that can be used by local gardeners for composting, but for little else.

The liquid tinctures are then filtered through various strainers and bottled with a simple bottling system Lee has developed over time. There's a bit of fine art in just how much plant sediment is to be left in these tinctures. They shouldn't clog the droppers, says Lee, but overly thin, overly diluted tinctures "are not what our customers want, and they really don't work as well in the body." I have noticed myself how some herb tinctures taste much more herb-like than others.

Pereira then adds droppers, a tiny piece of shrink wrap to form a tight seal, puts on the labels and gets ready to ship the now bottled product. The Herbalist puts up almost 150 single herb extracts plus 50 combination formulas to be used for help with specific health problems: Anti-Fungal, Lung-Mend, Tum-Ease, etc. Single herb extracts and combinations sell for $7.50 to $9.75 for a one ounce bottle.

Tierney's efforts to keep her customers well informed have to be a large part of her obvious success. She usually sends out four newsletters per year to some 15,000 people. "That ends up costing nearly a dollar per person per issue. I shut myself away for a couple of weeks to do one," she says, "as I want to make it as informative and interesting as possible."

Her web site is elaborate and also very informative. "At first we were getting over 300 requests a week for our catalog from the site," she says, but now they have put the whole catalog on the web, and ask people to print off the order blank for their first order. That first order triggers a newsletter and mail order catalog that will keep coming in the mail. A good way, it seemed, to weed out the serious customers from the mildly curious.

Sitting pretty? One might think so. But like everyone else who has spent the last 20 years teaching America about the value of herbal medicine, Tierney Salter is now getting ready for the big corporate herb business onslaught. Right in her own neighborhood.

A large national whole foods supermarket is moving into the area with a 50,000 sq. ft. store "and a huge tincture department." Both the nearby consumer co-op store and The Herbalist will be affected.

"I've had friends in the herb business around the country get knocked out by this," she says. "It can be just like a Wal-Mart invasion."

How many of her customers will remain loyal to the smaller, more personal store that has built its reputation with well trained, knowledgeable people and good service? Tierney Salter is not a romantic, or a fool.

"I and the other early herbalists didn't get into this business just to make a lot of money. We really believed in the herbs and what they could do for people's health," Tierney says. "I still believe that. I know that more people learning to use high quality herbal medicine can be a very good thing, no matter who sells the products."

She isn't sure just how much the good karma she has created with her shop will carry over into the more competitive environment she is now facing. "I actually do prefer," she says, "to shop in a small, more service oriented store, but we'll just have to see how many of my customers feel that way."

My own reaction to this is the deep sadness I always feel at seeing someone do a very, very good job in business, only to have it simply overwhelmed by an enormous capital investment that moves in to cream off the customers created by the hard work of others. Our American way of doing big business is pretty depressing sometimes.

I also know that the solid herb knowledge base and sharp business acumen that Tierney Salter has built up over so long will not let her fall very far—if at all. She was, after all, way ahead of the business world 20 years ago in seeing where herbs were headed, and out in front is just where I would expect to find her again when the dust settles in her neighborhood.

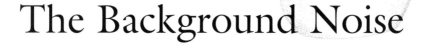

CHAPTER SEVEN

The Background Noise

"The U.S. Food and Drug Administration (FDA) claims that only by bringing botanical products under the same rules as synthetic drugs can the public be assured of their safety.

"Yet, according to the government's General Accounting Office, more than 50 percent of the drugs approved by the FDA as safe and effective have serious side effects that are discovered only after approval."

Rob McCaleb, president of the non-profit Herb Research Foundation, Herbs for Health, *1996*

U.S. Regulations

American medicinal herbs are regulated by the same agency (FDA) that was formed to oversee the Food and Drug Act of 1906. That important act came about because of rampant fraud, mislabeling, and adulteration of drugs. The act has been amended several times and, over many years, has come to fit itself around the drug manufacturing system that is primarily about creating biologically active, single chemical drugs.

New drugs, as you probably know, must always undergo expensive, state of the art tests known as randomized, double-blind, cross-over clinical trials. FDA approval then leads to a drug with a patent that the companies can sell in order to both regain the money spent on the trials, and to make a good profit.

The knowledge of the usefulness of herbal medicines, on the other hand, has come instead from long term observation of their uses around the world; three quarters of the world's population have never stopped using medicinal herbs. Now that herbs are becoming ever more popular in Europe and North America, all these new herb consumers are helping to create some of the conflicts and contradictions starting to play out in the corporate and regulatory offices of the U.S. and Canada.

As an example, let's consider what's going on right now around Prozac, the drug I mentioned in the Introduction. A very popular patented prescription drug that brings in a reported two and a half billion dollars a year to its manufacturer, Eli Lilly, Prozac is being challenged by that little yellow flowering plant from the medicinal herb world, St. John's wort.

Previously considered an invasive weed, the plant is easily grown, inexpensively processed (anyone can put it in a tea or simple medicine) and is now being promoted by magazines, books, television shows, and newspapers as being effective in treating mild depression—as effective, some say, as the more expensive drugs. German doctors, for instance, have long used St. John's wort as their primary drug for treating depression.

St. John's wort is also being recommended in the U.S. by the doctors working for large medical care corporations, doctors previously recommending the higher priced pharmaceutical. You can easily see, I'm sure, the high stakes battle that is being created over this one herb. And there are hundreds of herbs in the wings.

It was recently announced that the National Institutes of Health will now undertake a three year, four million dollar clinical study of hypericin, one of the main chemicals found in St. John's wort. Imagine the intense scrutiny such a study will get. We are no longer talking about our choice to go in and pick up an herbal remedy from the shelves of our local co-op, herb shop, or health food store. We are now talking about some of the larger financial interests in the world.

Previous efforts to fit the current FDA drug regulatory system around old fashioned herbal medicines have come to naught. In fact, regulatory actions over the years have left herb products hanging out in a strange limbo-land where they could be sold only as long as they didn't have any real consumer information on their labels.

The FDA had earlier given approval to a group of herbs on a Generally Recognized as Safe (GRAS) list, but many of the most popular medicinal herbs are not on the list; they didn't fit easily into the regulatory scheme of things. No one seemed to care very much, until medicinal herbs began to become very popular, first with the public, and now with large insurance and health care agencies looking to cut health care costs.

Like most other subjects involving large companies, the government, and lots of money, things can become quite political. They already have. In the early '90s, the FDA, following a few but very well publicized bad reactions to herbal preparations, saw that their duty to protect the public's health could be made easier if medicinal herbs were to be placed in a classification similar to drugs—that of food additives.

Putting medicinal herbs into this category would have meant virtually removing them from store shelves completely—and forever, as the herbs would have had to undergo tests as though they were drugs. Drug tests are shockingly expensive—more than two hundred million dollars per active ingredient, according to the experts. Every herb plant can contain many, many active constituents, and the herbs themselves are, of course, not patentable. Who could possibly be expected to pay for such research?

As this whole issue worked its way towards Congress in the early '90s, herb enthusiasts around the country mounted a large organized effort to challenge the idea of turning these ancient plants, first into drugs—and then into oblivion. In a remarkable public outpouring—the herbalists themselves can still barely believe it happened—Congress received more mail on this one issue than on anything else since the Vietnam war. Even people who never used medicinal herbs wrote to Congress insisting on their free choice to use herbs in their own health care.

Most of that energy went into pushing for a bill, sponsored by Democratic Congressman Bill Richardson (currently ambassador to the U. N.) and Republican Senator Orrin Hatch (senior Senator from Utah) in which herbal plant products would be placed under the same rules as supplements in a new Dietary Supplement Health and Education Act. The DSHEA (commonly called "DeShay") was signed by the president and became law in October of 1994. Herbs are now regulated within the same framework as vitamins, minerals, and amino acids.

The FDA and herb company representatives are still in complex negotiations over the details of the new regulations, but it now definitely looks like herbal preparations are here to stay. Present negotiations between the FDA and herb industry negotiators are taking place around key issues that may concern anyone interested in medicinal herb business issues: the establishment of good manufacturing practices (GMPs) for the manufacture of herb products, the possible establishment within the FDA of a natural products over-the-counter (OTC) drug review procedure, and continuing negotiations on labeling rules.

The subjects under GMPs by the way, can be quite extensive and could include the following manufacturing areas: premises, sanitation, samples, records, equipment, personnel, manufacturing control, quality control, raw material testing, product testing, etc.

For years, herb products have not been allowed to tell much of anything on their labels other than what they contained. That has led to great misunderstanding by the public who have not been able to learn much about the healing properties of herbs by looking at the products on the shelves. What is known as third party literature—information written by someone other than the product manufacturer, and not attached to the product itself—has been as close together as customer, product, and reliable herb information have been able to get.

Large food companies have long argued for putting health claims on labels about such ingredients as dietary fiber. This engagement with the FDA led Congress, in 1990, to pass the Nutrition Education Labeling Act, establishing the new "nutrition facts" panel on food packages. That act has also become a part of the current negotiations between herb product people and the FDA. But it should be remembered that these new dietary labeling laws only affect the larger companies. Smaller and start-up companies follow the simpler rules outlined in the chapter on herbal products.

The resource section on regulations will show you how to get detailed information about these particulars. This regulatory maneuvering and negotiating will no doubt continue for some time to come, both in the U.S. and in Canada, where there have also been recent changes.

Canadian Regulations

In Canada, a similar pattern has developed around medicinal herbs in the marketplace, in that medicinal herbs started out being sold more or less as foods, with no health claims at all allowed on the labels. Then, in 1994, as herbal medications became ever more popular, the Canadian government also began trying to put these herbal products into a different category.

Traditional Herbal Medicines, they said, were to be allowed as a new class of over-the-counter medications—for treatment only of certain illnesses. The product must be for a health problem amenable to self diagnosis and self medication. And it must be for something self limiting—not truly serious, such as what is known as Schedule A Diseases.

Producers of these Traditional Herbal Medicines, the government announced, would be allowed to apply for and purchase a drug identification number (DIN). These new products could also have health claims on the labels, as long as the claims could be substantiated by having been mentioned in journals. Not in scientific journals, which would only concern drugs, but writings about traditional herb uses—as in ethnobotanical journals.

For example, you could pay $750 and apply for and get a DIN for a single product made with echinacea, and claim on the label that it had traditionally been used for sore throats, because that's what traditional herb literature would show. But you couldn't refer to more recent, more scientific studies, showing echinacea's effectiveness in fighting colds, or as an immune system stimulant. That modern information might mean that it should be in the drug category.

Several problems, and a medicine cabinet full of confusion, came from these changes. For one thing, Schedule A Diseases, a list prepared in the '50s, includes not just cancer and diabetes, but also menopause and obesity—problems that are often very well treated with herbal medications.

Additionally, although the DINs were purchased and used by some herb companies, other manufacturers chose not to spend the money, simply leaving their products on the shelves under the former food classification. Not exactly a level playing field, and quite confusing for both retailers and consumers.

The government then announced that it would crack down on DINs, and must also initiate a new set of fees and licenses in a "cost recovery program"—to pay for the increased inspections its new DIN program required. This drove many small herbal businesses right to the wall, and many Canadian consumers to mount a strong public campaign against the government policies. Much of this occurred during a political year, and political things began to happen. The government backed down.

An Herbal Advisory Panel has recently been appointed by the government, with a mandate to identify all the issues involved and to make recommendations within a year. Canadian herb people are busy at the moment trying to gain the ears of the members of that panel and continuing the effort to keep medicinal herbs in the Canadian marketplace.*

Codex

There is one more regulatory subject worth noting briefly. For the last year or so, the subject of possible new worldwide herb and vitamin/mineral supplement regulations has worried some people—especially on the Internet, where so many ideas get kicked so quickly around the world.

In the whirlwind of new worldwide trade agreements—GATT, NAFTA, MIA, etc.—there has been a flurry of anxiety around the fact that at a '95 meeting of what is known as the Codex Alimentarius Commission on Nutrition and Foods for Special Dietary Uses, a proposal made by the Germans, and supported by others, would make recommendations for minimum and maximum quantities of vitamins and minerals in supplements, establish lists of acceptable or unacceptable ingredients, etc., etc.

The United States delegation opposed such an undertaking and is now busy trying to reassure Americans that we would not, could not, be party to such an agreement, should it "be in conflict with any statute, regulation, or policy under which FDA operates."

I can hear today's cynical reader's response to such reassurances from anyone in government. Meanwhile, the worldwide meetings have continued with proposals moving forward, being changed and developed, detail by detail, in an effort to get all the countries on board. At the last session of the group the issues regarding herbs were apparently dropped from consideration, at least for now. Rather than my trying to speak for or against, or even to explain, such a complicated issue, which is still a long way from resolution, the good old resource section will tell you how to follow up and keep an eye on this issue yourself.

---

*I am sincerely grateful to Allison McCutcheon, of the Canadian Herb Society, for helping me sort out the facts in this brief history.

Organic Growing Regulations

The American Herbal Association newsletter gives national and international coverage to herb issues. One newsletter reported on a 1996 fire near the Chernobyl nuclear power plant in the Ukraine that "filled the air with tons of nuclear ash that contaminated millions of acres of coriander."

Another piece told of the Singapore Ministry of Health banning three Chinese medicinal remedies in 1996 that all contained "enough mercury to cause vomiting, diarrhea, and fatal convulsions."

Serious examples, these, of the issues we have to concern ourselves with once we talk of taking more of our medicines again from growing plants, rather than from synthetic chemicals prepared in laboratories. We are living in a world now of nearly wide-open free trade, where buyers can seek best (as in cheapest) prices for their resources from almost any country in the world. We have long consumed spices and herbs from many countries; now those same kitchen commodities plus many new botanicals are being sold worldwide to go into the medicinal products suddenly in demand.

As more people learn about these contamination problems, the issues of safety and quality will be ever more important selling points for herb providers. Learning to grow plants organically is one of the important assets you can give your herb medicine marketing efforts. You can never compete on price with what is grown (or collected) in Malaysia and India, for instance. You can compete quite successfully in quality, safety, freshness, and service.

Organic growing is another one of those subjects very much in flux as we write this book. It is also a market area, like medicinal herbs, of tremendous growth—showing a 20% increase in each of the last seven or eight years. It is now predicted that organic foods will become a strong 10% of the U.S. food supply within the next few years. That's a huge dollar volume.

The U.S. Department of Agriculture is finally catching up with the American consumers who have been proving the appeal of organic products in the marketplace since the '70s. The USDA recently announced its intention to try to regulate how the term "organic" is used. The term has caused confusion in the past, but private certification programs have been running fairly well in many parts of the country, and some are now wondering if we would have been better off if the government had just stayed out of the whole topic because of very controversial issues it is ignoring in its proposals.

The Agriculture Department has recently placed hundreds of pages of proposed regulations on the Internet inviting electronic public comments. Most all of the comments so far have come from those wanting to urge that the following processes be named and excluded from the definition of organic foods: irradiation, gene-altering, fertilization with reprocessed industrial waste, and the use of antibiotics.

Some agricultural companies are arguing that because these processes are permitted under the law they should be allowed for organic food, too. Let us hope not. If this question is still open when you read this book, I urge that you add your voice to others on this subject. The addresses are listed in the resource section. These quarrels may keep the whole subject going far past the deadlines talked about now.

Unless and until this national question on organic standards is settled, medicinal herb growers must still depend on private certification. Tim Blakley covers this question in his section on growing, and some people feel the private sector will always be the best in this endeavor. There are over 40 private organizations that "certify" in the U.S.; the resource section lists ways to find out about them in your own area.

Herb Safety

Over the years, herbalists have been shaking their heads in discouragement and disbelief as the FDA and several so-called anti-quackery groups have put out endless "information" and warnings about the dangers in medicinal herbs.

The herb safety issue is a very serious one, but let's first put it in context. Between 1981 and 1993, there were zero fatalities recorded in the U.S. or Canada, as a result of anyone using a commercial herb product. During that same period of time, 100,000 people reportedly died from pharmaceutical drug fatalities. Today there are new reports in the news saying that estimate of drug fatalities is far too low. It's reasonable that we all keep medicinal herb safety in our minds as an important issue, but it has not been a major problem, especially considering the long worldwide use of medicinal herbs. They have a remarkable history of both safety and efficacy.

Two recent cases involving the use of unsafe herb products will show where I think the real focus should be on the subject of herb safety. In 1996, a young (age 20) college student, Peter Schlendorf, was vacationing with friends in Panama City, Florida. He took 8 tablets of a product called Ultimate Xphoria, complained shortly of not feeling well, stayed in his hotel room while his friends went out, and was found dead on the floor a few hours later. As far as I know, this was the first reported death from an American made herbal product, and the first case of a product containing an herb (Chinese ephedra, also known as ma huang) that was used as an alternative to street drugs,

The resultant media clamor was intense. The *N.Y. Times* and *Newsweek* said (incorrectly) that the product was Herbal Ecstasy (another street drug imitation containing ephedra), and the head of the FDA blamed the death on the 1994 passage of DSHEA. The *N.Y. Times* reported that the passage of that bill meant that the FDA "could not prevent the sale of the poisonous herb hemlock," that it could not act "until the bodies pile up."

The American Herbal Products Association, as early as 1994, had initiated a policy encouraging the use of both warning labels and limitations on any product with high ephedra (and other strong alkaloid) levels. They notified the FDA about their concerns over these first signs of herbs used as substitutes for street drugs, asking that the FDA consider stepping in to remove such products from the shelves, as the FDA has always had every right to do in the case of unsafe products.

"Sale of ephedra in products substituting for illicit street drugs cannot be condoned ... these products are an aberration," said Mark Blumenthal, executive director of the American Botanical Council, and editor/publisher of *HerbalGram*. The FDA did not respond. Following the Schlendorf death, efforts were made in different cities and counties to simply ban ephedra altogether—a plant drug long used, and long synthesized in the pharmaceutical industry.

The major media in America used the story in typical tabloid fashion: screaming headlines, shocking pictures, incorrect facts, and plenty of intimidation about all herbal products. Representatives from responsible herb companies and associations responded in measured, reasonable voices.

As it turned out, these imitation street drug products were unsafe in many ways. The packages had been completely and dishonestly mislabeled; some ingredients were adulterated; some contained ingredients no one could truly identify—something the mainstream press never reported, of course. They were totally unsafe products, and should have been recalled from store shelves—just as many bad products are recalled from store shelves every day of the year.

Since that time, I am happy to report, the issues between legitimate herb product companies and the FDA are being dealt with on a much more reasonable level. Perhaps because the herbalists held their own rather well in the public arena over that issue; perhaps because the passage of DSHEA has created more pressure on the FDA to find reasonable ways to deal with botanicals and phytomedicines. The FDA has now proposed that individual doses of ephedra be limited to 8 mg. per dose and 24 mg. per day, with new warning labels. The young man's family, by the way, has sued the producers of Ultimate Xphoria for two billion dollars.

The second case is a far more common problem with herbal safety that I hope everyone dealing with herbs will pay attention to and remember even longer than they might remember the tragedy of the young man in Florida.

As I write this chapter, a product called Chomper, made by a California company and sold as an herbal laxative, is being removed from store shelves across the country because the herb plantain (*Plantago major*) in the product was found to have been adulterated with the herb woolly foxglove (*Digitalis lantana*)—long used for a well known and strong heart pharmaceutical. No deaths have been reported in this case, but herb people everywhere are taking it very seriously.

So far in this incident, the FDA has found that at least 3,000 pounds of adulterated plantain were shipped from Germany and distributed across the U. S. to herb shops and herbal product manufacturers. This is serious business, and everyone involved in herbs needs to give this side of herb safety and identification their focused attention.

One of the important issues in the present FDA negotiations about good manufacturing practices is this question of herb identity and quality. It has been reported that had the proposed new GMPs for herbs been used by the companies involved in this incident, the Chomper case would not have occurred. Whether you are a grower of medicinal herbs, a seller of herbs and/or herb products, or just a consumer of medicinal herbs, this question of herb quality and identity has to be one of the utmost importance. If you are just getting into the herb world in a commercial way, you need to find a way to make absolutely certain that plant material identification is your very first safety priority.

Until the herb product industry and the FDA agree on a way to set standards and regulate the industry in a reasonable way, the people who dispense herbs must carry total responsibility for making sure that what they give out is what they claim it is.

So, how can you make sure that plant material you use in products or ingest yourself is, first of all, what you think it is, and secondly, of good quality? First by learning a whole lot about all aspects of medicinal herbs, and then learning some more about them. It is also obvious that the plants you grow and process yourself will always be the ones you can have the most faith in.

If you are going to be dispensing herbs as medicine—either as fresh dried herbs for a tea, or in tinctures, or in other herbal products, you will need to take further precautions. This is especially true if you will be using herbs supplied by others. Most reputable herb companies these days are turning more and more to chromatography equipment (their own or at commercial labs) for both identification purposes and to examine the specific chemical constituents in the plants.

But this can be expensive for small and start-up companies. They will have to rely at first on other less costly methods of plant identification. Microscopes are used by many small companies to make plant identification more certain, along with chemical assays of one type or another. Thorough herb plant knowledge by the person accepting delivery of the plant material for dispensing or manufacturing purposes is mandatory. Cut and dried herb materials can be difficult to identify depending on the conditions under which they were grown, harvested, dried, packaged, and shipped.

My own sense of smell often fails me in trying to identify herbs. Taste can also be misleading. I know I wouldn't qualify for the job of making a positive identification on herbs grown elsewhere and shipped into my shop or manufacturing lab.

The quality of the herbs can also be determined in the identification process, along with possible adulteration with extraneous matter. Besides careful visual inspection, companies also learn to do moisture tests, volatile oil testing, and/or chromatography. Either thin layer, high pressure liquid, or gas chromatography are used. The more processed the herb has been before delivery, the more difficult it can be to identify, dried powdered leaf being about the most difficult.

Luckily for those just coming into the commercial world of medicinal herbs, helpful information is now more available because of so much hard work done in the last twenty years by individuals and associations all across the country. I am ever grateful for their work.

The first American herbal monographs are just being produced and are available to all those with herbal interests. These long treatises, one for each herb, will help establish herb identity and quality criteria as well as therapeutic information. One of the first of these monographs, edited by herbalist Roy Upton for the American Herbal Pharmacopoeia, a nonprofit organization based in Santa Cruz, California, was reprinted in Issue 40 of *HerbalGram*. It is for the herb St. John's wort.

These monograms offer all possible names for one herb; a history of its use; a detailed botanical description; macro and microscopic descriptions; how and where the herb is collected, with details and pictures on processing, drying, storage, and preparations. They also offer constituent activities, methods of analysis, and pages of eye-glazing details of clinical studies, animal studies, in vitro studies, plus all the study conclusions; recommended dosages, contraindications, side effects, interactions, toxicology, and the regulatory status of the herb around the world. Whew!

This is the kind of concise, thorough information that has been long needed in this country and it will be welcomed by all. In the same issue of *HerbalGram*, the following list appeared showing which American Herbal Pharmacopoeia monographs are completed, and which ones will follow.

Completed monographs included: hawthorn, St. John's wort, valerian, willowbark. AHP monographs near completion included: ashwagandha, astragalus root, garlic, reishi mushroom, schizandra. AHP monographs in process included: billberry, black haw, chamomile, chaste berry, cramp bark, dandelion, dong qui, echinacea, ginger, ginkgo, ginseng, goldenseal, lemon balm, licorice, milk thistle, momordica, nettles, peppermint, saw palmetto, uva ursi.

North American herbalists have long known of the German government health agency Commission E monographs on which that country's large, well established medicinal herb industry is built. Those monographs are also all now becoming available in English for the first time in North America, and can help any serious herb person do a better and better job in the marketplace with herbs.

This kind of serious effort on the part of organizations like the American Botanical Council, the American Herbalist Guild, and the Herb Research Foundation must have also made a difference in the improving relationships with the FDA. The Chomper case is important because it seemed to mark a new spirit of cooperation between the herb industry and that federal organization. For years, the two have often been totally adversarial, with too many herb people squawking to "just keep the Feds out of our lives," and too many FDA people painting the herb culture as full of careless screwballs dispensing witch potions and mumbo jumbo. In the Chomper issue, the two sides worked together to get the word out and focus the attention where it belonged—on getting the adulterated product off the market and away from potential consumers. This is not to say there won't be plenty of new regulatory problems as medicinal herbs become ever more part of the American health care picture, but the picture is definitely becoming more positive.

Americans very much want choices in our health care and medications, and are rebelling against a seemingly paternalistic medical system that offers too many strong chemicals, with too many side effects. Herbal medicines have a more "natural" appeal to them and are seen by many as "virtually harmless."

Both these points are oversimplified, even overdrawn, but they lead to an important last point I want to make on the question of herb safety. America is an extremely litigious society these days. Those of us who want to work inside the new medicinal herbal pathway in America shouldn't forget that we have more lawyers and more lawsuits than we can reasonably stand. It's hard to see how we can continue to operate as a society with so many of them in our midst. But we have them anyway. So, just as for every other health care worker in the country, I think herbalists must remember the number one safety rule: First, do no harm.

Herb Standardization

"The whole herb is the balanced holistic shotgun mix with which our genes
co-evolved for thousands of years. I think the next millennium will see us
heading back to the Green Pharmacy, whole herb…and away from the more
toxic silver bullets."

James A. Duke, USDA, ret.

I can understand the push for standardized botanicals—from the sides of
both the producer and the consumer. After all, 25% of the ordinary medicines we now take are plant based, most of them in standardized products;
why not just more of the same?

On the producer's side, standardized medicines can eliminate so many
problems by simply taking the herbs apart, refining and processing only
the "most important and biologically active chemicals" of the plant, and
not having to deal with all that *warm and fuzzy stuff* that often accompa-
nies talk of the benefits of whole plants.

From the consumer side, standardized medicines can take away some
of the worry and uncertainty that have built up around the subject of
herbal medicines. "You can't really tell what's in them, or how much to
take," I often hear people say. Herbal products have simply been put out
there on store shelves without any real information on them, and consumers have had to learn to administer the potions to themselves, usually as a
result of a friend's recommendation. Not exactly a safe sounding recipe
for reasonable health care.

Right alongside the confusion have come what some others have described as the herbal "cowboy marketers" selling a wild panorama of remedies with claims that seem more appropriate for the early 1900s than for
the present.

I've thought quite a bit about this subject in the writing of this book,
and my own conclusions are, of course, strictly personal. I agree that some
sort of reasonable regulations have to continue to accompany the rise of
herbal medicines, but I have to come down on the side of whole plant
medicines rather than the standardized form that sounds, on the surface,
so much more like a better fit for our fast paced, fix-it-quick lives. For me,
as for many other people with a strong interest in plants, herbs are food
plants, and the best processing of my family's foods are those processes I
do in my own kitchen. The closer I keep my kitchen, food and herbs
together the better we seem to do. I seek herbal medication for a different
kind of health care, one that is more closely tied to the reasons I seek
whole foods.

The chemicals contained in plants and herbs are the chemicals our
bodies seek and need to stay healthy. Over eons of time, plants developed

these chemicals as a means of protecting themselves from insects, fungi, bacteria, viruses, and animals. When we ingest those plant chemicals, they offer us some of that same strong protection.

It is reading about these plant chemicals that has convinced me that whole plants and whole foods are the way to go whenever possible. A simple carrot, for instance, has at least 33 active chemicals, from aesculetin to vanillic acid, with lots of other weird sounding chemicals in between. And the common thyme plant, *Thymus vulgaris*, has 95 chemicals, from alanine to zinc. Garlic, I have read, has more than 200 chemical properties, many of these capable of safeguarding us against disease.

To study these chemicals and their biological activities is an astronomically expensive undertaking. It will be many lifetimes before reliable studies can be done on many of them—especially regarding their combinations, and how they might work together in the body. In the meantime, a lot of assumptions are being made about the special chemicals in some herbs and those are being isolated and sold as herbal cures in the single chemical forms we have all grown used to in both prescription and some OTC drugs. High in ginsenosides, says one ginseng advertisement; full of hypericin, say the ads for St. John's wort. Do herb customers need a degree in chemistry, I wonder?

Feverfew (*Tanacetum parthenium*) became a popular and successful herbal cure for migraine headaches in the 1980s. Parthenolides, it was reported, were the chemicals that caused feverfew's effectiveness. The feverfew products that appeared on store shelves soon were labeled *standardized to 0.4% parthenolide*. Very reassuring. Now it appears, in later studies, that parthenolides may or may not be the main cause of the herb's effectiveness in treating migraines. Other chemicals or perhaps the synergistic effect of several may be at work.

These days the herb label that says standardized on it is said be worth little more than "a good way to assure consumers that at least some of that particular chemical is in the product." It's also a way to produce a pill or capsule that can be familiarly marketed to those seeking a silver bullet to "just deal with the headache and let me get on with my life."

Where all this is headed is anybody's guess. My own simplistic answer to this chaos and uncertainty is to cling tight to whole plants grown and made into medicine as close to home as possible—sometimes even from my own garden, sometimes even at my own sink—most often from small companies in my region whose products I have learned over the years to trust.

For those wanting to start a small business in medicinal herbs, don't let this chaos and confusion on the sidelines deter you from the field. Whatever happens in the regulatory agencies, or in the chemical labs, is quite secondary to the continued and growing need for well grown or well collected medicinal herbs. The market that is opening so fast now can only get far larger as time goes by.

The consumer culture around what I call the "whole plant" medicinal herb world is happening in a very grass roots fashion—plainly visible in the herbal networks described in this book. It most resembles the whole foods consumer market. Herbs can be taken up rapidly by the mass market—and just as rapidly dropped. For those of us in the other, quality, whole foods world, medicinal herbs will only become more important as time goes by, and as the herbal networks spread.

Start learning more about these plants today; put some of them in your garden this season; learn how they are used and what's in them. Farmer Tim's section of the book that follows will get you started.

Good luck.

Part II

by Tim Blakley

*"Conservation through propagation is the key
to preservation."*
—Anon.

"In the garden of the senses lies the pathway to the spirit."
—Anon.

Acknowledgments

I've spent the last 20 years growing, selling, harvesting and teaching about medicinal herbs in preparation for writing this book. Along the way I've encountered many people who have helped me in my quest for knowledge and several who helped me specifically to write this book.

The person I have to thank the most is my wife, Heather. She typed much of the book as I dictated it to her after my recent shoulder surgery. She also edited the book and added many little phrases to it. She has also supported my need to grow herbs even in the rough times. (Heather likes to grow herbs as much as I do, but gets sidetracked by her goats!) I also must thank my parents, Joyce and Ray Blakley. Mom helped in editing, supplied a computer and a house when we desperately needed both. My sister Lesley Jay and her family also supplied me with a computer and a place to use it and I thank them also.

I would like to profusely thank Rosemary Gladstar, who was one of my first herb teachers and always inspired and encouraged me. Also all the other people I have met along my herbal journey, all with various amounts of plant and herbal knowledge, who all taught me something. These people are too numerous to mention but I will touch on a few. Mark and Marggy Wheeler of Pacific Botanicals, two of the sweetest, humblest herb growers ever, Richo Cech, Kathy K. Larson, Sunny Mavor, David Cavagnaro, Jane Bothwell, Kenny Collins, Autumn Summers, Ina Chung, Daniel Pinney, Kathi Keville, Snow and Bev dudes, and on and on and on. I probably forgot a few names as there have been so many people whom I've encountered along the herbal path. Please forgive me if I didn't include you.

Also I would like to thank Lee and Tal, without whose constant e-mails, faxes, phone calls, and letters this book might still not be in existence.

Tim Blakley

How to Grow, Process and Sell Medicinal Herbs for Fun and Profit

It has taken me many years of growing herbs to get to the point where I could write this book. I first started growing medicinal herbs in the late 1970s. At that time I was the gardener and a teacher at the California School of Herbal Studies in Forestville, California. Few people back then were using medicinal herbs and very few were growing them. There were no books available on growing medicinal herbs and I learned by doing. I made a lot of mistakes along the way.

I stayed at the herb school until 1991, eventually becoming a co-owner. I created and developed the botanical gardens at the school and taught classes on botany, horticulture, herb quality, herb conservation, and medicinal use of herbs. I also traveled around the country to various conferences and schools teaching similar classes. I also had a business growing and distributing medicinal herbs, culinary herbs, cut flowers, edible flowers, and wild greens. I left California in 1991 and moved to Iowa.

While in Iowa, I initially worked for Seed Savers Exchange. I then became the Land Manager at Frontier Herb Cooperative. At Frontier Herbs, I created and developed the botanical garden, and started their herb research and production farm. I left Iowa in the winter of 1993 and moved to Oregon in order to be the land manager at Herb Pharm.

At Herb Pharm I started with a relatively blank piece of land, 80 acres of it. The land had been heavily overgrazed for 60 years and was in very poor shape. I spent four years improving the fertility, planting crops and putting in several acres of display gardens. I planted 30 acres of row crops of medicinal herbs and raised about 100 species of medicinal herbs for harvest. In the botanical garden I planted over 600 species of herbs.

I'm now starting a new project for Frontier Herb Cooperative in Rutland, Ohio. The goal is to learn as much as possible about growing the many herbs that are presently being over-wildcrafted so they can be cultivated and thus saved in the wild. The information learned in the research will be passed on to farmers so that we can have a cultivated, organic supply of these herbs and reduce the pressure on the wild populations. Many of the herbs I will be carrying out my research on are already rare (Ginseng and Goldenseal) or on their way to becoming rare, like Black Cohosh and Blue Cohosh.

I've spent my whole adult life growing herbs. I've done other things in my life but few with the passion I feel for growing herbs. This book is a personal book and most of the information in it comes from my own experiences.

The purpose of this book is to convey as much information as possible on growing, harvesting, processing and selling medicinal herbs on small farms of a quarter acre or less, on up to big farms of a gazillion acres or more.

CHAPTER EIGHT

The Importance of Growing Medicinal Herbs

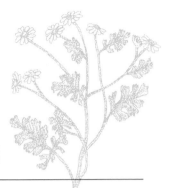

Most of the world's supply of medicinal herbs has traditionally come from wildcrafted sources. Wildcrafting is basically the harvesting of an herb from a non-cultivated source. Two of the major problems in our dependence on wildcrafted herbs are quality and quantity. Many wildcrafted herbs are of poor quality, and because of the incredible growth in the industry some herbs have become threatened or endangered.

Many people envision wildcrafted herbs as coming from some beautiful alpine meadow or from the center of an old growth forest. The reality is that wildcrafted herbs can come from just about anywhere. If you pick a dandelion growing in a crack in downtown New York City you are wildcrafting. Even though most herbs don't come from downtown New York City, many are picked along major highways, in polluted areas, in drainage ditches with farm runoff in them, and in other not so desirable locations.

Many herbs are picked in beautiful "wild" areas but that isn't necessarily a good thing either. Imagine someone going onto a beautiful piece of prairie land, somewhere in the midwest, and digging thousands of holes in order to harvest Echinacea *angustifolia*. In the process you can change drainage patterns, dig up other plants, eliminate an important food source (Echinacea seed) that migrating birds depend on, and basically compromise the ecological integrity of that little piece of prairie.

Another problem with wildcrafting that rarely happens with cultivation is the harvesting of the wrong species. It happens often with Echinacea where someone is trying to harvest Echinacea *angustifolia* and actually picks Echinacea *pallida* or *atrorubens*. At one point in the 1980s a large amount of the Echinacea supply was actually a plant called Wild Quinine Root (*Parthenium integrifolium*). Wild Quinine does not look even remotely like Echinacea.

Up to now I've only focused on some of the negative sides of wildcrafting. There are many wildcrafters out there who "ethically" harvest and in the process bring to the industry a good supply of quality herbs. The major problem is numbers. Too high a number for the demand; too low a number for the long term supply of some herbs.

The biggest problem facing the supply side of the herb industry today is the incredible growth the industry is having. Twenty years ago we were begging people to use herbs; now they are consuming them in such numbers that in many cases we cannot maintain the supply of certain wildcrafted herbs. Many herbs are being harvested at a rate that exceeds their ability to grow back. As demand for an herb goes up and the supply goes down several consequences will happen. First, the price will go up as pickers work harder and longer to supply the product. This in turn will cause the eventual demise of the population of that particular plant, perhaps causing it to become rare or even endangered. Two classic examples of that are American Ginseng (*Panax quinquefolius*) and Goldenseal (*Hydrastis canadensis*).

American Ginseng is the best example in this country of an herb that has been over-harvested to the point where it is now rare in nearly every part of its original range. Today, nearly all of the American Ginseng comes from cultivated sources. Wild Ginseng sells for very high prices and in my opinion should no longer be wild harvested. Goldenseal has the potential to be the next Ginseng. Supply seems to have recently been passed by demand and prices are going up. If we do not do something soon, in a few years Goldenseal may very well follow Ginseng into rarity.

United Plant Savers, a group founded in the early 1990s by Rosemary Gladstar, has as one of its goals the preservation of our native herbal resources. It recently put out a list of "at risk" herbs. Besides Ginseng and Goldenseal other major plants on the list include Black Cohosh, Bloodroot, Blue Cohosh, Echinacea *angustifolia*, Helonias root, Lomatium, Osha, and Wild Yam Root. There are many ways to help preserve the native populations of these plants. One sometimes overlooked way to help is to try, in whatever way possible, to eliminate the destruction of the habitats of these plants. For example clearcutting of a forest is a great way to eliminate species dependent upon shade for survival.

Another way to help is to facilitate the appropriate uses of these key herbs. It is a shame that a significant percentage of the Goldenseal harvested in this country is used by people who think it will help them pass a drug test. Goldenseal does absolutely nothing to help mask a drug test. Educating the public on appropriate herb use will help a great deal in easing some of the present harvesting pressures on Goldenseal.

Using a non-threatened species as a replacement can also help. One good example of this is the threatened Echinacea *angustifolia* versus the easy to cultivate Echinacea *purpurea*. Echinacea *purpurea* is used for the same reasons as Echinacea *angustifolia*. Since 99.9% of Echinacea *purpurea* comes from cultivated sources it would be a good substitute. Many herbs are unique in their particular actions though, and oftentimes a substitute just isn't the best course.

What other options are there? Finally we get to the whole purpose of this entire chapter. The best option is to cultivate herbs! By growing medicinal herbs we can produce a higher quality herb more consistently and we can guarantee the long term quantities necessary to continue to meet the public's demand for herbs.

I think that the most important aspect in producing quality herb products is to be able to use quality herbs. By growing high quality herbs we can insure they are grown free of noxious chemicals—and we can guarantee identification. First we need to select the most desirable species, sub-species and varieties with the desired constituent makeup. Then we need to grow healthy plants, harvest them at the best times, dry and process them correctly, and ship them fresh right after harvest (when appropriate).

I've always been an organic farmer and I think that growing herbs organically is a key factor in producing quality herbs. Nearly all herbs can easily be grown organically. If you are going to grow organically, then it would benefit you to certify your farm. There are many groups who will certify your farm, usually one or two in any area.

To qualify to be certified, your farm must be chemical free, according to your certifier's guidelines, for three years. You don't have to certify your land until you are ready to harvest your herbs. You can grow a crop for four years and then certify your land in the fifth year and harvest it. However, during that time you must follow the organic guidelines; otherwise your property would not be certifiable for another three years. In other words, you can save yourself certification fees until you are ready to harvest. The cost of certification can run anywhere from less than $100 to several thousand dollars, depending on the gross income of your farm.

Is certification worth it? You can nearly always sell your organic herbs for more money, and many of the best paying companies are seeking out high quality organically certified herbs. It definitely pays to be certified organic.

The herb industry is growing at an incredible rate and the demand for quality herbs is skyrocketing. At present there are only a few farms that supply nearly all of the organic herbs on the market today. We need more good herb growers now. Can you make money growing herbs? Definitely. Can you lose money growing herbs? Definitely. Can you have fun growing herbs? Most definitely! Growing any crop is always a risk. If the biggest hurricane in a generation goes right through your farm, then you

CHAPTER NINE

Getting Started

Once you've decided you are going to be an herb grower you have to make several important decisions. First and foremost you have to decide where you are going to grow your herbs. Several factors will be important in narrowing your choice of property. You need to consider soil, water availability, climate, drainage patterns, convenience to markets, and, most importantly, the cost and desirability of a particular area.

Since I have no experience with land out of this country (U.S.A.) I will focus on land here in the lower 48 states. Where is land "affordable" and is that a place where I would want to live? I've traveled quite a bit and looked at numerous farms throughout the country and I've found a few areas that seem desirable to many growers and would-be growers that are also reasonably affordable. However, what is desirable and attractive to me may not be your cup of tea. I'll leave the issue of desirability and cost to another author. Here I'll just focus on the basics.

Soil is the most basic ingredient in a farm. Without it you are going to have a difficult time making a living. With it you may still have a difficult time making a living, but at least you are on the right track. There are lots of good soils throughout the country and the world. The key is in finding them.

The place to start in the search is the local Soil Conservation District office or your County Farm Extension office. Every rural county has a Soil Survey book which contains maps and information on every bit of soil in that county. The Soil Conservation office has a copy and they will be more than happy to help you determine the quality of the soil in that county. It will have info on fertility, slope, drainage, and even the rockiness of the soil.

In general the herb grower is looking for a soil that is fertile, well drained, relatively flat, never sprayed, devoid of rocks, and south facing (most of the time). Does this perfect soil exist? If you look hard enough in the right place you can find some excellent soils that will fill the bill.

Fertility is important, but it is one aspect of the soil that is easy to improve. Still, it is much easier and cheaper to start with a fertile soil that doesn't need a lot of additives. How do you determine fertility as you walk a potential property? Look at the plants that are growing there. How tall is the grass? Are the plants green and healthy? Certain weeds are indicators of poor soils. If the soil was heavily grazed, then you will probably notice the warning signs like short grass, lots of introduced weeds, erosion, etc. I said earlier that you can improve a soil, but you don't want to start out with really bad soil or you will pay for it, in time, money, and bouts of frustration.

Drainage is determined by several factors including soil type, rock content, lay of the land, and proximity to moving water. Soil types can range from sandy to clay. For good drainage the preferred soils would be somewhere between a loamy sand and a loamy clay. I would prefer a soil closer to a sandy loam than a loamy clay because the worst thing to me is when a crop rots in the field in a wet winter or summer. It is possible to improve the drainage on a heavy clay soil, but it is a very expensive proposition.

The more rocks you have in your soil, the better the drainage. We are talking small rocks here. Large rocks are never a good ingredient in the soil—unless you are building a stone house, or a 21st century version of Stonehenge. Of course too many rocks cause other problems, like destroying your machinery.

When walking a piece of property and determining where the prime soils are, always take into consideration the slopes, low spots and surface water. If you plant in a beautiful field that unfortunately is also a flood plain, then you may not do too well when that 100 year flood comes. Those little swales you sometimes see in soils can also mean that you have water flowing through there during very heavy storms.

You are usually going to find the best soils in flat river valleys. Occasionally you might find good soils on somewhat flat hilltops. Avoid whenever possible trying to farm on a slope. Even the smallest slopes can create water problems, erosion problems, and mechanical problems. Those beautiful terraces in the Andes Mountains of Peru look beautiful and majestic but someone had to work awfully hard putting those rocks in place.

Most of your crops are going to need full sun, so generally a soil that is south facing is preferred. However, there are certain valuable crops that prefer shaded north slopes, so if you are going to be a Ginseng or Goldenseal grower, then you would seek out a north facing soil.

If you are going to be a certified organic grower, then you want to buy a property that has not been sprayed in the recent past. There are many ways to determine whether or not a particular property has been sprayed. The easiest thing to do is ask the owner if they sprayed it. Before purchasing your piece of land, you might want to take a soil sample to determine if any residual, harmful chemicals are present. Even if your certifier does not require a soil test, you may still, for your own piece of mind, want to do one. You can bet your sweet patootie that if the land was farmed and was not certified, then it was sprayed. A soil has to be free of chemical farming additives for three years before it can be certified. Remember, you do not have to certify your land until you are ready to harvest. If you want to harvest your first crop immediately, you should seek out land that has not been sprayed in the last three years.

There are several groups that provide organic certification services throughout the country. At the moment, they all have slightly different standards but in the very near future federal standards will be in place and all the regional certifiers will have to follow them. If you want to become certified, the best place to start is your regional certifying group. The best place to get information on this is to contact other organic growers in that area. My experience has been that not all certifiers are equal. Some are much more efficient and easier to deal with.

Certification is not cheap. All certifiers charge you according to how much gross income you made on the farm the previous year. In your first year even if you do not harvest a crop, you will still pay a minimum of anywhere between $100 and $250. The more you make, the more you pay. An inspector from the certifier will inspect your farm annually and make sure that you are following organic guidelines. Some certifiers require a soil test the first year to determine if there were any long term chemicals left in the soil. If a lot of DDT was sprayed 25 years ago it may still be present in the soil in significant quantities and you may not be able to be certified.

In some areas there may be more than one certifier. I would recommend you contact each certifier and see which one you feel the most comfortable with. Just like buying any other service, quality is everything. Of course you may also want to check their fees.

Now let's talk about the weather. The Department of Agriculture has divided the country into ten different climatic, or growing, zones. They range from 1 to 10, with 1 being the coldest and 10 being the warmest. Most of the United States is between zones 3 and 8. Zones 1 and 2 are found only in Alaska or extremely high altitudes. Zones 9 and 10 are found in the warm parts of California, the Gulf Coast, Florida, and Hawaii.

I've grown crops from zone 4 to zone 9 and although there are a few more species you can grow in zone 9 than in zone 4, anywhere in that range would be reasonable for growing medicinal herbs. Zone 3 is just a little too cold for a lot of crops, but if you don't mind wearing snowshoes in the middle of summer then zone 3 is okay for you.

Regionally, of course, there are lots of microclimates. It's nice to stay out of low areas in the valleys which tend to have both late and early frosts. In foggy areas, it's nice to avoid the areas where the fogs accumulate most. Generally speaking, microclimates have minimal effect on perennial crops so it's seldom a major issue when choosing your land.

In addition, along with soil, the most important factor in determining the growing ability of a piece of property is water availability. In much of the country, especially the area east of the Mississippi, water availability is not much of an issue. In the western United States water is everything.

In the western United States farmers have been fighting over water use for over a hundred and fifty years. In order to irrigate in most areas of the west you need to have water rights. Whether you are drawing water from a river, creek, pond, or well, you still need to have water rights if you are irrigating anything beyond garden size. New water rights are extremely difficult to come by; I have known some growers who waited up to 10 years to get water rights on a single well. It can be a bureaucratic nightmare and very costly.

It's better to buy a property with water rights already existing. The age of the water right is very important as the older the right, the less likely you are to ever lose the right to irrigate. In many areas, in dry years, water rights are simply terminated for parts of the growing season, according to the age of the water right. You can check with your local Watermaster, or other water official, to see whether or not a specific water right is good and not likely to be terminated at any point during the growing season.

One sometimes overlooked factor in determining if a property is suitable is its convenience to your market. When growing herbs, you need to determine where your most likely markets will be. If you are considering selling fresh herbs then you might want to be close to a major consumer. You can ship fresh or dried anywhere in the country. Still some companies would rather buy a product that is two hours out of the ground versus two days out of the ground. Dry herbs can be shipped anywhere in the country, so the distance to market is not as critical an issue.

CHAPTER TEN

Machinery, Tools and Equipment

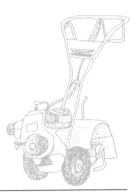

A whole book can be written about farm machinery, so I will simply try to pass on some basic information to get you started.

You can spend a lot of money on equipment or you can spend a little, depending on the size of your operation, your bank account, and whether or not you are willing to deal with old equipment. Under three acres or so you can probably get by without a tractor, though you might on occasion want to make arrangements for your neighbor to do some tractor work for you.

If you are going to try to do without a tractor then your equipment of choice will probably be a rototiller. The two major brands today are Troybuilt and BCS. Both make tillers of various horsepower (hp), from 3 hp up to BCS's 14 hp. For anything over half an acre I would opt for the 10 or 14 hp BCS. The BCS comes with the ability to add on a whole slew of attachments including furrowers, plows, mowers, spaders, and more.

One of the main advantages of the tiller is that it is a lot less expensive than a tractor, and cheaper to operate. A brand new 14 hp BCS tiller can be bought for around $4,000 with attachments being extra. They are easy to fix, transport, store, and operate. For small operations under three acres they are adequate for most of the jobs that need to be done. Bottom line though is that tillers do not have near the capabilities of even a small, 20 hp tractor.

One of the main advantages of the tractor is superior hp. With superior hp you can work more acreage in less time, pull heavier equipment, and work deeper soil depths. There is an incredible multitude of implements available for tractors, including tiller, plow, bucket, harrow, disc, root digger, transplanter, spader, mower, combine, blade, a variety of cultivators, and many more. And let's not underestimate the ability to sit while working. Working 10 acres on a 100-degree day is a lot easier sitting down on a tractor than walking behind a rototiller.

How big a tractor do you need, and how much is it going to cost? The size of your tractor needs is directly related to the size of your operation. A four-wheel-drive tractor is far superior to a two-wheel-drive of equal hp. I have used a 40 hp, four-wheel-drive for several years and it is capable of doing everything I have ever needed done—except making tea! A higher hp tractor, 60 to 80 hp and up, can go deeper into your soil with certain implements, which is beneficial at times. It can pull bigger implements and do the work in less time. The costs of a tractor can vary so much that it is hard to put down on paper. A new 40 hp tractor of a reputable brand might run $20,000 or so. You might be able to buy a nice used 40 hp tractor for a lot less. Remember, a tractor is the most important investment a farmer will ever make, so find the best way to balance quality and cost.

A lot could be said about the implements available for tractors; I will touch on my preferred implements. If I were to get one implement I would get a tiller first. A tiller enables you to turn under cover crops or heavy grass. Of all the implements, the tiller does the best job of prepping your bed for planting. The main disadvantages to a tiller include creation of a hardpan and its difficulty in working rocky soils. It also can have a negative effect on your soil structure, constantly pulverizing, so that it breaks up into particles that are too fine.

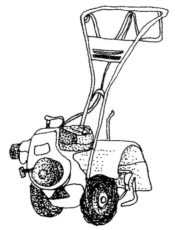

A relatively new implement that can be substituted for a tiller is the spading machine. It originated in Europe and its advantages over a tiller include not creating a hardpan, and not having such a negative effect on soil structure. There is even a spading machine designed to fit the 14 hp BCS tiller. Spading machines are becoming much more common in the States and most dealers sell them.

Next on my list would be a spring-tooth harrow or a disc. Both are capable of preparing the soil for planting. Both are capable of working in rocky soils without doing too much damage to the equipment. A spring-tooth harrow can work at greater depths, loosen the soil and not damage soil structure. A disc can break up rough soils with lots of vegetative matter, and is capable of preparing soil for planting. A disc will not work a soil as deeply as a spring-tooth harrow, so I won't use it for deep root crops. It is the most commonly used implement for farmers today. I like to follow discing with a drag line, made out of heavy duty wire with weight on it. This breaks down the large soil particles and ridges, making planting easier.

This is especially important when sowing seeds which often require a more uniform soil surface. When transplanting it is not as critical to have a smooth, uniform soil surface.

Many farmers would consider the plow the most important implement. I use a plow mainly to turn over heavily sodded fields, usually just the first time I work a field. Plows are easy to find at auctions and are extremely cheap. They do a good job but can cause some problems—such as creating a hardpan.

A good implement to use if you are looking to break up either an artificial or natural hardpan is a subsoiler. It is just a long curved shank attached to a tool bar that will go as deep as you can take it. The more hp you have the deeper you can go. If you are just trying to break up the soil for 10 to 12 inches, you might be able to run multiple shanks, but if it's depth you are looking for then one shank will probably be it—unless you get into a high hp tractor. Bars and shanks are very inexpensive and usually available used at auctions and farm sales.

For cultivation of weeds, most growers will use some combination of shovels, hoes, and sweeps mounted on a bar. They are easy to pull behind even a small tractor. They are very effective at cutting and churning up weeds in between the rows. You can get relatively close to your crop, if you are careful, especially when the crop is young and the top growth doesn't hinder the tractor and implements too much. Tool bars and cultivation implements are inexpensive and relatively easy to find used.

In the last few years, I've mounted my cultivation implements on an older tractor with a front mounted hydraulic that allowed me to look forward and down at the crop while cultivating. It makes it easier to see and thus get closer to your crop. It also eases some of that sore neck syndrome from constantly looking backwards on your tractor. The disadvantage of this type of tractor is that its main use is just cultivation of weeds, as you are not capable of operating most implements in that position.

Another implement for weed control is the multivator or multiple rototiller. It operates like a tiller but with multiple small tillers off a central bar that allow you to do several rows at once. They come in different widths and you can buy sizes that work for skinny rows or wide rows. They are great at dealing with the massive weed growth in the beginning of the season.

For transplanting starts out into the field it is nice to have a transplanter. They come with one-row planting capabilities on up to several rows. Two or three rows is all a small to medium size tractor can pull. The more rows you can plant at once the easier your cultivation will be later on because the rows are perfectly lined up with each other at whatever spacing you desire. Unfortunately a one-row planter won't help much for cultivation because each row will be slightly off in terms of width.

Transplanters can also be ordered with a fertilizer and water attachment. I've fertilized with water and fish emulsion which is dropped right next to the plant. Besides the fertilizer value, this also gives the plant that much needed watering to hold it over for another day or two until you either get your irrigation system on it or you have some wet or moist weather.

Transplanters cut down your planting time immensely. A two-row planter with four people working it (a driver, two planters, and someone walking behind) can plant 10 times faster than those same four people doing it by hand. They are expensive. A two-row machine will cost between $5,000 and $10,000. They can be purchased used especially in areas where there is a lot of vegetable production or tobacco planting.

If you don't have a transplanter then you can simply make a furrow and put your plants in. Even rototillers have an attachment for a furrower.

For harvesting, one implement you might want is a root digger. Commonly used for crops like potatoes and carrots, they can operate behind the tractor and dig your roots up and either drop them on the surface or directly into a trailer, via a conveyor belt. For doing large volumes of single crops they are very time saving. If you are growing small volumes of root crops then you can run a U-shaped bar under the crops to loosen them up or even run a shank under or next to the crop for the same effect.

Another harvesting machine is the combine. It can be used to harvest seed crops like Echinacea, or in some cases, modified to harvest crops like Chamomile. Unless you have multiple acres of seed to harvest, it probably would not pay to purchase and operate one.

There are numerous types of mowers and green choppers available. They are mainly used to chop or cut your cover crop or unused row crop tops into small pieces to hasten their breakdown. They are inexpensive and usually available used at auctions or used implement dealers.

For applying seed directly to the field you can go with several options. I use a rotary spreading seeder for my cover crops. I follow that with a drag line to work the seed in. I've also used a drill seeder which buries the seed and makes nice straight rows. For really small plantings of seed I've used a little hand pushed seed planter that buries the seed. It comes with a variety of plate sizes for the various size seeds you might encounter, and is usually used for vegetables but works well for herbs too.

One important implement that I haven't mentioned yet is the bucket. Having a bucket on the tractor allows you to do a lot. You can move soil and fertilizer, turn compost, scrape things level, move materials, etc. If you are going to have a tractor you have to have a bucket.

Besides the machine operated tools there are a lot of tools that are people operated. You can't have a farm without hoes, shovels, rakes, trowels, and pruning shears. I used to buy cheap tools but I think it is best to buy good quality tools and keep them in good shape, especially the ones you use a lot like pruning shears, trowels, and hoes. Lately I've seen more and more of the one-wheel push tools with various attachments for cultivating and even plowing. They take a lot of work but in good soils, where the sod has already been worked in, they can be effective tools. Of course there is always the old fashioned way of using horses and horse drawn implements. I've never used a horse for farm work but that is where we got the term "horsepower."

The herb farmer has to make a lot of choices about what tools to purchase. A farm can make or break by those decisions. There is a lot of good used farm equipment available today as we have fewer and fewer farmers. Auctions and used farm equipment dealers are a great way to buy good quality inexpensive machinery.

CHAPTER ELEVEN

Propagation

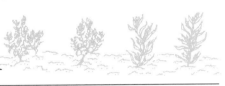

Most of the propagation done for field crops starts in the nursery area. I've found it is much easier to propagate in flats in the nursery and then transplant into the field than it is to direct sow seeds in the field. There are, of course, exceptions to this rule which I will cover later. Nursery propagation gives you more control over germination, weed competition, and temperature. When you do transplant into the field you won't have any empty spaces where seeds didn't germinate. Also, by utilizing the greenhouse you can extend your season, which is incredibly beneficial in areas where the growing season is short.

Almost anywhere in the country it is beneficial to have a greenhouse. Greenhouses can vary in size, style, shape, function, and cost. The simplest would be small cold frames or cloches that are unheated. The most advanced would be large ones, with fans, heaters, heating benches, tables, etc. The most important factor in determining what type of greenhouse you build is the climate in your particular region. If you live in an area with lots of cold and snow then a greenhouse structure capable of dealing with the snow and also capable of holding heat is essential.

An average freestanding greenhouse would consist of a metal framework, some wood siding and end pieces, two layers of plastic, vents and some form of heat. A 30' x 50' greenhouse without heat would cost between $2,000 and $3,500 in materials, depending on its style and the quality of materials you use. They are relatively easy to put up and can be purchased from a greenhouse supplier in your region. In areas of extreme weather, greenhouse suppliers from that region would be able to give you the best advice on what type of structure can best deal with the elements. They could also advise you about what size heater you might need. The cost of the heater would be dependent upon the size and type of fuel it uses (electricity, gas, propane, etc.) with costs ranging from $300 up. Heat is not always necessary in many parts of the country. One thing you can do to minimize the need for heat is use a double layer of plastic with a little fan blowing air in between the layers. This provides an insulation factor of R-3 and is very helpful in conserving heat.

I have seen greenhouses where people have used wood stoves, kerosene heaters, and various solar collection devices to minimize their heating cost, which is by far the most expensive aspect of operating a greenhouse.

I have built and seen numerous greenhouses attached to other buildings including houses, barns, and other outbuildings. In most cases they are simple lean-to structures built off one side of the existing building. They are easy to construct and usually cheaper to build and operate than a standard, free-standing greenhouse. When attached to a house they both give and receive heat to and from the house.

Though *Northern Exposure* was a great TV show, it made for a lousy greenhouse setting. When determining where to locate your greenhouse in virtually every part of the country (except maybe the desert or other super hot, sunny areas) sun exposure is everything. When attached to a building it would preferably be on the south side, and when freestanding it would hopefully be in an area where it gets full sun.

If you do live where summers are extreme and you still need to use your greenhouse because of space or severe thunderstorms, then shade cloth over the roof is one alternative to reduce sun exposure and temperature. It's very effective in cutting down the temperature inside the greenhouse. Also the more you vent the greenhouse the cooler it will be in summertime.

Inside the greenhouse a variety of possibilities await you. Some people like to propagate directly on the ground; I prefer to use tables. It makes it easier to work and it minimizes the amount of lifting and bending. I personally like to use tables that are 4' x 8' and generally constructed of 2 x 4s

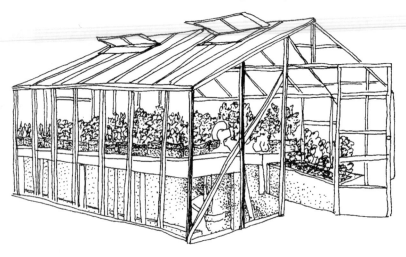

and wood lath. I have some tables like this that have been in use for over 15 years.

Some greenhouses utilize bottom heat especially for cuttings. Bottom heat is when you run either electric cables or hot water in pipes underneath the area you are planting. I think hot water in the long run is far less expensive than electric cables. The cost can be several hundred dollars for a single heated table either way you do it. Heating cables are available from nursery supply companies, whereas the hot water system you can construct yourself using a hot water heater, regulator, thermostats, and pvc piping.

What to start your seeds and cuttings in? I prefer to use cell-packs with between 96 and 256 cells per flat. One wonderful grower I know likes to use 432 cells per flat. It depends somewhat on personal preference, but most importantly on the type of plants you are growing and the amount of time the plants are going to stay in the cell-packs. The smaller the cell size, the quicker you need to transplant. The larger the cell size, the longer it can stay in the cell. Some plants adapt well to cell-pack life and can stay in them for even a year with no significant impact on their health. Other plants, especially those with sensitive taproots, need to be transplanted relatively quickly. On my 4' x 8' tables I am able to fit 20 flats. As I usually use 200 cell-packs for seeds, I can get 4,000 plants per table.

For cuttings, I like to use 96 cell-packs which can be broken down into eight 12-cell pieces. Usually when I do 96 cell-pack cuttings I will be potting them up into larger pots before planting them out. Sometimes I'll use 200 cell-packs for certain cuttings that I will then transplant directly out in the field without potting up. This only works with really hardy plants that root well from cuttings like Gotu Kola. This allows them to be transplanted with the transplanter instead of being hand planted. I try to avoid planting anything in large pots because they need to be hand transplanted and they take up too much room and materials in the greenhouse.

I would say I do about 95% of my plants from seed, most of the rest from cuttings, and a rare few from divisions.

For potting mix I have used tons of combinations over the years. Ingredients have included soil, compost, perlite, vermiculite, peat moss, sand, bark, and a variety of organic fertilizers. The last few years I have focused mainly on a mix of perlite, vermiculite, peat moss, and bark. These are easy to mix, and are more or less sterile with no weed seeds or significant pathogens present. When using soil or compost, I always sterilize it using a steam sterilizer. Because soil and compost are cheap I will still sometimes use them for potting up plants into large pots, but generally for seeds I use the sterile mix.

I vary the mix somewhat according to the weather and the moisture requirements of particular plants. For root crops, I try not to use perlite because it tends to attach itself to the roots. When you harvest them several years later, you can have a difficult time washing the perlite from the roots. My average mix would be 40% to 60% perlite/vermiculite, 30% to 40% peat moss and 10% to 20% bark. It's very important to thoroughly mix your ingredients. In the last few years I have done this using a 55-gallon drum that can be rotated with a handle. It has a door cut into it, for putting in and taking out materials, and was designed by my friend Don.

For cuttings I use coarse sand that is relatively sterile and weed free. Many times I have just gone down to the local beach and dug it up.

One thing I have noticed over the years is that people do not realize the water requirements of nursery plants. I have had too many plants killed by underwatering and even overwatering. It's important to monitor the water in your nursery area and as the season progresses and heat and sun amounts change, you need to change your watering schedules to adapt. Even if you put automatic sprinklers on timers, you still need to react to changes in light, heat and differing needs of the varieties of plants you will be growing. It's important with young seedlings not to apply the water with such force that it moves the soil and disturbs the seed or plant. With cuttings you will need to apply more water more often until the root system is developed. Most cuttings die from too little water.

Fertilizing of your nursery plants can be done either with a solid fertilizer mix (bloodmeal, cottonseed meal, shrimp meal, crab meal, etc.) or with a liquid mix applied through your irrigation (fish emulsion or manure teas). I usually use fish emulsion applied through the irrigation system. Liquid fertilizer injectors can run anywhere from $15 to $300 and are easy to install and use. I try not to use too much fertilizer because I don't want to get too much leafy growth. Depending on the plant, I fertilize every two weeks. I add solid fertilizers to my soil mix or, if the plant's been in the pot a long time, I might top dress by applying fertilizer on the surface of the pot. One of the main advantages of a liquid fertilizer is that it gets utilized by the plant very quickly, whereas a solid fertilizer can take a long time before it's taken up by the plant. The disadvantages of fish emulsion are that it is somewhat expensive and it does stink.

In all the years I have been farming I have had very few major pest or disease problems. Most of the problems I encounter are in the greenhouse (or driving in L.A. traffic) with the worst problems being damping off and aphids. Damping off is a fungal disease that affects very young seedlings and can easily wipe out tables full of plants. It is best controlled by using a well drained potting mix, not applying too much water, having good air flow and sanitation. Always make sure that you adequately clean any nursery flats or pots before reusing them; I generally use diluted bleach, steam or hot water. Sulphur is the only approved organic product that I have found to be effective against damping off.

Aphids are easily controlled by spraying soap on the areas of the plant affected. Many organic growers use Safers soap which can be purchased at any garden nursery. Other growers simply use liquid Ivory hand soap diluted anywhere from 20 or 30 parts water to one part soap. It is usually applied with a small hand or backpack sprayer. You can also put ladybugs into your greenhouse and they will feed on the aphids. They are somewhat effective over time and can be purchased at a garden nursery center or through the mail. Many pests you might encounter in the greenhouse can be somewhat controlled with a variety of predators that can also be purchased.

Most of the herbs I've planted from seed take between eight and 16 weeks from time of planting until they are ready to be transplanted into the field. Herbs that can grow in cooler conditions, or slower growing herbs, are usually seeded in the greenhouse first. Depending on where you live, that could be anywhere from mid-January to mid-March. I like to get my plants into the field in the early part of the growing season, but it doesn't always work this way. I do try.

When seeding into cell-packs you can either do it by hand or use a mechanical seeder. Mechanical seeders are faster and somewhat affordable, but I still do most of my seeding by hand. Another good idea is to conduct germination tests on your seeds to determine their germination percentages. If your seed only has a 50% germination factor you will want to double up on the number of seeds per cell, to ensure fuller flats, and not end up with a half empty greenhouse. Also, seeds from different years have different germination rates. Just because you have new seed does not mean it will be better than your three year old seed. Keep each year's seed pure and test it to see which will be best to use. It's important when seeding not to plant the seed too deep; this is by far the biggest problem I've encountered in the seeding process. Many seeds are light-dependent for germination and they simply won't germinate if they are planted too deep. Another important thing is to label each flat as you seed it, with its name and date of seeding and any other information that you think pertinent.

Some seeds need a period of cold, or stratification, in order to germinate. These are usually seeds that are native to areas of cold winters. Stratification is accomplished by either seeding the seed outdoors in the fall, so it can get a natural cold treatment, or by placing the seeds in a sealed, plastic bag with a little damp bark, peat moss, or sand. Put the bags in a refrigerated setting, with a temperature between 35 and 40 degrees, for anywhere from four to 16 weeks. A few herbs benefit by placing the seeds in the freezer for a short time, usually one to three weeks. A lot of plants need to be stratified in order to germinate. Whenever you don't know, it is always best to stratify. A few plants need a short warm spell followed by stratification, and then more warmth before they will germinate. But I have encountered very few seeds that need this.

Scarification is a rare technique that I have very rarely used, so I will not go into details. It basically is a process of scarring the outer seed coat, which I have done using sand paper. One plant family where this is sometimes necessary is *Fabaceae*, the pea family.

Not all plants you will start from seed will be easy. Some germinate very slowly taking as long as two years, and others germinate at extremely low percentages. It is best to know whether or not you are dealing with a difficult to germinate seed. If you are it is best to apply numerous seeds per cell pack and put the flats in the "be patient" area of the greenhouse. One of the most difficult herb seeds to germinate is Siberian Ginseng; it usually takes two years to germinate. Fortunately most of the seeds you will plant, like Echinacea *purpurea*, will germinate quickly and easily.

I propagate a lot of the plants I use for landscaping by cuttings but very few of my row crops are done that way. Those that I do by cuttings are herbs that do not do well from seed and can easily be done by cuttings. Examples would be Gotu Kola, Chaste Berry, Rosemary, Wormwood, and Elderberry. I usually do tip cuttings using the top two to six inches of growth. You need at least two nodes (area where leaves emerge from the stem), one node to go below the surface and one above, in order to have a successful cutting. Generally the more nodes the better. After you make your cuttings it is best to get them into your cutting medium and watered as soon as possible. Don't let them dry out and wilt.

I use pure sand for most of my cuttings though I also will mix sand and perlite together. Before putting the cutting into the sand, strip off all leaves that will be under the surface and eliminate as many large leaves that will be above the surface as possible. The more leaves you have exposed the more the cutting will transpire, lose moisture, and will have more difficulty rooting. I'll do some cuttings where I have no leaves showing at all. After you put the cuttings into the mix, water them immediately. Too little moisture is the reason for most cutting failures. Many light waterings a day is the best way to water. Cuttings will benefit from bottom heat. Most cuttings will root without it but with it they will root faster and at a higher percentage.

Not all herbs will root from cuttings. Others will but only with a lot of difficulty. Commercially many nurseries will use a rooting hormone to facilitate root production. Many of these substances are not accepted by organic certifiers, so you need to find out before using them. I simply do not use them anymore. So far, any herb I've needed to grow from cuttings, I've been able to do so with the help of bottom heat.

Herb cuttings will take root in two weeks to two months. Fast growing, spreading herbaceous plants usually root faster, and woodier plants usually root more slowly.

The best time to do a cutting is usually when the plant has some nice new growth but before it sends up its flower stalk. This is usually in late spring but you can do cuttings almost any time during the growing season—though you may have to cut off flowers or look harder for nice new growth. These are known as softwood cuttings. Some plants are propagated by hardwood cuttings, which I don't do for any of the crops I've grown.

Another type of cutting is a root cutting. This is a technique where you cut roots into shorter pieces and then put them into soil and they grow. I use this technique for both Comfrey and Horseradish. I generally cut them into two to four inch pieces and put them into a three to four inch pot with my normal potting mix (not cutting mix). They will usually put up leaf growth and develop more roots in a few weeks. It is important, when doing this, to always put the root cuttings in the same up and down position they were in when they were dug up; otherwise the top will have to grow down and the bottom up which confuses them and makes it more difficult for them to grow.

Most cuttings (after they produce roots) I will pot up into a larger pot like a three to four inch size. A few herbs I will transplant directly from the cutting flat into the field. This saves both potting time and transplanting time. This is only practical with herbs that root really well and that fill up the cutting pot so that when you pull them out the soil and roots don't break up.

I don't do any row crops by division though I propagate many of my landscape plants this way. It is an easy way to get a few plants right away, but you can't get very many as it is a slow process. It is accomplished by digging a plant up and pulling it apart, making sure you have root growth in each section you pull apart.

There are a few herbs that I will sow directly into the field. I don't like to do this because of weed competition, poorer seed germination, and less environmental control when the plants are in their most susceptible stage. The herbs that I do sow directly are herbs that do not transplant well at all, that grow quickly and easily in the field, and the seed is inexpensive. Examples would be beets, corn, and oats.

In some cases there are herbs which do not grow well from seed and you may need to buy roots or plants in order to get started. From these original plants you can later do cuttings or divisions. A good example is Goldenseal. In order to get it started you will have to buy some roots from a reputable grower or wildcrafter.

I usually collect all my seed for replanting. Seed collecting is both very easy to do and rewarding. It is most important to ensure your seed is pure and has not crossed (for instance *E. angustifolia* will readily cross with *E. purpurea*). After collecting, clean, dry, and label your seed and store it in airtight, moisture proof containers. An advantage to collecting your own seed is that you can develop a "line" of seed that does well for your particular growing situation.

When purchasing your seed always try to buy it from a company that knows herbs and sells you a quality product for a good price. Nearly all medicinal herb seeds are available in bulk at reasonable prices. I cannot tell you how many times I have found companies selling mislabeled seeds. A lot of Echinacea *pallida* seed is still being sold today as Echinacea *angustifolia*. I visited several farms this year alone that thought they had *angustifolia* but actually were growing *pallida*. Licorice seed has been mislabeled by many companies for years though it does seem that most are getting it correct now. Some companies sell seed of poor quality or seed that is too old. Oftentimes when seed doesn't germinate it isn't the grower's, but the seed company's fault. There are many good seed companies out there. We recommend several in the resource section; I often use Horizon Herbs, in Williams, Oregon.

CHAPTER TWELVE

Planting and Cultivation

Most of the time I recommend planting your crops from nursery transplants, rather than direct sowing. This gives you better control over weeds, allows for a longer growing season, and enables you to fill all the space in your rows with viable plants.

Most of the field planting is done in late spring/early summer. The reason for this is to allow enough time for your nursery starts to mature. If you get your greenhouse planting started in February or March you will have enough time for the plants to mature. It will also enable you to get your plants into the field before the hottest part of summer, and allow for the longest growing season possible.

There are several ways to transplant your crop into the field. They include: 1) running a string line, hoeing a furrow, and dropping the plants in and covering them; 2) making a furrow with a tractor or rototiller, dropping the plants in by hand and covering them; 3) using a transplanting machine on a tractor which does everything.

Running a string line to plant your crops is simple, but very slow. You have to hand hoe a furrow which is a lot of work. Using this method a crew of four people could probably plant a quarter acre a day. It is still an effective way to plant if you have no machinery.

Making a furrow with a tractor or rototiller takes away the work of hoeing. If you are capable of making multiple furrows at once, that will enable you to cultivate weeds much easier later on. You will have more rows lined up with each other, with uniform spacing allowing you to cultivate in multiple rows without destroying plants. You will still have to cover the plants by hand with soil. Using this technique a crew of four could plant about a half an acre or more in one day. One advantage of these two techniques is that you can easily apply a solid based fertilizer directly to the base of each plant, in the furrows.

Using a transplanting machine is by far the easiest and most productive method. A transplanting machine and a crew of four can plant several acres a day. A transplanting machine sits behind the tractor and runs off the tractor's PTO. You can buy a machine with either a single row transplanter, or multiple rows; the bigger the tractor the more transplanting rows you are capable of pulling. A 40 hp tractor is capable of two rows, a 60 hp tractor is capable of three rows, etc. The more rows you do, the faster you go, and the easier it is to cultivate later on, as the rows are more uniform. In order to operate a two-row transplanter you will need a minimum of four people. One to drive the tractor, two to sit on the transplanter and operate it, and a fourth to walk behind the transplanter and make sure the plants are correctly planted in the rows. A transplanter first makes a furrow, then drops the plants into the furrow, waters and fertilizes the plants, and then packs the plant down into the rows. The transplant operator(s) sits on the transplanter with flats of plants; the plants are dropped one at a time into a revolving cylinder that then drops the plants into the rows. The fertilizer is in the water and each plant is fertilized and watered as it is planted (I use fish emulsion). Transplanting machines can be purchased new or used. A new two-row transplanter will cost over $5,000.

Occasionally, in areas of high rainfall or very poor drainage, it may be necessary to utilize raised beds in order to reduce disease from too much moisture. Usually with raised beds several rows are planted in one bed. The rows are planted closer together than with conventional planting. One of the difficulties with raised beds is that they are more difficult for utilizing machinery. A transplanting machine can still be used but it is more difficult as the rows are closer together in each raised bed. You would also be planting into already made beds that are not perfectly uniform. It can be done, but most raised bed plantings are done by hand.

Occasionally you will plant crops in other seasons. For instance, bare root trees like Ginkgo, Hawthorns, and Elderberries are planted in late winter/early spring. Some root divisions can be planted in the fall or early spring like Goldenseal, Black Cohosh, Blue Cohosh, and Bloodroot. Late summer/early fall planting of many perennials can be done, but the growing season is short before winter and the plants won't be as established. In really warm, dry areas, fall planting is more common, especially for landscaping. This allows the plants to develop a root system during the wet winter season and better prepares them to survive the next dry season.

How many plants you plant per acre depends totally on the type of spacing you choose. The distance between the rows depends on a couple of factors: the type of cultivation you are going to use and the size of the plant. For most plants a spacing of 24" to 30" between rows is appropriate. For a few larger plants like Wormwood, you may have to go 36" to 48". Within the row itself the spacing between plants is usually 12" to

24", with 12" being the most common. Using Echinacea *purpurea* as an example, planting on 24" row spacings and 12" centers, you can get approximately 20,000 plants per acre. The more plants you get per acre, the higher your yields per acre. For the record, an acre is approximately 43,500 square feet, and there are 2.4 acres per hectare.

Though I tend to steer away from sowing seeds directly into the field, there are some plants that I regularly direct sow, and some growers will direct sow a lot of crops that I don't. Crops that are sometimes best field sown include plants with long, quick growing taproots like Echinacea *angustifolia* and Burdock. Seeds can be sown either with a walk-behind push seeding machine, or from a tractor mounted seeder. The advantages to direct sowing seed include less transplant labor, less greenhouse need and time, and less cost of materials. Unfortunately you also spend more time thinning, weeding, and replanting.

It is critical that the plants and seeds have adequate moisture immediately after planting. In areas where irrigation is used you should water within 24 hours of planting. I have lost more plants to underwatering after planting than for any other reason.

In most of the western United States, irrigation is essential for the production of medicinal herbs. In the midwest, south, and northeast, irrigation is not essential—although it is sometimes helpful in ensuring that your crops do well. Even in the areas of the country where summer rain is common there are occasional droughts. If it's planting season and the soil is dry with no rain in sight, you could be in trouble if you do not have irrigation. Even in northern Iowa I had a small irrigation system set up for such dry scenarios.

Irrigation can be accomplished in several ways. Methods include: overhead irrigation, drip irrigation, and flood irrigation. All three have their advantages and disadvantages.

Overhead irrigation can be done in many ways. You've probably all seen a variety of very large irrigation systems that run on mechanized wheels and cover many acres. For smaller operations, under 100 acres, smaller overhead systems are used consisting of either set or movable metal pipe that sits on the ground. The advantage of this system is that it is somewhat inexpensive and easy to set up and operate. The "hand lines" as they are sometimes called, can be moved from field to field, thus saving the expense of buying pipe for every field but increasing labor costs. Depending on the source of your irrigation water, plus the size and quality of the pumps you choose, a system like this can cost a little over $1,000 per acre. Some growers use a system of single irrigation guns which can be rolled from spot to spot. There are many other types of overhead irrigation combinations which I won't cover, but they all have the same advantages and disadvantages. The advantages include ease of installation, the ability to water broad areas and the potential to elevate the humidity significantly in the area around the plants. Disadvantages would include overwatering and subsequent soil erosion—especially on hillsides—and the fact that you apply water to the space between the rows which is relatively useless and contributes to weed growth.

Drip irrigation has been around for a few decades and is becoming very popular. It consists of long stretches of black poly pipe running off your main lines, with thousands of feet of "T-tape" running off the black poly pipe. It is similar in cost to movable hand lines. Its main advantage is that it saves a lot of water—up to 75% compared to an overhead system. It can also be used on hillsides with less chance of erosion. Disadvantages include it getting in the way of cultivation, and the labor to install and operate it; that it cannot significantly raise the humidity around crops; its effectiveness is limited to crops planted in rows, rather than crops that spread such as Red Clover, Skullcap, Peppermint, etc. Another disadvantage is that, at some point, the T-tape must be replaced due to wear and tear. The cheapest T-tape is used for just one or two seasons; the best quality T-tape can last up to ten seasons. Drip irrigation is mainly used in the dry parts of the country where water is scarce.

Flood irrigation, although once common, is now rarely used. It is a very inefficient use of water in most situations and it can cause significant soil erosion. In certain areas though it is cheap and can be done without any electricity.

How much you should water depends on the crop, your climate, your soil, cultivation practices, and a slew of other minor factors. Obviously, in the western U.S., you need irrigation for nearly every crop, whereas in the rest of the country you can probably get by without it for most years and for most crops. Throughout the sections on specific plants, I mention the dry west when referring to irrigation needs. The west is a big place with some areas dryer than others; some areas, like the Olympic rain forest, are extremely wet. When I refer to the dry west I am generally including areas where there is little or no rainfall during a major portion of the growing season. In simplistic terms, if your crop is wilting then it needs water. It is easier to say that than to spend several pages talking about the intricacies of plant water needs.

Next to water I would have to say that soil fertility is the next most important factor in growing successful crops. As I mentioned in a previous chapter the easiest way to get a good quality soil is to buy land with good soil to start with. Still you will have to fertilize even the best soils at some point.

In organic farming the basis of all fertilization programs should be cover cropping. Cover cropping is a technique whereby you plant your land in certain crops that will, in one way or another, improve your soil. These crops are field sown and usually not planted for harvest. They are allowed to grow for a certain period of time before they are tilled into the soil and allowed to decompose in the soil. You can keep planting cover crops until you feel your soil is healthy enough to sustain your crops. Usually I'll cover crop after harvesting any perennial crop. This increases the organic content of the soil which makes for a healthier soil by balancing out drainage, air flow, and increasing nutrient exchange amongst other things.

Cover crops can be planted any time throughout the year in warm areas, but in extreme cold areas cover cropping is more limited. Generally, in the warm areas, you can plant a cover crop in the fall, have it over-winter and then turn it under in spring when it is starting to flower. It's important to turn under your cover crop before it goes to seed; otherwise you have a lot of weeding to do. Summer cover cropping starts soon after you turn under your winter cover crop and continues until it's time to plant your fall cover. In areas with long growing seasons you can sometimes plant more than one summer cover crop. Generally, different types of cover crops are planted in the summer season than in the fall season. Summer covers include Summer Oats, Buckwheat, most Beans, Sudan Grass, and many others. Winter covers include Winter Oats, Winter Rye, Winter Wheat, Crimson Clover, Field Peas, Vetch, and others.

Cover crops are usually divided into those that fix nitrogen and those that are mainly grown just as green manures. Nitrogen fixing plants are found mainly in the legume family but the term also includes several plants in other families. The nitrogen fixing is done through small bacteria nodules located on the root surface. These are capable of converting atmospheric nitrogen into solid nitrogen. Commonly used nitrogen fixing cover crops include Crimson Clover, Vetch, Field Peas, Alfalfa, Red Clover, and most Beans including Soy Beans, Green Beans, and Fava Beans. If you haven't planted legumes in your field yet, it's best to buy an inoculant which supplies the bacteria necessary to fix nitrogen. The inoculant comes in small, plastic bags which need to be refrigerated. You apply it to the seed before planting. Once bacteria have been introduced into the soil you generally do not need to use the inoculant again, but it's inexpensive and it doesn't hurt.

Green manure cover crops are used for several reasons, most importantly to add organic matter and nutrients, but also as a way of diminishing the weed population in fields. Buckwheat is widely utilized as a summer cover to reduce weed populations. Generally speaking the bigger and bulkier the cover crop, the more green manure it adds to your soil.

Usually you will want to add more than one type of plant to your fields. My favorite combination for fall planting is a mix of Crimson

Clover, Vetch, and either Winter Oats or Winter Rye. For summer covers I prefer a mix of Summer Oats, Vetch and/or a type of Bean. The only cover I generally will use alone is Buckwheat which grows well with minimal water in hot areas and does a great job of smothering weeds. Most of the cover crops I've mentioned are annuals and will not take over your fields, as long as you turn them under before they go to seed. The exceptions are Red Clover and Alfalfa. Red Clover and Alfalfa are generally planted as long term cover crops to build up exceptionally poor soils—especially those that are highly eroded. They are usually left for three years or more and then turned under; they will sometimes come back and will need to be turned under again. The Red Clover flowers can even be harvested.

If you have a soil with extremely low fertility you will need to fertilize it even before you plant your first cover crop; otherwise the cover crop will be stunted and not produce enough green manure or nitrogen.

How do you know if your soil is good or bad? One simple technique is to look at the plant growth and types of plants in your field. If the plants are stunted, yellow, or generally look poorly then your soil fertility is probably low. Certain species of plants are dead giveaways for poor soils. These species vary from area to area and if you talk to local growers you'll know soon enough what they are.

The best way to determine the fertility and overall health of your soil is to have a soil test done. In most states you can have this done through your local Farm Extension office. They are relatively inexpensive and can tell you just about everything you need to know about your soil. Soil tests can be simple or complex; the more money you spend the more you can find out about your soil. Get soil tests from all your different soil types. The Farm Extension office will usually have someone available to help you determine from your soil report what you can do with your land. Realize of course that most of these agents are not into organic farming. You can get your soil tests interpreted by a private company or individual who specializes in organic farming. Fortunately more and more Extension agents are realizing the value of organic farming. I know some Extension agents who have organic farms of their own.

Once your soil is tested, then you have to decide how you are going to improve it. We've already talked about cover cropping but inevitably you're going to have to add fertilizer to your soil. The question is what type of fertilizer to add?

The most commonly used organic fertilizer is animal manure. It can come from cows, horses, chickens, pigs, goats, or even elephants. The manures all vary somewhat in terms of their fertilizer value. Generally speaking, they are well balanced fertilizers that supply both macro-nutrients (nitrogen, phosphorus, potassium) and micro-nutrients (magnesium, manganese, calcium, sulphur, iron, boron, etc.). Animal manure is probably the best value for the dollar. It's available in virtually every part of the country and is easy to apply and incorporate into your soil. My personal favorite is chicken manure which is extremely high in nitrogen and generally free of weed seeds. Chicken manure, where it's available, generally costs about $10 to $12 a ton. You can fertilize an acre of land with between $100 and $300 worth of chicken manure, depending on your soil needs. Cow manure is cheaper and generally more available but it has lower fertility value and it often has weed seeds in it.

Other good fertilizers should contain large concentrations of macronutrients. These would include fish emulsion, blood meal, bone meal, kelp or seaweed, shrimp meal, crab meal, cottonseed meal, and many others.

Liquid fertilizers like fish emulsion or kelp are my preference for my nursery plants. Unlike most solid fertilizers, these liquids are readily available to the plants and are used almost immediately. I rarely use them in the field because they are expensive and easily washed away from the plants. However, I do use fish emulsion with the transplanter, which is capable of dropping the fertilizer right at the root zone. Kelp is a very balanced fertilizer that contains all the micro-nutrients and I often add it to my fish emulsion mix (10 parts fish to one part kelp). I also use kelp as a foliar fertilizer with some crops that need immediate fertilizer in the field. Plants can absorb fertilizer through their leaves, so I can take a backpack sprayer and apply liquid kelp. When doing foliar fertilizing, try to make sure rain isn't due soon, and don't irrigate right away: you'll just wash the fertilizer right off.

Of the solid, organic fertilizers, my preferences are cottonseed meal, shrimp meal, or crab meal. Cottonseed meal is affordable and a very balanced fertilizer with a high amount of nitrogen. It has gotten a bad rap from organic certifiers because of the chemical sprays used on cotton crops. Just recently a significant amount of organic cottonseed meal has been made available at a reasonable price. When hand planting, I apply it by simply putting it at the base of each plant. It can also be applied with a fertilizer attachment on a tractor that drops the fertilizer along the edges of your rows. Shrimp meal and crab meal are very affordable near the coasts—more expensive in the interior. They are very balanced fertilizers and, though they stink, I like using them. Like virtually every solid organic fertilizer they are slow to break down, taking up to two or three years to totally release their nutrients. Animal manures also take up to three years to release all their nutrients, depending on the conditions. Heat and moisture are the two most important factors in determining the rate of nutrient release of most organic factors. The hotter and wetter it is, the faster the nutrients are broken down and made available to the plants.

There are literally hundreds of possible fertilizers to use, probably good ones at good prices in each region of the country. If I lived next to a chocolate factory, for instance, I would definitely use cocoa bean hulls. Thoroughly investigate possible fertilizer sources in your area before choosing what you are going to purchase and use. I strongly believe that the best thing you can do for your soil is to cover crop, cover crop, and cover crop some more.

Last but not least another great way to fertilize is to use compost. There are numerous excellent books on compost making and I recommend that any serious grower purchase one. I'll just try to pass on some basic information here. As a grower, the most important factor in making a compost pile is finding inexpensive ingredients with which to make the pile. It is sometimes possible to find free ingredients like old hay, animal bedding material mixed with manure, waste from various industries like fish scraps, grape pomace, rice hulls, or sawdust, leaves, and many other ingredients. I like using as many ingredients as possible as it tends to bring in more diversity of nutrients. It is best to use shredded materials as they break down much faster. It is important to turn your compost pile frequently. Small piles can be turned by hand (talk about hard work) or with a tractor bucket. Commercial piles are turned with special machines that can turn piles quickly. These piles are usually long and narrow. Compost requires heat and moisture to efficiently break down. Piles don't do much in winter when it is cold. Moisture is important but if your pile is exposed to heavy rains you will lose nutrients from runoff. I think it is best to cover piles during rainy times. Compost is a wonderful addition to the farm and I love good compost but it is more expensive than cover cropping as a way to improve the soil on large acreage. One advantage of compost is that you can apply it to crops already in the field as a top or side dressing. That is its main advantage over cover cropping.

There are whole books written on soil fertility and I would strongly recommend the purchase of a good book that has lots of information on organic fertilizers.

Another factor that determines the growth of your plants is the pH of your soil. The pH ranges on a scale of 0 to 14 and represents the percentage of hydrogen ions in your soil. Soils under 7.0 pH are considered acidic, and those over 7.0 pH are considered alkaline, with 7.0 being considered neutral. However, most farmers would consider a pH of under 6.0 to be an acidic soil. The majority of soils are between 5.0 and 7.0 pH. Most crops like soils between 6.0 and 6.5 pH. Most of the alkaline soils are found in dry, desert regions; acidic soils are found in forested, wet boggy areas with heavy rainfall. Lowering your pH is usually accomplished by adding a significant amount of organic matter to the soil. To raise your pH add dolomitic limestone, bone meal, wood ash, or oyster shells. It's very inexpensive to raise your pH.

Weeding is the bane of all farmers. It seems like you always have too many weeds. The old fashioned way to weed is to use a hoe and I still use one today. I also use a lot of machinery to weed. The most important weeding is usually done in springtime. I go between the rows of my perennials with either a multivator or rototiller. After that, whenever necessary, I run some sort of cultivating tool down the rows throughout the growing season. (As I mentioned earlier there is a wide range of weed cultivating tools available to use on a tractor.) This does not get rid of all the weeds though, and you must still hand hoe the weeds around the plants themselves. Weeding is an ongoing process, and it's best not ever to let the weeds get out of control. Crops can be lost by being overtaken by weeds.

Before planting a field, there are several things you can do to reduce the number of weeds you will have. As I mentioned earlier, cover cropping is a great technique for reducing weeds. Also, turning under your weeds before planting will hopefully eliminate many of them. Try to get as many weed seeds to germinate and grow before you turn the soil under and plant. Sometimes irrigation can facilitate weed seed germination. For some weedy fields you may have to turn under weeds several times before planting—especially if the field has not been planted before. Too often I've made the mistake of planting before eliminating my weed problem.

Another technique for weed control is mulching; it's seldom used in farming but it is quite common in smaller gardens and landscaping. Mulching is simply putting some substance on the surface around an existing planting. That accomplishes several things: reducing weeds, retaining moisture, and reducing temperatures around the plants. It can also be used to protect plants from extreme winter cold, and to occasionally even raise temperatures around the plant. Mulch eventually adds fertilizer and organic matter to the soil, reduces erosion, and adds aesthetic beauty to landscapes.

The most important use of mulch is to reduce weeds. It is important to use plenty of mulch; the biggest mistake most growers make is in not using enough. My favorite mulches for weed control are newspaper and sawdust or wood chips. Now that over 95% of the newspapers use soy based ink, organic certifiers now have okayed it. Most still say not to use glossy paper. Newspaper can usually be obtained for free in a variety of ways. Applied thickly it will keep out most weeds for about two years before breaking down. I like to put sawdust on top of the paper for both aesthetics and to hold it down. Newspaper won't work for every weed and I must confess that I have found nothing that totally smothers Quack Grass. Some growers use black plastic to control difficult weeds like Quack Grass and it can be extremely effective. Transplanting machines can be set up to lay down plastic and plant directly into it. The problem I have with plastic is that when it starts to shred and lose its usefulness, it is hard to pull up without making a mess and having pieces of plastic blow away.

Other mulches I've used include hay, alfalfa, grass clippings, leaves, rice hulls, compost, plastic, cocoa bean hulls, and even rock. I was in Hawaii recently, with Heather and friends Dave and Kathy, and found a garden in an area of low rainfall where they were mulching numerous plants, including Kava, with volcanic rock. Cocoa bean hulls are my absolute favorite. Though expensive, on a small scale they are both effective and make your garden smell like chocolate.

Mulching is rarely used on a farm but I've found it to be useful for a few crops including tree and shrub plantings where cultivation close to the plant is difficult. Also with water loving valuable crops like Goldenseal and Ginseng, it is worth mulching them in the dry west with leaves or some other mulch. Ginseng growers in the west like to use sawdust.

Fortunately, herbs are very hardy and are rarely subjected to major insect infestations. I have occasionally had problems with aphids, mainly in the greenhouse. Aphids are easily controlled with a soap spray. I have had some problems in the field with cucumber beetles, blister beetles and a few other chewing bugs. Rarely have they significantly damaged a crop. One substance that is often used by organic growers to kill certain insects is Bt, *Bacillus thurengenensis.* It comes under many trade names and is available at most nurseries. It is applied to the surface of the plant where the insects eat it, get sick, and eventually die. It doesn't work for all insects, unfortunately. There are many other stronger organic pesticides available including Pyrethrum, Rotenone, Sabadilla, Neem and others. These are broad spectrum poisons that should only be used when a crop is being overrun by an insect infestation.

In some cases you can introduce predatory insects to kill the pests that are attacking your plants. Most nurseries will either carry or will order predatory insects for you. They don't always work and they are expensive, but oftentimes they are worth the effort.

Some of the simpler methods of insect control include hand removing the insects, or using a variety of companion planting techniques—even using a simple Garlic or Cayenne spray. When dealing with pests, it's best to seek out as much professional advice as you can. Like any other aspect of farming, it's always helpful to find out what the locals are doing.

I've rarely had any problems with disease in my herb crops. What little disease I've had has almost always been in the greenhouse, which I've already talked about. In the fields the main problem has come from root rot, caused by too much water on plants that don't like it. Always try to plant crops that require good drainage in areas where they get good drainage. One of the most common mistakes is to plant a crop in an area which you find out later is poorly drained, and have that crop rot in the ground. There are herbs that prefer wet areas, and herbs that prefer well drained areas, so match the herb to your soil drainage. There are some techniques you can do to improve drainage, such as raised beds and building curtain drains, but it is easier to plant crops that naturally would thrive in your particular soil conditions.

CHAPTER THIRTEEN

Harvesting, Processing, Drying and Selling

Now the fun begins. Harvesting and selling has always been my favorite part of growing medicinal herbs. I love handling the herbs while I pick them and when I set them in the dryer. I love the smell of the drying room with all the different herbs. At the end you get to sell a quality product to someone who really needs it. And then you also get paid for it.

Harvesting might include leaves, some stem, flowers, seeds, root, fruits and/or bark. Some growers focus more on the tops, others on the roots, but most do a little bit of everything except barks. I don't grow any herbs for bark harvest so I won't be including any information on bark. Ideally you would harvest leaves and flowers after the dew has dried. Unfortunately the day is only so long and sometimes you have to pick first thing in the morning, when the plant is still wet with dew.

Leaves are usually harvested with the flowers just as the flowers are opening; this I call "top harvest." You don't want to wait too long and have some dead flowers with your harvest. However, because all the plants in a row don't flower at the same time you generally pick when the earliest flower is just at its peak and all the others are either perfect or just about perfect. Some herbs are picked with just the leaves and no flowers. A good example would be Mullein, where the leaves are picked one season and the flowers another. Also some herbs are usually picked without flowers, like Sage and Rosemary, but sometimes they might have some flowers on them. Most medicinal buyers will accept that. One big question is whether or not to include the stems with the leaves.

Most top harvests include some stem; it is easier and obviously gives you more weight. The problem is that with many plants the stems are lacking in the constituents you are looking for. Generally the succulent part of the stem, which is usually near the top of the plant, is still "active." The rest is relatively inert. In many plants, like Echinacea, Motherwort, and Lemon Balm, etc., you might as well use it for firewood. Some companies want just the best quality part of the plant so you will have to separate the leaves, flowers, and succulent stem from the dry woody part of the stem. You can either do this as you harvest or you can do it after the herb is dried. I do it when I'm harvesting, as much as possible, so I don't waste drying room space. If I'm worried about bruising though, I might do it after drying. This process is called garbling.

Occasionally some leaf crops accumulate enough dirt that they need to be rinsed off before either drying or shipping fresh. It is generally not a good idea to get the crop wet before you are going to dry it, but sometimes it is a necessity. The two ways to do this are to dunk the plants into a bucket of clean water, or gently spray with a hose, then lay the plants to air dry in a shady spot before shipping fresh or moving to the drying room.

Companies that want the best quality herbs usually pay top price and it usually pays to spend the extra garbling and washing time when selling to those companies.

When harvesting tops I do it by hand, using high quality pruning shears. I have always sold medicinal herbs to companies looking for the highest quality and that means picking by hand. You eliminate the possibility of incorporating low quality or rotten plants into your harvest when you pick by hand. You also eliminate severe bruising which happens with many herbs that are machine harvested. It's also easier to reduce heat build-up and decomposition by quickly putting your harvest in the shade, making sure that it is not piled up so thick that it starts to heat up. Also, I'll often have to strip off the lowest leaves which sometimes have already yellowed, or died back, and eliminate them from the harvest. Most top harvesting is done between mid-spring and late summer.

You may talk to some people or see references about commercial herbs where the terms "leaf" and "herb" are used. They are commonly used in the herb trade. I don't like to use them, especially "herb" because it is too all inclusive. "Leaf" in those circumstances refers to either just leaf, or leaf and part of the stem. "Herb" refers to everything above ground that was picked including leaf, stem, flower, seed, and fruit.

I also do flower harvests by hand, sometimes literally with my hands for Calendula and Red Clover, for instance. I use pruning shears for plants like Goldenrod, Elderberry, Arnica, Lavender, and Passionflower. For Chamomile, I either harvest by hand or with a blueberry rake. The blueberry rake is faster but it does give you quite a bit more stem with the harvest. Flowers are usually harvested as they open or when they are fully open. Many flower crops, like Calendula and Red Clover, are continually harvested throughout their growing season. It's important not to let these flowers mature too much, or you reduce the quality. You have to stay on top of these crops, constantly picking them at their peak, several times a week. Occasionally, if they get ahead of you, you'll need to dead-head the developing seed head in order to ensure that they continue to produce at their maximum rate. There are some growers who machine harvest some of these crops. This incorporates both leaf and stem with the flower, which usually lowers the quality of the herb. Of course it is a lot more productive and less expensive to harvest.

Seed harvest is usually done in the fall when the plant is in seed. Seeds that I harvest for medicinal use, as opposed to harvesting just for replanting, include Echinacea, Chaste Berry, Oat, Stinging Nettle, Khella, Fennel, and Burdock. Echinacea can be harvested with a combine or by hand, but all the rest are harvested by hand. Some plants like Oats are harvested well before they reach maturity. Others, including Chaste Berry and Fennel, are sometimes harvested just before they reach full maturity, depending on the company you are selling to. Still others are harvested when they are totally mature. The most important factors for seed quality are: harvesting at the appropriate time and when the seeds are dry—not wet from rain or irrigation.

Seeds can be processed, or cleaned, in a variety of ways. The simplest way is to crush the seeds by hand and winnow out the chaff by exposing it to wind or blowing on it. Seeds can also be cleaned by forcing the heads through various sizes of screens until you separate the seed from the chaff. On a large scale most seeds are cleaned with an electronic seed cleaner. These seed cleaners basically do it all and can be purchased new for from $1,500 to much more. Used seed cleaners are available in many parts of the country from used farm equipment dealers or at auctions.

I don't harvest very many fruits. I do harvest Hawthorn and Elderberries. In a couple of cases, I might be technically harvesting the fruit but most people would think of them as seed or seed pods. Fruits are generally harvested by hand when they are totally mature. Some, like Hawthorn, are easy to harvest and easy to handle because they are somewhat dry on the tree. Elderberries, on the other hand, are juicy and more difficult to deal with. They are also much more difficult to dry.

Root harvest is usually done in the fall, winter, or early spring with the majority of it being done in the fall before rain or cold weather makes harvesting impossible. It's always a rush in the fall to harvest as much as possible before the weather turns bad. In warmer areas, if the rain is delayed, you can sometimes harvest right into winter.

Roots can be harvested in a variety of ways. The simplest way is to use a spading fork or shovel. With a tractor you can either use a root digger or a variety of implements which will loosen up the root and make it easier to pull up. For large root harvests a root digger is by far the most efficient. It goes underneath the root and can either deposit it on the surface or deposit it in a trailer, via a conveyor. Root diggers cost between $5,000 and $10,000 new, but used root diggers are available. Depending on the size of your root digger, the size of your tractor, the type of soil you have, and the size of your crew, you can harvest up to several acres a day.

After harvesting your roots, you need to clean them as soon as possible. This can be accomplished by shaking as much soil off as possible, and then applying pressurized water to the root. This can be done with hoses, or with a mechanized root, or barrel, washer. Conventionally barrel washers are used for washing vegetable roots like carrots and potatoes. They are available either new or used. Barrel washers are much more efficient than spraying by hand, but a lot of hand labor is still involved. You still need to pre-rinse the roots in most cases, and with some knobby roots, like Valerian, you will have to rinse them again at the end.

Now that you have harvested, you need to either ship it off fresh, or dry it. When shipping fresh it's important to ship as soon as possible after picking. Be extremely careful not to pile it up so that it starts to generate heat and ruin the herb. Be sure the recipient of the herb knows it is on its way so the herb does not sit and spoil. Depending on when and what you ship, ice packs may be necessary. Shipping in the height of summer is the most dangerous time—for the obvious reasons.

Herbs can be dried in a wide variety of scenarios. Some growers dry them in their house, some in their barn, and some in a special drying room. I even visited one very creative grower who dried herbs in a greenhouse. Though some growers still dry herbs outdoors I do not recom-

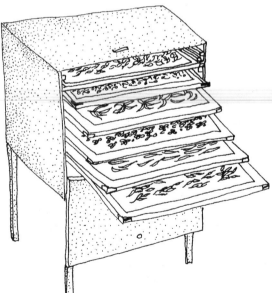

mend it at all. There is too much temperature variance and in most areas way too much moisture in the air. You also want to avoid direct contact with the sun as it may cause the loss of volatile constituents and degrade the herb's appearance. The most important factors in drying herbs are a relatively steady heat, lots of air flow, a low humidity, and an area sealed from rats, mice, bats, elephants, and other animals.

Steady heat can be generated by whatever type of heating method you choose.

Ideal temperatures range from 80 to 100 degrees, or more, depending on the crop and drying method you use. Too much heat and you destroy some of the more volatile constituents in the herb. It is especially important not to heat it up too quickly as you might dry the external surface too rapidly and make it more difficult to pull moisture from the center of the herb. Too little heat and you might promote bacterial and fungal growth in the herb. Roots and barks generally need a little bit more heat than leaves or flowers; some growers will raise the temperature up to even 120 degrees. In the summertime of many areas, artificial heat may not be necessary, but be wary of cold moist nights. Care should be taken to eliminate any possibility of fire. One major herb grower lost an entire drying room to a major fire recently.

Air flow is extremely important; it's almost impossible to have too much air flow. Air movement is usually created by the use of a variety of fans. I prefer a system where the air is flowing directly underneath and through the individual herbs. Air flow is something that is important winter, spring, summer, and fall. Air flow can also be combined with heat, and together they can be blown underneath the herbs.

It's important to construct your drying facility so that it is animal proof. Many growers use drying facilities which are accessible to mice, rats, and bats and other animals which might leave deposits on the herbs. Ideally your drying facility would be animal proof, but it is not always possible so you simply have to do the best you can.

High humidity can greatly decrease the quality of your dried herbs. It's important to have a humidity percentage under 40%. I prefer a humidity of 25% to 30%, or less, in my drying room. The most effective way to reduce humidity is by using an electric dehumidifier. Even in the most humid parts of the country a dehumidifier, when used with proper air flow, will reduce the humidity level. One side benefit of a dehumidifier is that it also gives off heat, thus helping to heat your drying room.

You can dry your herbs on a variety of surfaces including wood lath, burlap, window screen, cotton sheets, or you can simply hang your herbs upside down. I prefer using window screen because it's easy to clean, sturdy, and sanitary. Burlap is very inexpensive and easy to set up, but not as easy to clean as window screen.

Herbs can be dried in a single layer system or you can build a multi-layer rack system. A multi-layer system will give you more drying ability for the floor space used. If you use a multi-layer system, more care needs to be taken that you have adequate air flow. A system can be set up using ducts and vents where air flows under each rack layer.

The percentage of water content varies greatly from herb to herb. Leaves and flowers range from 65% to 95% water content. The highest water content I have encountered is Watercress, which is about 95% water. An herb that has a water content of 75% will have a dry down ratio of 4 to 1. This means that for every four pounds of fresh herb you start with, you end up with one pound of dry herb. Roots range from 45% to approximately 75%. Though roots usually contain less water than leaves or flowers they dry more slowly due to the way the water is immersed in the herb. Herbs should be crisp when dry, not brittle. The moisture content should be approximately five to 10%.

A fast drying herb will be dry in three to five days. A slow drying herb, under the same conditions, can take as long as two weeks. Most leaves will take about five days. Roots average seven to 10 days. All of this depends of course on your drying conditions. This is an average time if you use some fans and a dehumidifier and keep the heat between 80 and 100 degrees. You can definitely reduce this time with more heat and air flow but I believe that dries the herb too quickly. In the plant section, I list a drying time for each herb.

More and more buyers of herbs are buying the herbs before they are processed or cut up. The reason for this is that herb quality degrades much more rapidly after an herb has been cut up. Many companies prefer to buy the whole herb and do the processing themselves. Whenever possible it usually benefits the farmer to sell whole herbs. Despite this trend many growers still have to process their herbs before they can sell them.

The most commonly used machine to process herbs on the small herb farm is the hammermill. It is capable of cutting herbs into a variety of shapes and sizes depending on the cutting blades and screens you use. It works by forcing the herb into a chamber where it is worked by blades until it is forced through the screen. Various sizes of screens can be employed in order to supply the appropriate size material to your customer. Hammermills come in various shapes, sizes, and quality and can be purchased from a variety of machine manufacturers throughout the U.S.

Milling adds a whole new side to the medicinal herb farm. It can give you a wider market to sell your product to but it also takes time away from the field. One option might be to ship your whole herbs to someone who will process them for you. There are several herb companies who will do this for growers for a fairly reasonable fee.

After milling you might need to sift your herb through a variety of screens in order to make it more uniform. This can be done in a variety of ways including running it through a seed cleaner.

There are a variety of ways that herbs can be "cut." The most common is the cut and sift. Most herbs are sold this way. Roots are sometimes sold as chip which leaves them between one and six inches long. Powdering is extremely common because it allows for easier extraction if companies are making liquid extracts. It also is the form used in pills which in our society are quite common. Between whole herb and the smallest powder size there are many possibilities; if you get into milling you will have to work with your customers to ensure they are happy with your product.

After drying you will need to store your herbs. I prefer to use large polypropylene bags surrounded by a burlap bag which won't allow light in. Burlap by itself is still commonly used but the burlap does shred off into the herb, doesn't seal the herb in as well, and isn't as sanitary. Your herbs should be stored in a cool room that is relatively animal proof.

Most whole herbs, if properly handled, can be stored for six months to a year without significant loss of quality. There are a few herbs, like Feverfew, which lose their major constituents quickly and should be sold as soon as possible. Milled herbs break down much more readily than whole herbs and should be sold in a much shorter time frame depending on the herb. Some herbs like Echinacea and Valerian break down rapidly when milled. Others like Goldenseal hold their medicinal qualities relatively well for up to a year or longer. There is not enough information at the present time on shelf life and loss of major constituents of dried and/or milled herbs. Communication with your buyers is important so that they know how you are dealing with the quality of your herbs. It is also important in the herb industry always to keep up on new information which means reading the latest books, going to conferences, communicating with other people in the industry, and getting subscriptions to the key magazines.

Now that you have a product ready for sale you need to find someone to buy it. There are numerous outlets for herbs. You can sell to companies that make medicinal products, sell to stores that sell bulk medicinal herbs, sell directly to retail customers by mail or at farmers' markets, sell to an herb distributor, or make your herbs into your own product line.

The herb industry is booming and will continue to grow at a fast pace for several years. There are hundreds of companies looking for medicinal herb farmers to supply them with product. Many of these companies are looking specifically for the best quality organic herbs available. You will usually get the best price by selling fresh herbs to these companies but the fresh market is somewhat limited. If your farm is located near a large manufacturer that uses fresh herbs in their products then you have a ready and willing customer. Fresh herbs can be shipped all over the country but if I were a manufacturer and I had the choice of receiving them within hours of harvest or second day air, I would obviously take the former. These companies are also looking for dried herbs and they will generally pay you a reasonable price for your product.

When getting started you need to get out there and meet the herb buyers of these companies. You might meet them at herb conferences or you might have to go visit the company, but direct contact is always beneficial in starting a relationship. If necessary you can obviously do it over the phone, and many of your connections will be that way, but I still believe in face to face meetings whenever possible. If a company is located nearby have them come visit your farm and dazzle them with its beauty. I would not recommend a farm tour in January, unless you live in Hawaii, in which case everyone will want to visit you. Convince them of the quality of your product, and most importantly assure them that you will supply the product on time, and that you will be capable of filling the entire order. I can't tell you how often buyers will talk with growers who will agree to supply a certain quantity of herbs and then not have it. Your first shipment is critical to a company. Make sure you can meet their demands in terms of quantity and quality.

You can locate these companies in a variety of ways. You can look in trade magazines for advertisements, look at products in health food stores and write down addresses, look in phone books, word of mouth, or a slew of other ways. When calling always ask for the herb buyer.

Many stores in the country sell bulk herbs. Most of the time they buy from distributors but often they would love to buy direct from the farmer. Store people especially love to visit farms so try to arrange a visit if it's a local store. If it is a chain store then you might impress the local buyer, who then might tell the regional buyer how wonderful you are, who then tells the national buyer, who then tells the international buyer, who then tells the intergalactic buyer and before you know it they are using your herbs on Star Trek where your herbs will boldly take them where no herb has gone before. You get the picture.

Selling to distributors is an easy way to sell large amounts and often they will do the processing for you. The main negative in selling to distributors is that you probably won't get a great price. You can make deals with distributors to contract grow a crop with them. You can do this with any company and there are advantages, most importantly, like knowing your crop is sold ahead of time. A disadvantage is that if it is a three year crop the price may go way up in that time and you will have to settle for the price in the contract.

Some growers sell directly to the public which is rewarding in many ways and frustrating in others. You get a good price for your herbs but you have to deal with the fickle nature of the American consumer. It is easy to get started in this sales mode. Just get the word out in your community, send your brochure out in the mail, and hope that the word gets out. Word of mouth is amazing in its ability to advertise a product. You could also rent a Goodyear blimp and fly around with an advertisement message. I haven't seen an herb grower try it yet, but you never know. If you could get yourself on the cover of *People* magazine, I guarantee you would get a lot of business.

Some growers are now making their own finished products like extracts, salves, oils, etc. It would be a completely different company but some growers are attempting it. Also, some growers are not just selling their crops but they are buying other growers' crops and becoming distributors. It would once again be a completely different business but it is closely tied to what you are already doing.

I'm often asked by potential herb growers, "How much can I make?" You can make a lot, a little, or you can go bankrupt. Farming is never easy and it rarely makes you rich. Still herb farming has the potential to net you enough money to make a living on fewer acres than most other crops. I know people who have made a reasonable living on less than five acres. So many factors go into determining how much you can make that it is hard to give even remotely accurate numbers as to what you might gross or net per acre. Growing herbs is not like growing corn. Suffice it to say that the herb industry is growing and we need more quality growers now. If someone is a good grower and likes selling a quality product then they will be able to make money.

It is important when deciding which crops to grow to see if you can't find some unfilled niche in the market. Many companies are looking for organic herbs and at the present time they can only find them from wildcrafted sources. A lot more species of herbs will be cultivated in the near future and if you can grow and supply something new, then you have an in to the market. The question of endangered herbs is becoming a big issue and companies would love to find cultivated sources of over-harvested herbs like Goldenseal, Blue Cohosh, Black Cohosh, Echinacea *angustifolia*, Wild Yam, Osha, Yerba Mansa, Arnica, Collinsonia, and many more. Gather as much information you can before you decide what herbs you are going to grow. One single herb choice can make or break your farm. In the next section I have a category for each herb called selling. In that category I list an average price for that herb per pound. The price that I give is the average wholesale price. If you sell retail you would make more per pound, but if you sold to a distributor, or broker, you would make less than the price I list.

Reading this book is a great way to learn about growing herbs but the next step is to go out and visit farms and see what others are doing. Some growers are secretive and won't show you their place but others, myself included, will show you around and help out as much as possible. You might want to get a job on an herb farm for a while or maybe apprentice with a grower for a season. I think apprentice programs are a great idea for both the grower and potential grower. There is no better way of learning than by actually doing it. Many apprenticeships may also include general herbal knowledge which is very helpful if you are going to be a grower. You need to understand herbalism and know how to talk "herb talk" with your customers.

I can only encourage the would-be grower. This is a great time to get into medicinal herb growing and I can't think of a better way to make a living.

Medicinal Herbs
A to Z

ANGELICA

Angelica archangelica   *Apiaceae*

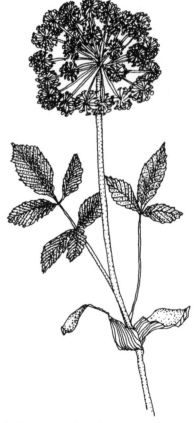

DESCRIPTION Up to 6 feet in height in flower and 3 feet in width. Before flowering the immature stems are about a foot high. Leaves are green and large with finely toothed edges. Stems are hollow. Flowers are greenish white and shaped in a spherical umbel. Bloom time is usually late spring or early summer.

PROPAGATION Usually done from seed, although older plants can be divided somewhat. Seed loses viability in a short period of time; when 6 months have gone by the seed is pretty useless. The viability time can be lengthened by freezing or refrigerating the seed. The seed germinates best when it is fresh, but it will germinate to a reasonable degree after cold storage. The big question is whether to sow it direct or in nursery flats. I've always sown it in flats, and despite the fact it has a taproot it transplants well. I have found that when sown directly it does grow a little quicker and you avoid the transplant shock. It can either be sown outdoors in the summer or early fall or you can store it in the fridge and sow it in the spring. It germinates in 2 to 4 weeks. It can self sow itself quite easily. Division is difficult because it usually only produces a single stem from the root though older plants can sometimes be divided a bit.

PLANTING If you seed directly outdoors it can be done with either a small seeder or by hand. I prefer to sow it in spring. In flats it takes 12 to 16 weeks before it can be transplanted. It is easy to transplant either by hand or with a transplanter. It can be sown at one foot spacings in the row, and 2 to 3 feet between rows. If you are planning on harvesting it the first year you need to plant early; otherwise plant it later in the season and harvest it the following year. It is very cold hardy and can be planted outdoors very early in the season.

CULTIVATION Biennial or short lived perennial. Hardy to Zone 3. It will usually continue to live as long as you cut the flower stalks off well before they go to seed. I've had plants over 5 years old that way. The deep roots need a deeply tilled soil, a pH of 4.5 to 7, and preferably a relatively rich fertile soil. It likes a lot of water and can thrive in wet soils that would kill other herbs. In areas where irrigation is necessary it needs to be watered a minimum of once a week with a deep soaking. It prefers to grow in a cool situation which means if you live somewhere with a hot summer you will have to provide a little shade and regular water. In the cooler areas of the country it will grow in full sun. The first year it is in the field the cultivation is done like any other herb in which you have open space in the row. If you wait to harvest it the second season of growth it will fill in the row space eventually so early season weed control is essential. I have had no major pest or disease problems with it.

HARVESTING Generally it is the root that is used. Although there is a small market for the seed and dried leaves I've never sold any. Depending on when you plant it the root is harvested in the fall/winter of the first year, the early spring of the second year, or the fall/winter of the second year. I prefer to plant it right after the seed has ripened in June and then harvest it the next fall/winter. It can be harvested by hand or with a root digger. The roots can be quite large, up to 3 pounds per root fresh. It can yield over 1,000 pounds of dry root per acre.

PROCESSING AND DRYING Being a taproot it is relatively easy to wash. It is a large root and thus needs to be cut up in order to facilitate drying. The root is approximately 80% water. It should be dried at relatively high heat and should take 5 to 10 days.

SELLING IT Internationally most of the Angelica harvest is turned into essential oil. There is a small market for the dried root in the United States. Prices vary greatly with a high end price of $15 per pound down to as low as $1.50 per pound. I don't foresee any major rise in its use in the near future.

MISCELLANEOUS Stinging nettle, when planted as a companion plant, is said to increase oil content by up to 80% (Foster, 1993).

ANGELICA
A. Sinensis

Generally called "Dong Quai," this an extremely popular herb used in Chinese medicine and is now used in western herbal medicine. Grows under similar conditions as Angelica. For many years there were no viable seeds for sale in this country. Now several herb seed companies have secured a source of good seed. The seed takes up to 4 months to germinate and likes to be kept very damp.

ARNICA
Arnica montana   *Asteraceae*

DESCRIPTION Grows 1 to 2 feet in height. The leaves form a flat rosette at the base with a spread of 6 to 12 inches. The leaves are arranged in opposite pairs up the hairy stem. It has a dark cylindrical rhizome. The flowers are vibrant yellow and appear in late spring or early summer. It is native to central Europe though many related species are native to North America.

PROPAGATION It is generally propagated from seed though mature plants can be divided. The seeds are difficult to germinate and must be stratified for 8 to 12 weeks. Germination is slow and sporadic, 30 days or more and at very low percentages, less than 30% for me. Time to transplant size is approximately 3 to 4 months. Divisions are easily done in spring and mature plants will yield several healthy divisions.

PLANTING Transplants can be planted in the field in late spring from a very early seeding. Spacing is 12 inches in the row, and 24 inches between rows. Because the leaves are in a very flat rosette they are somewhat difficult to pull out of the flats so if using a transplanter the planters will have to hustle. It is easy to plant by hand. It should be watered immediately as it will dry out quickly.

CULTIVATION Perennial, hardy to Zone 4 or 5. Grows best in a rich, well drained soil. Likes regular moisture during the growing season but can easily be killed by too much water, especially during the dormant winter season. I've had plants rot in their pots from having too heavy a potting soil in a wet winter. In hot dry areas it must be irrigated every 7 to 10 days. I don't think it likes extreme heat so I would irrigate it overhead in order to keep it cool. It prefers full sun. It grows slowly the first year so weed control is critical. Once established it is pretty hardy. No major pest problems. The major disease problem is root rot from too much water.

HARVESTING The flower is the most used part of the plant though the leaf and root are both sold on a smaller scale. The flower is harvested as it starts to mature. Easily picked by hand. It breaks down quickly so if you are going to sell it fresh it should be kept cool. Leaves are usually harvested at the same time, with the roots harvested in the fall. It will not produce a significant harvest until year 3 but should continue to produce after that. Division of older plants might be advisable at some point.

PROCESSING AND DRYING Arnica is sold both fresh and dried in the U.S. The market is larger for the dried but there is a significant market for fresh Arnica. The flowers break down quickly so if they are sold fresh they must be cooled and shipped immediately. I've seen fresh flowers arrive second day air and they were partially black and well on the way to decomposition. Flowers harvested for drying should be kept shaded until they are put into the dryer. Drying time is 5 to 7 days. Much of the dried Arnica I've seen is of marginal quality; most comes from Europe. The fresh Arnica is from native species in the Rockies, Sierra Nevada, and Cascade Mountains.

SELLING IT A lot of Arnica is sold in the U.S. and the market for it will continue to grow. I believe it would be a good crop for an organic grower as much of the supply is either wildcrafted or of only fair quality. The main difficulty is propagating it and having the right soil.

MISCELLANEOUS Arnica is on the United Plant Savers (UpS) secondary list. In the long run I don't believe we can continue to meet our needs from wildcrafted sources without some environmental consequences. I believe we need a good quality domestic organic supply. Arnica is a nice plant for the perennial flower garden with its attractive, sunny flowers.

ASHWAGANDHA

Withania somnifera *Solanaceae*

DESCRIPTION Evergreen shrub, 2 to 6 feet in height, spreading 1 to 3 feet. Lush green ovate leaves. Tiny green to yellow flowers are followed by red berries containing yellow seeds in a papery balloon-like calyx. Flowers bloom in mid to late summer. Native from India to the Mediterranean and Africa.

PROPAGATION From seed or cuttings. Seed germinates readily and at high percentages. Easy to grow in flats. Ready for transplanting in 12 weeks. Cuttings done in mid to late summer root easily. It is possible to take cuttings in late summer in cell packs and then transplant them the next spring directly. Or you can take cuttings from large greenhouse plants in early spring and transplant into the field in summer. Very leafy growth requires adequate moisture and fertilizer.

PLANTING Do not plant until weather has warmed up significantly as it will not grow in the cool spring season. June or July is a good time. Can be planted by hand or with a transplanter. Spacing is at 12 inches with row spacing at 2 to 3 feet.

CULTIVATION Perennial, usually grown as an annual. Hardy perhaps to Zone 8 but seems to rot in wet winters. Best grown as an annual. Needs a well drained soil with good fertility. Grows in full sun. Seems to grow best with greater than average irrigation, but can survive with a lot less water than I imagined; it looks and grows like a tropical plant. Grows quickly once it gets hot and is very weed competitive. It will fill in the row within a couple of months. Cultivate early before it fills in. I've had no major pest problems, other than aphids, but it is susceptible to rot if the soil or planting mix is not well drained.

HARVESTING Root is what is used; it is harvested in the fall of the first year. Can withstand some frost so I usually harvest it after the first frost in order to allow it to grow as much as possible. Can be harvested by machine or by hand. Grows to the size of a large carrot in one season. Seed will only mature if you have a long growing season.

PROCESSING AND DRYING Used both fresh and dry. Clean the root thoroughly of course. Easy to dry; cut it into smaller pieces and allow about 7 to 10 days to dry. Easy to ship fresh.

SELLING IT Ashwagandha is a major herb in Ayurvedic medicine used mainly in India. Many herbalists expect Ayurvedic herbs to become quite popular in the U.S. in the future. For now, the market is still small and only a small number of growers have it. Its name in India translates somewhat like "smell of horse urine."

ASTRAGALUS

Astragalus membranaceous   *Fabaceae*

DESCRIPTION Three to 6 feet in height spreading on top to 3 feet. Compound leaf with 12 to 18 pairs of leaflets. Yellow pea-like flowers, up to an inch long, bloom in early summer. Seed pods are up to 6 inches in length. Native to eastern Asia. Over 2,000 species in the genus, perhaps the largest genus in the world.

PROPAGATION Easily propagated from seed. Germination in about 4 weeks with up to 12 weeks to transplant size. Must be in an extremely well drained potting mix. I've lost lots of Astragalus plants due to rot.

PLANTING Plant in late spring/early summer either with transplanter or by hand. Plant on 1 foot centers with rows at 2 to 3 feet.

CULTIVATION Perennial and deciduous. Hardiness unknown for sure but I think it is hardy to Zone 4. Requires an incredibly well drained soil of minimal fertility. Too much water is its chief nemesis. Needs better drainage than nearly any other row crop I've grown. Average to low irrigation needs in summer. Tall and spreading, it will fill in rows in the middle of the season. Cultivate before then. No pest problems I've encountered but lots of root rot. Would not attempt to grow it in a heavy soil with lots of rain. Raised beds might be appropriate in some situations.

HARVESTING Long root is harvested in late fall after 3 or more years of growth. Machine or hand harvested.

PROCESSING AND DRYING Clean and dry the root. To dry it should be cut into smaller pieces to facilitate drying in 7 to 10 days.

SELLING IT One of the most popular Chinese herbs in the U.S. Popularity is growing perhaps due to its use as an "immune system herb." Used mainly dry with a very small fresh market at the moment. Prices as high as $15 for dry root. Only a few growers in the U.S., so I think it is an herb worth trying.

MISCELLANEOUS Often "cooked" before it is made into a product. Excellent tasting, can be eaten in soups or stews. The North American species, *A. americanus*, is very similar. Although interesting, Astragalus is not especially attractive in the flower garden.

BLACK COHOSH
Cimicifuga racemosa   Ranunculaceae

DESCRIPTION Up to 8 feet in height when in flower and spreading up to 3 feet. Leaves have toothed margins and are divided into 3 lobed leaflets, very lush and beautiful. Flowers are cream colored, fragrant, and gorgeous. Flowers bloom late spring to early summer. Roots or rhizomes are thick and knotty, and very dark. It is native to the North American eastern woodlands. Fifteen species worldwide including *Cimicifuga foetida*, which is used in Chinese medicine and called "Sheng ma."

PROPAGATION Seed or division. Seed matures in the fall and it seems that it does best when planted immediately so it can get some heat before the cold season. It will germinate in spring. I have had zero success up to now with the seed but several growers I know have grown it easily from seed. If stratified in the refrigerator it will germinate in approximately 4 weeks. Divisions are easy to do on mature plants and can be done in either fall or spring. Plants grow quickly once divided, it being best to plant them directly into the ground.

PLANTING From seed it takes about 3 to 4 months to reach transplanting size. Best done by hand. Divisions can be planted directly in either the spring or the fall with spacings of 18 to 24 inch centers and row spacing of 3 feet.

CULTIVATION Deciduous perennial hardy to Zone 3. Grows best in humus rich fertile soil, though I've seen it grow in poor rocky soils. In its native environment it grows under heavy to light shade but it seems to need only light shade. I've even seen it grow in full sun in cooler climates. I think it lends itself well to large scale cultivation in cool, wet summer areas with minimal shade, or maybe even full sun. It requires regular summer water and seems to like a high humidity. Cultivation for weeds is difficult once it is in flower so cultivate early before it gets too large. I've not encountered nor heard of any problems with pests or diseases.

HARVESTING The rhizome is what is used medicinally and is harvested in the fall or early spring. Could be done by machine though I don't know of anyone growing it on that kind of scale yet. It is easily harvested with a spading fork. You can harvest it and divide it and then replant some of your harvest.

PROCESSING AND DRYING Must be chopped up before cleaning. Somewhat difficult to clean because of its knotty nature. Drying time is 5 to 10 days.

SELLING IT A relatively popular herb with the potential to become a major seller. Nearly 100% of the supply now comes from wildcrafted sources. Many companies would love to have organic Black Cohosh. We don't have enough data on its productivity in cultivation but it is worth the risk. I plan on growing this plant the next few years to collect data. Rhizome is sold both fresh and dried with dried being the larger part of the market. Prices are low for wildcrafted root, between $5 and $7 per pound dry, but I think a good price could be secured for organic rhizomes.

MISCELLANEOUS This plant is on the UpS primary plant list and we need to start cultivating it soon. Some companies are already starting research plots and small plantings for harvest. Black Cohosh is one of the best plants for the shaded landscape with its lacy foliage and stunning flowers.

BLESSED THISTLE

Cnicus benedictus   *Asteraceae*

DESCRIPTION One to 2 feet in height and spreading 1 to 2 feet. Leaves are lanceolate, prickly, grayish-green in color, with pale veins, and short sharp spines. Flowers are yellow, concealed by leaves somewhat, and surrounded by sharp spines. Root is a taproot 4 to 6 inches in length. Blooms in mid-summer. Only species of its genus.

PROPAGATION From seed. Easy to grow. Germinates without stratification in 7 to 15 days. It will flower from direct sowing in the field in 60 to 80 days, a little longer if transplanted. From the nursery it is ready in 30 to 50 days for transplanting.

PLANTING Either direct from seed or by transplants. Transplanting can be done by machine or by hand on 1 foot centers and 2 to 3 foot rows.

CULTIVATION Annual. Grows in poor, well drained fields with minimal fertilizer requirements. Requires minimal water; without it, plants are smaller and less productive. Likes to grow in full sun. Growth is quick so a single early weed cultivation is all that is necessary. I've had no problems with pests or disease. Very easy plant to grow.

HARVESTING Harvest when plant is beginning to flower in mid-summer. I've always harvested the entire plant above ground by hand. In Europe they sometimes use mowers and loaders to harvest. It should be dried immediately as it decomposes quickly. If you harvest the tops but leave about 6 inches of growth it will flower a second time and allow for another harvest. Plants are spiny so gloves are beneficial when harvesting Blessed Thistle.

PROCESSING AND DRYING No cleaning necessary if carefully harvested. Put into dryer immediately but don't pile too thick either as you harvest or in the dryer. Dries in 3 to 5 days. Dried herb should be light green.

SELLING IT Very small market in the U.S. but larger in Europe where it is used by the liquor industry in certain drinks. I would only recommend growing it on a small scale, and even then only if you have a buyer for it. I don't anticipate any major growth in its use in the near future. It presently sells for $4 to $7 per pound dried.

MISCELLANEOUS It is considered one of the best herbs for increasing breast milk production. Also, it was very popular with monks in medieval Europe. Like most thistles the stems are edible if stripped of leaves.

BLOODROOT

Sanguinaria canadensis
Papaveraceae - Poppy Family

DESCRIPTION Grows up to 8 inches in height with about the same spread as height. Green lobed leaves wrap around the flower, then after the flower blooms they continue to grow. A single leaf per flower. As they age they spread and produce more leaves and flowers from deep red rhizome. Flowers bloom before leaves open and are white to pink and absolutely beautiful. Only species of its genus.

PROPAGATION Seed or divisions. Seed matures about a month after flowering ends. When seeds are ready they just drop one day. Close monitoring is necessary to collect the seed. Difficult to germinate. Planting seeds immediately after harvesting is probably the best way to germinate them. Seed may not germinate until the next spring. Divisions are done in the fall. When you cut the rhizome up make sure you have a minimum of one growing bud or node with each cutting.

PLANTING Plant divisions in the fall on 6 inch spacing. I've never grown them in rows and don't believe it has been done on any scale yet. Seedlings are probably best planted in late spring after leaf has come up.

CULTIVATION Perennial hardy to Zone 3. Native to North American eastern woodland region. Likes full shade with a soil rich in humus. Grows best with significant moisture but relatively well drained soil. Little is known about its cultivation at the present time but test plots are in the works and some growers are attempting it on a small scale.

HARVESTING Rhizome is best harvested in the fall. Easily done by hand but it is brittle. Time from planting to harvest is unknown though I would estimate about 4 to 5 years from divisions and longer from seed. Yields are unknown but I've seen projections as high as 1,000 pounds per acre (Foster, 1993).

PROCESSING AND DRYING Must be carefully cleaned. Use gloves when touching it as the root is somewhat caustic. Dries easily in 7 to 10 days.

SELLING IT Small market at the moment but it is growing due to its ability to prevent dental plaque from adhering to the teeth. Wildcrafted rhizomes sell for $12 to $16 per pound dry. Some companies are now making toothpaste and mouthwash using it as the active ingredient. Many companies would love to buy it from organic growers. The big questions are, how easy is it to grow and how productive will it be?

MISCELLANEOUS Bloodroot is poisonous. It can cause extreme irritation to mucous membranes. When using the extract as a mouthwash spit it out afterwards. Best to rinse mouth soon thereafter as it will stain your teeth red with regular use. It is on the UpS primary plant list and its cultivation may be essential in order to ensure a long term supply without over-harvesting it in the wild.

BLUE COHOSH

Caulophyllum thalictroides
Berberidaceae - Barberry Family

DESCRIPTION Grows 12 to 30 inches in height with a width of 1½ feet. Each plant produces one bluish green leaf with 2 to 3 leaflets. Leaflets are oval shaped and lobed. Flowers are yellow green, star-shaped and bloom in mid to late spring. They are followed by beautiful bluish-black fruits. Rhizome is dark and knobby. It is native to the North American eastern woodlands with heavier concentrations in the central and northern regions.

PROPAGATION Seed or divisions. Seed can be planted after it matures; it will germinate the next spring or it can be immediately stratified until spring planting. Germination after stratification is about 4 to 8 weeks but very sporadic and of low percentage. Young plants grow very slowly and may not be ready for transplanting until fall. Divisions are done in fall or spring and are very easy to do.

PLANTING Seedlings are incredibly slow growers and should be planted by hand in the fall of the first year after the leaves have died back. Divisions can be planted immediately after dividing the rhizome or after purchasing them. Spacing is on 18 to 24 inch centers. I don't know of anyone growing it on a large scale.

CULTIVATION Deciduous perennial hardy to Zone 3. Blue Cohosh grows best in a humus rich, well drained soil with shade. It grows naturally in mixed hardwood forests of approximately 75% shade. It likes a moist humid growing condition. If you are growing it in the west you will need to irrigate it frequently, preferably with overhead irrigation to raise the humidity. Very slow growing. When young it is delicate so weed carefully. It is susceptible to root rot so take care with adequate drainage. Like all shade loving plants it could be grown under shade cloth but its value on the market is not worth the expenditure in shade cloth.

HARVESTING The rhizome is dug up in the fall, winter, or early spring. Due to the slow growing nature of the plant I believe 6 to 7 years is a reasonable period of growth before harvest.

PROCESSING AND DRYING The root is knotty and somewhat difficult to clean. Nothing difficult about drying it after it is chopped up just a bit.

SELLING IT The price for Blue Cohosh is low, $6 to $9 per pound dried, and the market is relatively small. If you could find a company willing to buy it organically cultivated and at a much higher price then it might be worth growing. It is generally sold dry.

MISCELLANEOUS Blue Cohosh is on the UpS primary list. It has the potential to become a popular herb and be over-harvested. In the long run we must cultivate it. It is a beautiful plant in the shade landscape with exquisite leaves, a subtle but interesting flower and beautiful berries.

BONESET
Eupatorium perfoliatum   *Asteraceae*

DESCRIPTION Up to 5 feet in height and spreading 2 to 3 feet. Very erect growth with lanceolate deep green leaves. Beautiful white flowers open in mid-summer. Related to Joe Pye Weed (*Eupatorium purpureum*).

PROPAGATION Easily propagated from seed or cuttings. Seeds will germinate reasonably well without stratification but will germinate better with it; up to 80% to 90% germination is typical. Germination time is 2 to 3 weeks, with nursery seedlings ready to transplant in approximately 2 to 3 months. Cuttings are easiest when plant is not in flower, ideally in late spring or early summer. Cuttings root readily and can be potted into larger pots in about 4 to 6 weeks. Older plants can be easily divided in early spring.

PLANTING Plant as soon as seedlings are ready in late spring/early summer. Cuttings can be planted when ready. Easy to plant with transplanter. Plants should be on 18 to 24 inch centers with row spacing 24 to 30 inches. Boneset seedlings require a lot of water so either irrigate immediately or plant when rain is expected.

CULTIVATION Perennial, hardy to Zone 3. Prefers a rich, moist soil. Can grow in full sun with adequate moisture or partial shade if moisture is somewhat scarce. Regular water is important; irrigate deeply at least once a week, if necessary, with either overhead or drip. Somewhat competitive with weeds. Because of its size, early cultivation is important. I've never had any pest problems with it. Plant can be harvested year after year in same location. If it is left in the ground for many years it must be fertilized annually with a balanced fertilizer.

HARVESTING Aerial portions are harvested when flowers are starting, usually in mid-summer. A second fall harvest is sometimes possible. I harvest by hand and immediately put it into the shade as it starts to decompose quickly if it gets too hot.

PROCESSING AND DRYING It bruises easily and starts to decompose quickly so careful handling is important. It is best to get it into the dryer as soon as possible with care being taken not to pile it too thick. The plant should be dry in 4 to 6 days.

SELLING IT Once a popular herb for colds and flu, it is now making a comeback. Though still not a major herb, it is commonly traded. All the supply comes from wildcrafters in the midwest. It sells for $8 to $10 per pound dried. I think several companies would like to have an organically cultivated supply.

MISCELLANEOUS Grows in wet areas of the midwest which are often areas of major farm runoff. Organic supply would guarantee a clean, non-polluted source. It is a nice plant for the perennial landscape. Name comes not from its ability to set bones, but because it was used to help "bone setting" chills for people with severe fevers.

BURDOCK

Arctium lappa   *Asteraceae*

DESCRIPTION A very large herb with gargantuan leaves. Grows up to 8 to 10 feet tall, and can spread 3 feet. The flowers are purple and thistle like, and bloom in mid-summer. The fruits are covered with spines that

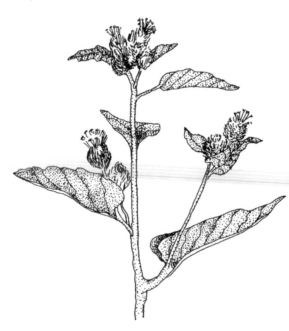

allow them to readily attach themselves to any passing object. The leaves are dark green above and downy gray underneath. The root is long; if planted in North America it will grow all the way to China, and vice versa. Actually it will usually grow down to 3 feet. A related species, *Arctium minus*, grows wild throughout the U.S.

PROPAGATION Always from seed and very easy. Seed germinates in 1 to 2 weeks. The tap-root grows quickly so it is best to sow it directly into the field. Don't put seeds out until the soil has warmed up in mid-spring. Once the seeds germinate I like to thin to 6 inches in rows spaced at 24 to 30 inches. One quarter ounce of seed will plant 100 row-feet (Cech, 1995).

PLANTING   Plant seeds directly into the field in spring, thinning to 6 inches. You can use a commercial seeder or do it by hand. Very large seeds can be planted relatively deep.

CULTIVATION   Biennial, hardy to Zone 3. Capable of growing well in poor soils, it will thrive in rich soils. Grows best in full sun but can grow in partial shade. Using a rotational planting with cover crops in between harvests it should never need fertilizing. Requires reasonable moisture and grows wild in many parts of the U.S. If it doesn't grow wild in your area it is probably because it is too dry in summer so you will need to irrigate it. Occasional deep irrigation in dry areas is essential. Plants should be cultivated when they are very young before the leaves become too large, making cultivation very difficult. I've never encountered any pest problems with Burdock.

HARVESTING   Roots are harvested in either the fall of the first year or the spring of the second year. If it is going to be used for culinary use it should be fall harvested, but if it is to be used as medicine it can be harvested in either fall or spring. As little as 3 months will produce a healthy sized root but if you leave it until late fall you will get a larger root. Roots weigh between ¼ and 2 pounds averaging about ½ pound fresh weight; they are approximately 75% water by weight. Roots can be harvested with a root digger or by hand. The root digger will not harvest the entire root even at maximum depth, which is usually no more than 12 inches. Roots that are broken off occasionally grow new plants but they are easy to cultivate out. The seeds are harvested in the late summer/fall of the second year. Extreme care should be taken when harvesting them as the small hairs can be terribly irritating to any body part. I strongly suggest wearing coveralls that seal tightly at the neck along with a respirator and goggles.

PROCESSING AND DRYING   Roots should be carefully washed by hand or in a root washer. In order to facilitate drying you must cut the root longitudinally in several pieces. It dries slowly and should have higher heat than most other herbs. The seed pods are broken up with a hammermill and then run through a seed cleaner.

SELLING IT   There is a pretty good sized demand for Burdock root. Most of it is sold dry though there is a very small fresh market. I've seen it sell direct for as much as $14 but more typically it sells for less than $7 per pound dried. There are several Burdock growers in the U.S. but I believe it is possible to sell to ever expanding markets. There is a very small market for the seed.

MISCELLANEOUS   It is commonly said that the person who invented Velcro got the idea from Burdock seeds. The Japanese call Burdock "Gobo" and most of the commercial seed comes from Japanese cultivars. Many herbalists consider it the best herb for skin problems.

CALAMUS

Acorus americanus   *Araceae*

DESCRIPTION Yellowish-green Iris like leaves are followed by a spadix that contains many small yellowish-green, sweet scented flowers that bloom in summer. Can grow from 1 to 6 feet in height and can spread a foot or so. Rhizome is large, cylindrical, loaded with small roots, and very aromatic. Confusing taxonomy with the *americanus* species sometimes listed as *Acorus calamus var. americanus, Acorus americanus* is distinctly different from *Acorus calamus* in its constituent makeup.

PROPAGATION Easily grown from rhizome divisions made in fall or early spring. When dividing it is best to cut pieces into 1 to 2 inch lengths. Older plants produce many divisions.

PLANTING Plant the divisions in either early spring or fall right after harvest. You'll have to hand plant them. Plant on 12 inch centers with rows at 24 to 30 inches. Don't allow the rhizomes or roots to dry out after dividing or after planting.

CULTIVATION Perennial, hardy to Zone 3. Can be grown in standing water. However, I grow it in a rich, often watered soil with a pH range of 5 to 7.5. Prefers full sun but I've grown a few plants in partial shade. If irrigating you need to water it every few days, especially if you have a well drained soil in a hot climate. Cultivate early and often. After it starts to multiply it gets more difficult to weed in between the plants. I've never had any pest or disease problems; in fact, it has historically been used to repel insects. The greatest difficulty in growing Calamus is giving it the necessary amount of water without overwatering all your other crops. It is best to plant it with other water lovers like Blue Flag, Yerba Mansa, Stinging Nettle, and others.

HARVESTING Rhizome is harvested in the fall or early spring. It can be harvested by hand or with a root digger. Can be harvested after the second or third year of growth. As it ages the oldest part can become hollow and rotten, so I think two years of growth is ideal.

PROCESSING AND DRYING After digging the rhizomes the leaves should be cut off at the crown. Clean the rhizomes thoroughly before cutting them and drying them. They are easy to dry although they are approximately 75% water, which is on the high side for a root crop. Very aromatic as they dry. They are fun to dry in the kitchen where they leave a nice smell.

SELLING IT There is a small market for Calamus either fresh or dried. Even though it has a multitude of uses I don't anticipate any major increase in consumption. It sells for $8 to $10 per pound for dried, wildcrafted rhizome.

MISCELLANEOUS The European species, *Acorus calamus*, contains a carcinogenic substance known as B-asarone which caused cancer in laboratory rats, but through its long use by humans, it has never been implicated with any cancer increases. In North America, Calamus was commonly used by numerous Native American Indian peoples. Calamus is a very useful medicinal plant that is wonderfully aromatic and definitely worth growing in the garden.

CALENDULA

Calendula officinalis   Asteraceae

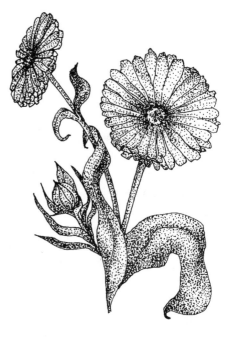

DESCRIPTION Grows up to 2 feet with a spread of 1 to 2 feet. Pale green oval leaves 2 to 6 inches in length. Many-petaled flowers are orange or yellow, large, and will continuously bloom for several months. The fruit is a brown, curved achene with a prickly surface. The root is a long spindly taproot that penetrates deeply into the soil. There are many cultivars available but I prefer the original. I always check for resin content whenever I plant a new batch of seed. Orange flowers will often mutate to yellow and vice versa.

PROPAGATION Easily grown from seed which germinates in about 7 to 10 days at a very high percentage if the seed is of good quality. I prefer to plant them in flats in the nursery and then transplant them out about two months later with a transplanter. You can also sow them directly and then thin them. The young seedlings are susceptible to damping off so take care to have good drainage and ventilation.

PLANTING I do an early planting in February that I try to get outside in early May. After my initial greenhouse planting, I continue to plant a new crop in the greenhouse every month through June. I transplant by hand, or with the transplanter, with spacing of 6 inches in the row, and 24 to 30 inches between rows.

CULTIVATION Annual that is somewhat frost hardy. I've over-wintered it in Northern California when temperatures dipped into the teens. It prefers a moderately healthy soil with average drainage and a pH of 5 to 8. I grow it in full sun, though it can be grown in partial shade. Irrigation needs are on the high side so I recommend watering once or twice a week depending on the temperature, humidity, and soil type. Cultivation should be done soon after transplanting and probably one more time before it becomes unnecessary due to the short life of the crop in the field. I've had several pests attack the flowers when they are open including blister beetles, aphids, and cucumber beetles. The best way to deal with pests is to pick the flowers often so there is little time for the pests to feed. Cucumber beetles are extremely difficult to deal with except with strong botanicals like rotenone which I don't like to use. I've had a lot of problems with damping off on Calendula seedlings in the greenhouse but never in the field.

HARVESTING Flower harvest can start as early as late May in warm areas if you get your plants out early. I like to pick a particular planting three times a week until productivity goes way down, which is usually after 6 to 8 weeks, though I've picked many plantings for up to 12 weeks. Harvests start to diminish in the late plantings after the first frost. I harvest with my hands picking as fast as my two hands can pick. The difficult aspect of Calendula harvest is that the flowers are at that perfect height where your back bends the most! I pick the entire flower and I pick anything with color at each picking. The best time to pick is in the heat of the day when the resins are highest and the water content the lowest. The resin content seems much lower in the morning before the heavy sun hits the plants. The resin sticks to your hands. Never let the flowers develop to the point where the seed is forming or you will greatly diminish your harvest totals. Continual picking will guarantee a healthier and larger harvest.

PROCESSING AND DRYING The flowers should be dried as soon as possible as they tend to heat up and decompose if kept in the sun or in your harvest bucket. I like to continually send someone down to the drying room as often as possible as we are picking especially on a 100 degree afternoon. The petals dry quickly but the receptacle does not so you can expect a total drying time of 10 days or more at 90 degrees or so. Some growers advocate quick drying at high temperatures of 120 degrees which dries them in 5 to 7 days. Flowers should retain their color if dried properly, but take extra care to make sure the flowers are totally dried before storing them or they may mold later. They must also be stored carefully as they suck up moisture readily. Dry flower yields of 400 to 600 pounds per acre can be expected.

SELLING IT Calendula is a popular herb that is growing in popularity. Nearly all of the market is dry though a few extract companies use it fresh. A lot of the organic Calendula is now being shipped from Europe. I have seen several samples from there and have not been impressed with its quality. It is a good herb for the American grower. The main difficulty is finding a crew to harvest it. An acre would require a crew of 3 to 4 picking nearly every afternoon for 3 or 4 months. Prices on the high end are near $20 per pound and on the low end about $10. At $20 it could be a profitable crop, but at $10 you are hardly going to make enough to pay for your massage and chiropractic care.

MISCELLANEOUS Once used as a poor person's substitute for Saffron. Flower petals are beautiful in a salad. Medicinally it has many uses especially to help heal wounds and as an anti-inflammatory for swollen tissue. It is a very common ingredient in salves. A very common landscape plant for the annual flower bed.

CATNIP

Nepeta cataria   *Lamiaceae*

DESCRIPTION Erect, square stemmed, branched woolly stems up to 4 feet in height and spreading 2 feet. Heart shaped leaves are toothed around the edges, grayish-green, downy soft, and almost white underneath. Flowers are white to pink with small red dots that grow in dense whorls and bloom in summer. Native to Europe, it has naturalized in eastern North America. Related to several different species of *Nepeta* commonly called Catmint.

PROPAGATION By seed, cuttings, or divisions. Seeds germinate easily in 2 to 3 weeks. I plant in nursery flats and then transplant into the field in 2 to 3 months. Softwood cuttings are done in late spring or whenever you have new growth and no flowers. They are relatively easy, and ready for transplanting into the field in 8 to 12 weeks. Divisions can be done from older plants but only if you want just a few plants. Catnip will readily self sow itself if allowed.

PLANTING Transplants are planted as soon as ready in late spring/early summer with a transplanter or by hand. Cuttings can be planted in late summer or fall. Spacing is on 12 inch centers and 2 to 3 feet between the rows.

CULTIVATION Perennial, hardy to Zone 3. Capable of growing in any well drained soil. Prefers full sun though it can grow in partial shade. Can tolerate minimal water but will become lush and more productive if given a regular dose of water. I irrigate it every 7 to 14 days in the dry west. It prefers a pH of 5 to 7.5. I grow it for 3 years and then replace it as it becomes less productive. It does well with constant cultivation. I've never had any pest or disease problems, other than from cats who love to nibble on or roll in it, and gophers who love to munch on the roots.

HARVESTING Leaf and flowering tops are harvested when flowers are just starting. Much of the Catnip on the market includes the stem which makes up 60% to 70% of the total dry weight. If you include the stem it would be possible to harvest it with a mower. I harvest it with pruning shears, strip off the leaves and tops from the stem, and then discard the stem. Catnip stems are like kindling and of poor medicinal quality. I can usually get a second harvest in the late summer/early fall in the second and third year. The first year it is possible to get a small harvest, the second year is the best and the third a little less. I replace it at that point with new plants. Yields can be as high as 3,000 to 4,000 pounds per acre if the stem is included. Tops and leaves alone should yield approximately 1,500 pounds dry per acre at peak production.

PROCESSING AND DRYING I separate the stem as I pick so as not to fill up the dryer. The leaves will dry in 5 to 7 days. The leaves and tops are about 75% water. If shipping fresh just ship tops, don't strip off the leaves as the bruising might cause serious problems in shipping.

SELLING IT The market is pretty large as it is both a popular medicine and a tasty tea. I've seen prices as high as $10 to $12 per pound for quality stuff, and as low as $2 or $3 a pound for the run of the mill, low quality stuff. It is an easy herb to grow and probably worth growing, but because it is so easy there is a lot of it out there. There is a small fresh market but only a few companies are buying it.

MISCELLANEOUS Cats love Catnip. I had a cat, Herbie, who ate some every day and then would run around like a mad cat for 10 to 15 minutes before he would crash and sleep. Herbie was an addict. Unfortunately, it does not affect humans the same way and for some reason many cats are unaffected by it. It is very popular in children's formulas for its nervine and carminative actions.

CELANDINE

Chelidonium majus   Papavaraceae

DESCRIPTION Grows up to 1 to 3 feet in height with a spread of 12 to 18 inches. The leaves are yellow-green, pinnately divided with pairs of oblong leaflets ending in a large terminal leaflet. The stems are very brittle and along with the leaves exude an orange sap when broken. The yellow four-petaled flowers are followed by linear seed capsules with small black seeds. The root is a thick, multi-branched taproot. It is the only species within the genus and though there are also a couple of cultivars, they are very rare.

PROPAGATION By seed or division. Seed germinates readily in 2 to 3 weeks at a high percentage. I propagate in flats and transplant into the field after 12 to 16 weeks. It can be sown directly into the field but it is not a fast grower so weeding becomes difficult. Divisions can be done in early spring from older plants but few divisions are possible. Celandine will self sow itself readily.

PLANTING Transplants are planted in the field in late spring/early summer. A transplanter can be used; however, the plants are difficult to pick up from the flat without breaking, so the larger they are the better. Also, the transplanters should wear gloves as the sap is somewhat acrid and can cause a slight burning or irritation of the hands. Divisions are planted as soon as they are dug up in spring. Plant on 9 to 12 inch centers with rows at 24 to 30 inches.

CULTIVATION Perennial, hardy to Zone 4 and maybe Zone 3. Can grow in virtually any soil but like many herbs it flourishes in rich soil. Can be grown in full sun or even medium shade. Celandine likes water and if it is grown in full sun it needs a regular watering, once or twice a week in the west. It is a brittle plant so cultivate it somewhat carefully. I have had no pest or disease problems with it.

HARVESTING The surface part of the plant is harvested when it is in flower in summer. Some companies also like the root which is dug up with the tops. The tops are cut by hand. If you are harvesting the root then you dig up the whole plant with a spade. Again, when harvesting be sure to wear gloves as a barrier against the somewhat acrid sap. Do not scratch or touch your eyes when working with this plant. The orange sap will stain any clothing you are wearing, so do not wear your "Sunday best" to harvest in!

PROCESSING AND DRYING If you are selling it fresh, you will have to wash the plant whether you harvest the tops or the tops and the root. Care should be taken once again to avoid getting sap on your skin or eyes. If you are going to dry it, just harvest the clean tops so you don't have to wash it. The lower part of the plant invariably has dirt on it. Dry it in thin layers as it heats up quickly and has a high water content, approximately 85%. Drying time should be 4 to 7 days.

SELLING IT The market for Celandine is small though growing. Because some of the medicinal qualities diminish with drying many companies purchase it fresh. The fresh herb sells for up to $6 a pound while the dry herb sells for between $10 and $15 per pound.

MISCELLANEOUS Native to Europe, western Asia, and North Africa, Celandine has naturalized in parts of North America. Some of the supply comes from wildcrafted sources and some from a couple of growers. Fresh Celandine sap is commonly used to eliminate warts.

CHAMOMILE, GERMAN

Matricaria recutita   *Asteraceae*

DESCRIPTION Grows 12 to 24 inches in height and spreads 4 to 15 inches. Many branched stems with finely divided leaves giving it an almost feathery look. The small daisy like flowers have white petals surrounding a yellow center and bloom in early summer. The seeds are grayish-white and very small, over 30,000 seeds per gram. Several cultivars exist which have been developed in Europe which seem to have both higher productivity and also a higher essential oil content. This plant is not to be confused with Roman Chamomile, *Anthemis nobilis,* which is a low growing ground cover with a very different taste and use.

PROPAGATION Easily propagated from seed which germinates in 7 to 14 days. I like to plant the seeds in nursery flats and transplant them into the fields approximately 8 to 10 weeks later with a transplanter. They can be field sown but they tend to crowd and produce shorter, less productive plants that are more difficult to harvest.

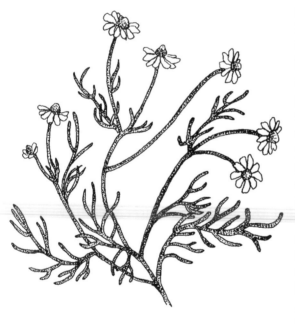

PLANTING I've planted in both spring and fall. Spring is most common and the earlier you get the plants in the field the better. They prefer growing in the cool weather of spring. I've also planted in the fall and allowed the young plants to over-winter; then they grow to maturity earlier the next spring. These fall plants seem to grow a little taller making harvesting easier. This technique would not be successful in the colder parts of the country but it will work in Zones 7 and above and maybe even in Zone 6. I like to plant on 6 inch centers with row spacing at 24 inches. If you choose to direct sow them into the field, plant them as early as possible in spring or in the fall in either rows, double rows, or in 2 to 3 foot wide beds. I prefer 3 foot wide beds with the seeds scattered and then lightly raked in. These planting methods are used when harvesting is to be done by hand. If a machine harvest is planned then the field would be sown with a seeding machine in tight rows much like cereal crops.

CULTIVATION Annual that can be grown anywhere. Chamomile can grow in the worst soils though it does benefit somewhat from a reasonable amount of nitrogen and potassium. Generally though I would plant Chamomile in my worst soils as long as they have adequate drainage, then add about 50 pounds of available nitrogen and 50 pounds of potassium per acre. Chamomile prefers full sun. Though it is somewhat drought tolerant when it is mature, it needs plenty of water to germinate and develop when it is young. I irrigate overhead if needed in late spring but try not to irrigate within 24 hours of harvesting. Weed control is essential with Chamomile to insure that you don't harvest weeds with the flowers. Whatever technique you employ for planting make sure to eliminate as many weeds as possible beforehand. If planting in rows from transplants, cultivate several times when the plants are young, but use caution; the young roots are somewhat sensitive. I've had no major pest problems or disease problems with Chamomile.

HARVESTING The flowers are harvested as they open. A planting will continue to produce for a few weeks and I generally harvest once or twice a week. The more open the flowers the better for both production and quality. I harvest either with my hands or with a blueberry rake with care taken to pick only flowers and not too many stems. In some areas machine harvesting has started. I haven't seen the machinery myself but I think they are using a modified grain combine harvester. A yield of 300 to 500 pounds of quality dried flowers should be expected per acre. The flowers are about 80% water.

PROCESSING AND DRYING Chamomile heats up quickly so care must be taken to get it to the drying room as soon as possible. If you are shipping fresh it is best to harvest and pack it before the heat of the day. It dries easily in 5 to 10 days and the drying room smells of Chamomile for a long time; in fact the whole farm smells like Chamomile on harvest days.

SELLING IT The market for Chamomile is very large and growing. There is a fresh market for it and the price is reasonable, between $8 and $12 per pound. Selling dried Chamomile would only be feasible if you harvested it with machinery as labor costs are too high in this country. Much of the dry Chamomile comes from Egypt.

MISCELLANEOUS I'd recommend growing it in your garden so you can harvest some for your own use. Home grown Chamomile is an absolute delight. Chamomile has a wide range of medicinal applications and I believe it will become an even more used herb in this country in the near future. It would be nice if we could meet our domestic needs with home grown certified organic Chamomile.

CHASTE BERRY

Vitex agnus-castus   *Verbenaceae*

DESCRIPTION Deciduous shrub growing 6 to 18 feet in height with a spread of up to 15 feet. Palmate leaves with 5 to 9 leaflets up to 4 inches long, dark green on top and gray underneath. In summer small lilac flowers are borne on long spikes followed by little red-black fruits. The entire plant is aromatic, especially the flowers and fruit. It is one of the last plants to leaf out in spring. I once made the mistake of thinking a plant was dead, but it was just its normal slow self. There are numerous species in the genus *Vitex* but in this country you will probably only find *agnus-castus* and *negundo*. There is one popular cultivar of *agnus-castus* called "Alba," which has white flowers.

PROPAGATION From seed or cuttings. Seed germinates readily with no pre-germination treatments in 14 to 28 days. Cuttings root easily, though like many cuttings they do much better with bottom heat and misting. Cuttings are difficult to do once flowering starts so I suggest you do them in June before flowering. They can be overwatered so use a well drained soil medium. Cuttings take about 8 weeks to reach healthy transplant size and I think they are easier than propagating from seed.

PLANTING I plant 4 inch pots or gallon size plants from summer to fall. I plant on 6 to 8 foot centers. I put in a small amount of balanced slow release fertilizer when I plant.

CULTIVATION Perennial shrub, hardy to at least Zone 6 and maybe parts of Zone 5. I've seen young shrubs die in a Zone 5 winter, so if you are going to try it there plant a gallon size plant in spring so it can mature a bit by winter, and make sure it is in a somewhat protected spot and then mulch it. Chaste Berry is incredibly hardy; it can grow in near desert conditions as well as in the fertile and lush parts of the midwest. It is also, from my experience, totally deer proof. I only fertilize it when I plant it. It prefers full sun but I've seen it grow in the fog belt near a Redwood forest canopy with a lot of shade. Once established it only needs irrigation in the dry, hot west; even there maybe a handful of waterings a summer in a normal non-drought year. Drip irrigation is ideal as is a mulch around the base to keep down weeds and reduce evaporation. I like to keep it trimmed to about 6 feet to make it easier to harvest. I've never had any problems with pests or disease. *Vitex* is about as easy as it gets.

HARVESTING The fruit is harvested in the fall after the second or third year and will continue to produce for the next century or so. The fruit (also called a berry) is already dry on the plant and you just strip it off the stalk with your fingers. Harvest it before the fall/winter rains come so as not to decrease the quality.

PROCESSING AND DRYING It requires no work other than maybe a few minutes to clean out a few leaves or stems that you might accidentally harvest.

SELLING IT There is a large and growing market for Chaste Berry. Most of the supply comes from wildcrafted sources in the Mediterranean. Prices vary from $6 to $10 per pound. I think a lot of companies would love an organic source and it would be easy to sell. I still haven't determined a reasonably accurate yield per acre but due to the ease of growing it I think it would be worth growing in certain areas of the country.

MISCELLANEOUS It gets its name from the fact that at one time it was used as an anti-aphrodisiac but alas it does not work. It is used extensively for menstrual and menopausal disorders.

COLTSFOOT

Tussilago farfara   *Asteraceae*

DESCRIPTION Creeping, 4 to 8 inches high, heart shaped to round leaves, green leaves on top but grayish-white underneath. Leaves are slightly toothed. Flowers appear on woolly, scaly stalks before the leaves in very early spring. The flowers are similar to a Dandelion and are followed by a Dandelion-like seed head. The underground stolons spread rapidly.

PROPAGATION Seed or divisions. I've never grown it from seed as the divisions are incredibly easy, just about any time of the year but especially in spring. A one year old plant will yield a dozen or more divisions.

PLANTING Divisions are best planted in spring with a spacing of 12 to 18 inches. It is not feasible to plant it in a traditional row as it will spread so rapidly, so it is best to just make a bed of it, maybe 3 feet wide or so.

CULTIVATION Perennial, hardy to at least Zone 3. Grows in any soil though a soil that holds moisture is preferable. With a rich fertile soil it will spread rapidly and produce more. If you harvest it for several years you will need to fertilize it. Irrigate once or twice a week in dry areas. Can be grown in full sun to heavy shade. Once established it will smother most weeds. Difficulty is in keeping it from spreading too much. I've had no pest or disease problems with it.

HARVESTING Harvest the leaves in late spring and then again once or twice more when you get enough leaf growth to cut. Harvest with pruning shears.

PROCESSING AND DRYING Leaf is easy to dry and will take 5 to 10 days. The leaves are large so you will have to turn them at least once.

SELLING IT The market is small and not growing much. The price is around $5 to $7 per pound.

MISCELLANEOUS Do not confuse this plant with Western Coltsfoot (*Petasites spp.*) which is native to the western U.S. Though it has some similarities in looks, they have different medicinal uses. Coltsfoot has a long history of use in cough formulas to help soothe coughs. Some smokers put it in their mixes to ease the harshness of tobacco. The leaves contain pyrrolizidine alkaloids and may cause veno-oclusive liver disease when taken in large regular doses.

COMFREY

Symphytum officinale   Boraginaceae

DESCRIPTION Grows 2 to 3 feet in height, and spreads 12 to 24 inches, and beyond if allowed to. Leaves are long, pointed, lanceolate, dark green, covered with hairs, and have distinct veins. The flowers are funnel shaped, purple to white, grow in drooping clusters, and bloom in late spring/early summer. The roots are thick, fleshy, dark on the outside but white inside, branched, and can go down several feet and spread out several feet. There are numerous species of Symphytum in the U.S. besides *officinale*, with *Symphytum x. uplandicum* being the most common.

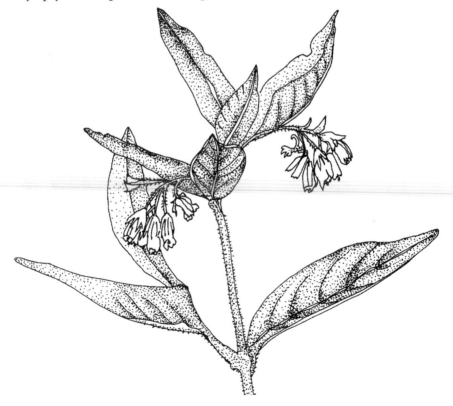

PROPAGATION Comfrey is propagated by root cuttings and on rare occasions by seed which is usually sterile in *S. officinale* and is not sold commercially. The roots can be dug up at any time of the year and cut into one inch pieces and then replanted. Plant the pieces about one inch deep in the same vertical position as they were in the ground.

PLANTING Plant cuttings immediately after you do them with spring or fall being the best time. Plant on 12 inch centers with 24 to 30 inch row spacing.

CULTIVATION Perennial, hardy to Zone 3. Prefers a fertile, rich, and moist soil though Comfrey will survive in almost any soil. If you are harvesting the tops a regular fertilizer program will be essential for continued high productivity. A balanced fertilizer with extra nitrogen on the side should do it. Regular water is essential for high productivity; a deep watering once a week should do it. Comfrey grows best in full sun but also does well in partial shade. Soil must drain somewhat or you might get some root rot, but it can take a pretty wet soil. I've encountered no major pests other than gophers and no disease problems. Once you plant Comfrey in a spot it will be there forever as even the smallest piece of root will grow into a robust healthy plant. Be very careful when selecting its permanent home.

HARVESTING Leaves are harvested up to 10 times a year starting in spring. The longer the growing season and the richer the soil the more harvests you will get. Leaves can be cut by hand or with a tractor mounted mower. If you are cutting with pruning shears it is advisable to wear gloves as the leaves can be irritating. The leaves contain pyrrolizidine alkaloids (PA) which may cause a type of liver disease if consumed on a regular basis. It has been found that the first cutting of leaves is highest in PA whereas the later cuttings and mature leaves have a very small amount; some cuttings or perhaps even plants have none at all (Keville, 1991). The first cutting should probably be put into the compost pile and the subsequent cuttings allowed to mature a bit. Leaf harvests of 2,000 to 3,000 pounds of dried leaf per acre are possible. The root is harvested in the fall or spring and can be accomplished with a root digger or by hand. You will never get all the root so just take what you get. The root is very high in allantoin, a cell proliferator that helps heal many types of injuries and is partly responsible for Comfrey's amazing healing powers. The root is also high in PA, maybe 10 times higher than the fresh leaves. The root can be harvested on an annual basis but if you do harvest the roots the plant spacing will soon be non-uniform. Of course, in time, the Comfrey will take over anyway, so who cares.

PROCESSING AND DRYING The leaves break down quickly and definitely should never be allowed to dry in the field or they'll blacken quickly.

In the drying room the leaves tend to mat together so they must be turned several times. The leaves are 80% to 90% water and take 5 to 7 days to dry. If shipped fresh, care should be taken to avoid the heat by picking and shipping early in the day. Roots need to be thoroughly cleaned and then cut in order to dry. They are very mucilaginous and slow to dry. I would recommend higher heat, over 100 degrees when drying Comfrey root.

SELLING IT There was a time when Comfrey was one of the biggest selling herbs in the country; that was before the PA scare which almost destroyed the Comfrey market in the U.S. Internal use has diminished but externally it is totally safe to use and still is one of the main ingredients in healing salves and oils. Leaf price varies from $5 to $10 per pound while root prices go from $6 to $12 per pound. I would not recommend planting Comfrey as a cash crop at this point unless you have a contract to sell it. I would recommend you have it in your garden as it is one of the most healing herbs in the entire world.

MISCELLANEOUS There is no doubt that long term, regular consumption of Comfrey can lead to veno-occlusive disease of the liver. Toxicity is cumulative and difficult to diagnose. Yet it is extremely rare and medicinal doses of Comfrey internally have been used for over a thousand years with relative safety. I wouldn't graze on it but I wouldn't eliminate it from my herb garden or cabinet either. Comfrey was the first herb I ever intentionally used for healing myself and it, of course, worked incredibly well.

DANDELION

Taraxacum officinale   *Asteraceae*

DESCRIPTION Everyone knows what dandelion looks like! Grows 1 to 2 feet in height and spreads up to 2 feet. The leaves grow in a basal rosette and the plants are stemless. The leaves are green and up to a foot long with toothed margins. The flowers are solitary, bright yellow and followed by an incredible puffy seed head that when you blow on it helps make all your wishes come true. The flowers bloom mainly in spring but can bloom nearly all year. The taproot can grow a foot deep or more. All parts of the fresh plant, when broken, exude a milky sap.

PROPAGATION Seeds or divisions. Seeds germinate easily in 10 to 14 days and can be grown in nursery flats or sown directly into the field. If sown in flats they should be ready to transplant in 8 weeks or more, either with a transplanter or by hand. If sown direct do so in the fall or early spring. Divisions of older plants are easy but only practical for getting a few plants.

PLANTING Transplants should go out in spring or summer for harvest the next spring for whole plants, or the next fall for roots. Spacing at 6 inches in the row and 24 inches between rows. Direct sown seeds should be thinned out early and can be planted by hand or with a seeder.

CULTIVATION Perennial, hardy to Zone 3, though I'm sure it has spread to the planet Pluto by now. Will grow in virtually any soil but produces best in a fertile, rich, and well drained soil. Dandelion seems to appreciate phosphorus and may turn somewhat purple if phosphorus deficient. Likes full sun but can grow in partial shade. I irrigate it one to two times a week depending on the soil and temperature. It can survive with very little water but productivity diminishes. Cultivate and weed as soon as possible after planting. Though Dandelion can obviously compete with weeds it does better if it has space. I've had no major pest problems or disease in my Dandelion fields.

HARVESTING Many companies prefer fresh Dandelion. I harvest the fresh leaf, flower and root all together in the spring of the second year when it is in full flower. If they want just leaf, then harvest it just before flowering and then later in the summer. Root is harvested in the fall of the second year. When harvesting the whole plant, it should be dug up carefully to avoid damage to the tops. Leaf is harvested with pruning shears. If you are harvesting leaf off the same patch for more than one season you will need to fertilize it. The root can be harvested with a root digger or by hand. The average whole plant weighs up to 1 pound fresh. The root alone weighs ¼ pound to ½ pound, depending on the age.

PROCESSING AND DRYING Fresh top harvest must be carefully washed as the leaves hold a lot of dirt and sometimes slugs. The root should also be washed before drying. If drying the leaves, washing is probably necessary to eliminate excess dirt but it makes it more difficult to dry. If there is little dirt present don't wash the leaves. The leaves dry in 5 to 7 days and are 80% to 90% water, the roots about 75%.

SELLING IT There is a good market for Dandelion leaf and root. There is a fresh market and if you can find a buyer the price is good, about $6 to $7 a pound. Dried root goes for $7 to $12 per pound. Dandelion is an easy crop to grow and worth growing though it might be somewhat difficult to find a market.

MISCELLANEOUS You know you are into herbs when you cultivate Dandelion. Dandelion has so many uses both culinarily and medicinally. If I had to pick a handful of herbs to have with me when I fly to the far reaches of the galaxy in search of a class M planet, Dandelion would definitely be one of them.

ECHINACEA

Echinacea spp. Asteraceae

DESCRIPTION Stately plant growing up to 4 feet in height with a spread of 1 to 2 feet. Leaves are ovate to lanceolate, hairy, and 3 to 6 inches in length. Flowers are purple and daisy-like with an orange center, and bloom in summer. Most species have taproots but *E. purpurea* has a fibrous root system. There are 9 species of Echinacea all native to North America. The three most commonly used medicinally are *E. purpurea, E. angustifolia,* and *E. pallida. E. purpurea* and *E. pallida* grow up to 3 to 4 feet while *E. angustifolia* only grows 12 to 18 inches.

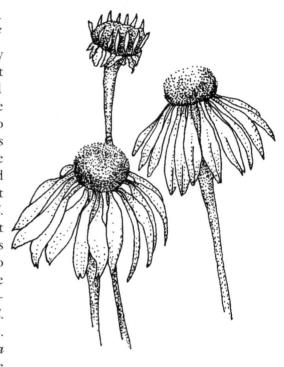

PROPAGATION Seed or divisions. Seeds on *E. purpurea* germinate easily without pre-germination treatment. They germinate in 10 to 20 days and are ready for transplanting in 8 to 12 weeks. A pound of *E. purpurea* seed should produce enough plants for close to 3 acres if growing starts in a greenhouse. Other Echinacea species need to be stratified for 4 to 12 weeks, with *E. angustifolia* liking a long stratification period. *E. pallida* germinates at about 50% after stratification, while I've rarely gotten more than 50% germination from *E. angustifolia. Echinacea angustifolia* germinates best when it is soaked for 24 hours after stratification and immediately before planting. Divisions can be done from mature plants in the fall or early spring, using pruning shears to cut the buds from the crown.

PLANTING Seedlings are planted in late spring or early summer with a transplanter or by hand. *E. angustifolia* does not transplant well and if done in cells it should be in deep ones. It can be sown directly. The difficulty with sowing it directly is that it germinates poorly and grows slowly so it doesn't compete well with weeds. Try to eliminate as many weeds as possible before planting. It can either be fall sown or spring sown from stratified seed. Seed might benefit from a 24 hour soaking before planting. Divisions from all species can be planted immediately after dividing them, which is usually during fall harvest, or they can be over-wintered in sawdust and spring planted. Spacing is 12 inches in the row and 24 to 30 inches between rows.

CULTIVATION Perennial, hardy to Zone 3. *E. purpurea* likes a fairly fertile soil with a pH of 6.0 to 7.0. Manure and cover crop the year before planting if your soil is poor. It likes to be irrigated every 7 to 10 days from either overhead or drip irrigation. It grows in full sun or partial shade. Weed control is important the first year as the plants get established. Cultivate when necessary. By the summer of year two the plants are too tall to run a tractor over them, so cultivate early. The same applies to year three.

E. angustifolia will grow in less fertile soils and needs excellent drainage and minimal water. It does not like the wet winters of the Pacific northwest or the southeast. It grows naturally in the driest parts of the great plains. It likes a high pH, 6.5 to 8.0. Apply lime if necessary. It needs little irrigation even in the west but does need some, once every 2 to 3 weeks from either drip or overhead. It is slow growing and not very weed competitive. Weed early and often. It needs full sun to thrive. A field of *E. purpurea* is absolutely gorgeous in flower whereas a field of *E. angustifolia* is interesting. If growing it in relatively wet areas it would probably be best grown in raised beds.

E. pallida has needs similar to *E. purpurea* but it requires full sun and likes a slightly higher pH.

HARVESTING With *E. purpurea*, the whole plant is harvested; with *Echinacea angustifolia* it is the root and the seed; and with *E. pallida* it is mainly just the root that is harvested with a very small amount of seed harvested. It is possible to get a small leaf and flower harvest from *E. purpurea* the first year if you plant early. The second and third years you definitely get a leaf and flower harvest. Harvest when the flowers are just starting to open, cutting the plants at the point where the first healthy leaves are growing. A full size *E. purpurea* plant has fresh tops weighing close to 2½ pounds with about half of that being stem. Some companies will buy stem, others will not. The seed is harvested in years two and three if you didn't harvest the tops. The seed can be harvested by hand or with a combine if you are doing a large amount.

E. purpurea root is harvested in the fall of the second or third year and can be done using a root digger or by hand. Production is greater if you wait until year three but not much greater so if you need a fast crop then harvest after year two. Average root weight is one-third to two-thirds of a pound fresh depending on year harvested and the health of the field and the plants. In general a fresh yield of 8,000 to 10,000 pounds of root per acre is average. The roots average 70% water thus giving you a yield of around 2,500 to 3,000 pounds of dry root per acre.

E. angustifolia root is harvested after year three. The root is a taproot and the root digger might cut the bottom off. I don't have any accurate yield numbers on *E. angustifolia*. The root is about 60% water.

E. pallida root is harvested after year three and is larger than either *E. purpurea* or *E. angustifolia*.

PROCESSING AND DRYING Echinacea is sold both fresh and dry. Fresh roots ship easily but some care should be taken when shipping tops as they can heat up and decompose. Harvest early and don't pile too thickly as you pick, and keep it in the shade. Some companies want just leaf and flower so it needs to be garbled with the stem discarded. If you are shipping fresh and garbling you will have to start early; garbling is slow. The water content of leaf and flower is about 75% and dries fairly easily; however the flower is slow to dry due to its thickness. Roots should be chopped up a bit and then thoroughly washed. Roots dry fairly easily. Seed heads need to be broken up in a hammermill with at least a one inch screen. They are then run through a seed cleaner. For any significant amounts it is best to use a seed cleaner; ship your seeds to someone else to clean if you don't have one. On a small scale you can clean the seeds yourself by running them through small hand held screens, ¼ inch to start and then a smaller size to eliminate dust. After that you need to separate out the seed from the seed sized chaff. Use a fan and let air help you out or go outside on a windy day. This is slow but you will get pretty clean seed.

SELLING IT Echinacea is the biggest selling herb in the U.S. Sales will continue to grow and there is room for more growers. The market is dominated by one very large grower but smaller growers are entering the market. The key, as with all crops, is selling it. *Echinacea purpurea* is easy to grow almost anywhere in the country so producing it is not the problem. *Echinacea angustifolia* is difficult to grow and I would recommend it only if you want to take a small risk. The seed is expensive, over $200 per pound, and germinates poorly so there is an initial investment. Also it is difficult to grow, especially in areas of heavy rain and less than good drainage. If I lived in the areas where it grows naturally, like the dry western parts of the midwest, I would grow it for sure. The return is high and it obviously grows well there. If I lived in a wet area I would not grow it myself; I'd let others take the risks.

Echinacea purpurea leaf sells for $5 to $10 per pound dry and $2 to $4 fresh. *E. purpurea* root sells for $18 to $27 per pound dry and $6 to $10 fresh. Seed sells for $20 to $55 per pound. All prices are for certified organic.

Echinacea angustifolia root sells for $30 to $40 per pound dry for certified organic and less for wildcrafted. Seed sells for $150 to $300 per pound.

The market for *E. pallida* is small in the U.S., though somewhat larger in Europe, specifically Germany. I would not suggest planting it unless you feel assured you have a buyer. *E. pallida* root sells for $18 to $23 per pound dry.

MISCELLANEOUS Nowadays, whenever I travel and teach, everyone I encounter seems to know Echinacea. Even my mother's friends know of Echinacea and use it. It is a beautiful herb, one of my favorites in the perennial flower garden. When it is blooming on the farm it is indescribably gorgeous. *Echinacea purpurea* exists in only small patches in the wild and nearly all of the world's supply comes from cultivated sources. It should not be picked in the wild.

Echinacea angustifolia is still mainly picked in the wild and the populations are diminishing rapidly. It is now on the UpS primary plant list. We need to grow it now and stop wildcrafting it. Another problem with wildcrafting *E. angustifolia* is that a lot of pickers harvest the wrong species. Quite often they pick *E. pallida* and sometimes pick *E. atrorubens*, which is somewhat rare and should never be picked. In the process of wildcrafting *E. angustifolia*, a significant amount of damage is done to the environment. The bottom line, in my herbal opinion, is that we should stop wildcrafting *E. angustifolia*. *E. purpurea* is as effective medicinally and if you have to make a choice between organic *purpurea* and wild *angustifolia*, I urge you to use *purpurea*.

I think that other species of Echinacea will be used medicinally in time especially *E. tennesseensis*. *E. tennesseensis* is on the federal endangered species list and only a few populations exist in the wild. It can be easily cultivated though.

There is a lot of Echinacea seed being sold that is mislabeled. One reason is that Echinacea species cross pollinate readily so if they are growing within a mile of each other they have probably crossed. Most of the *tennesseensis* I've seen is from hybrid crossed seed. A lot of so-called *E. angustifolia* seed is actually *E. pallida*. I visited several farms this year that thought they were growing *angustifolia* but were actually growing *pallida*. If it grows easily it probably is *pallida*. *Angustifolia* only grows up to about 18 inches at the most whereas *pallida* grows up to 3 to 4 feet. A taste test of the root or seed will also give it away, as *angustifolia* will have that "buzz" or tingling sensation in your mouth when you chew it that results from its high concentrations of isobutylamides. *E. pallida* has only tiny amounts of isobutylamides so it won't give you that tingling sensation in your mouth.

I grow and use more Echinacea than any other herb, I absolutely love it, and it is definitely going with me as I boldly cross the galaxy in search of the ideal land for growing.

ELDERBERRY

Sambucus nigra, S. canadensis
Caprifoliaceae

DESCRIPTION Shrub or small tree growing up to 25 feet with a spread of 6 to 15 feet. Light green leaves are pinnately compound consisting of 5 to 7 leaflets up to 3 to 4 inches in length. The flowers are yellow-white in large saucer-like umbels. The fruits are black, juicy, and very tasty. The bark is green at the ends of the branches but grayish-brown everywhere else. It is native to Europe, western Asia, and North Africa. Several species are native to North America; some are often used interchangeably with *S. nigra*, most often *Sambucus canadensis* in the midwest and east and *S. caerulea* and *S. mexicana* in the west. Numerous cultivars are available for both berry production and for landscaping. High berry and flower producing cultivars include York, Adams, Johns, and Nova which are from *S. canadensis*.

PROPAGATION Seed or cuttings. Seed is planted right after harvest in the early fall in flats and allowed to get fall heat and winter cold before it germinates in spring. Young seedlings can be planted the next fall. Softwood cuttings root easily and are best taken in late spring/early summer before flowering, though late summer cuttings are also possible. Cuttings can be transplanted into the field in the fall.

PLANTING Fall planting of seedlings or young cuttings is best. If you purchase plants they will probably be bareroot and will be available in late winter/early spring. Bareroot plants do well but should be watered early and often. I plant on 8 to 10 foot centers with the idea in mind that I will keep them trimmed to small shrub height, about 6 to 8 feet.

CULTIVATION Perennial, hardy to Zone 5. *Sambucus canadensis* is hardy to Zone 3. Prefers a rich soil with adequate moisture but also decent drainage. Compost around the base of the plants is ideal for continued health and productivity. Prefers a pH near 7.0 but will grow in slightly alkaline or acidic soils. Regular watering is a must in the dry west, a deep watering once a week, though young plants may need more. Drip irrigation is ideal for Elderberry. Can grow in full sun in moist areas but in real dry areas it might do better in partial shade. I like to keep the plants trimmed to 6 to 8 feet which is the average height of *S. canadensis*, but *S. nigra* will need to be trimmed annually. I've had no pest problems or disease with Elder.

HARVESTING Flowers with the supporting peduncle are harvested as they are just starting to open, usually in early summer. They should never be harvested soon after they have gotten wet as this will cause them to blacken. Flowers are harvested with pruning shears. Fruits with the peduncle are harvested in the fall by hand when they are ripe and juicy. A harvest is usually possible the second or third year after planting.

PROCESSING AND DRYING Flowers should be dried carefully with as little bruising as possible. Bruised flowers that are stuffed too much while harvested can turn brown. Drying time is 7 to 10 days. Flowers are about 80% water. After drying, if you want just flowers, they are garbled and separated from the peduncle, which is discarded. The color should be the same yellow-white that existed when they were harvested. The berries are dried with the peduncle in place, so as not to lose juice, and then garbled like the flowers. The fruits are approximately 75% water.

SELLING IT There is a solid and growing market for both flowers and berries. Flowers sell for between $9 and $15 dollars per pound, berries average $9 to $10 per pound. I think it is worth growing on a small scale as a perimeter plant around your farm.

MISCELLANEOUS Elders are absolutely beautiful shrubs in the landscape. One cultivar, *S. nigra "Variegata"* is perhaps my single most favorite plant. Elder has a long history of use for colds, flus, fevers, and sinus infections. Recent studies verify that it is indeed anti-viral and anti-inflammatory. *S. pubens* (with red berries) should not be grown for medicine as it is poisonous.

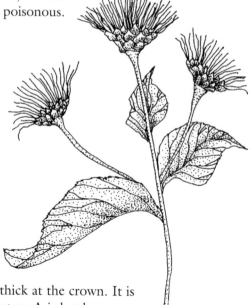

ELECAMPANE

Inula helenium   Asteraceae

DESCRIPTION Striking herbaceous plant up to 7 feet in height and spreading 2 to 4 feet. The leaves are pointed, toothed, up to 1 to 2 feet in length. They are dull green with a velvety underside and very hairy stems. The flowers are yellow and daisy-like, up to 3 inches across, and bloom in summer. The root is up to a foot in length with many laterals spreading up to a foot, and very thick at the crown. It is native to southern Europe and western Asia but has naturalized in parts of eastern North America.

PROPAGATION Seeds or divisions. Seeds germinate in 3 to 4 weeks at a reasonable percentage. Seedlings grown in flats are ready for transplanting in 8 to 12 weeks. Divisions can be done in fall or spring; you can get a dozen divisions or more off a two year old crown. Just take a knife or pruning shears and slice vertically making sure to include a bud with leaf growth. Length is about 2 inches. You can do this after harvest by cutting the top 2 inches of the crown to propagate from, and using the rest for harvest.

PLANTING   Seedlings are transplanted out in late spring/early summer by transplanter or by hand. Divisions are planted in early spring. If harvesting in the fall I prefer to over-winter the root in sawdust, and then plant in spring, to better control the weeds. Spacing in row is 12 to 18 inches with rows at 24 to 30 inches.

CULTIVATION   Perennial, hardy to Zone 3. Grows best in a rich soil with a pH of 4.5 to 7.0. Grows best in full sun though it can grow in partial shade. Requires good drainage and deep irrigation about once a week to thrive. I've seen neglected plants survive for weeks without water in the west—they are very tough—but they didn't thrive. Mature plants are fairly weed competitive but spring weeding is important to allow for maximum growth. I've had no pest problems other than occasional gophers and a few insects who work the roots. I've never had any disease problems.

HARVESTING   Roots are harvested in the fall of the second year. After the second year they get pithy and insects will attack them more readily. The roots are large and the root digger may not get the whole root. If digging by hand watch out for the lateral roots, make sure you get them all. Yields of 2,000 to 3,000 pounds per acre of dry root are possible.

PROCESSING AND DRYING   Roots need to be chopped and washed thoroughly. Drying is facilitated by cutting the roots into smaller pieces; the section near the top should be cut vertically several times. Drying time is 7 to 10 days.

SELLING IT   The market is small and I doubt it will grow much. The price for dry root is between $10 and $13 per pound. Fresh root goes for $4 to $6 per pound but the market is very small. It is such an easy crop to grow with a high yield that it is worth growing if you think you can sell it.

MISCELLANEOUS   A nice plant for the perennial flower landscape. Best to put it in the background and cut off the flower stalk after it blooms. In the flower garden it is best to divide it every 3 to 4 years. It was the most often mentioned herb in the popular book *Clan of the Cave Bear*.

FALSE INDIGO
Baptisia tinctoria   *Fabaceae*

DESCRIPTION Grows up to 4 feet and spreads up to 2 feet. Compound pea-like leaves are deep green. The small yellow pea flowers bloom in early summer and are followed by interesting brown pods. The roots are large, deep, and very bitter. There are several related species which are also native to eastern North America.

PROPAGATION Seeds, cuttings, or divisions. Spring planted seeds germinate in 2 to 4 weeks at somewhat low percentages, around 50% or less. Germination improves with mild scarification and soaking of the seed for 24 hours. Transplanting into the field is possible in 12 weeks or more. Cuttings root okay and are best done in late spring or in late summer. Cuttings are ready to be put into the field in about 12 weeks. You can get hundreds of cuttings off a mature plant. Divisions are done in fall or early spring off mature plants but are not easy and result in few plants.

PLANTING Roots do not like to be transplanted, and nursery seedlings are best grown in deep flats or even small pots. Direct seeding might be the best way but the seeds are slow to germinate and slow growing at first so weed control will be a problem. Cuttings are a great way to go and can be planted whenever they are ready. Divisions should be planted after fall or spring harvest. Spacing in the row is 18 to 24 inches with rows set at 30 inches.

CULTIVATION Perennial, hardy to Zone 3. Grows in full sun or partial shade in very well drained soils. Can grow in an average to rich soil. Irrigate every 7 to 10 days in the west. Weed early and often so the young plants can get established. Once mature they are very competitive. Plants grow quickly after the first year so cultivation should happen early in the year. I've had no pest problems with *Baptisia*. Root rot will definitely occur in poorly drained soils.

HARVESTING Large roots are harvested after the third season either by hand or with a root digger in the fall or early spring.

PROCESSING AND DRYING Roots should be chopped and then thoroughly washed. Drying time is facilitated by breaking off the lateral roots and dividing the crown. Root is about 50% water.

SELLING IT Though not a big seller at the moment it has a lot of potential because it is an immune system stimulant and very effective at fighting a wide variety of illnesses. The dry root sells for up to $20 per pound. There is also a small market for fresh root. All of the False Indigo supply now comes from wildcrafting and a successful grower could easily sell their crop.

MISCELLANEOUS All *Baptisia* species are beautiful in the perennial flower bed.

FEVERFEW

Tanacetum parthenium
Asteraceae

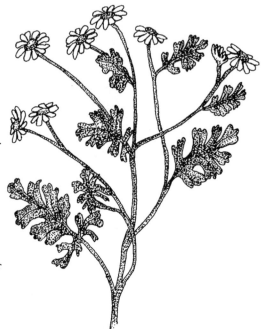

DESCRIPTION Grows up to 30 inches with a spread of 12 to 18 inches. The yellow-green leaves are pinnately lobed and up to 3 inches in length. The clusters of daisy-like flowers appear in summer. The whole plant is strongly aromatic. There are many cultivars available: gold leaves, double flowers, and even a dwarf cultivar. Native to southern Europe, it has naturalized in parts of North America.

PROPAGATION Seed or cuttings. Seeds germinate easily in 10 to 14 days. Make sure the small seed is very lightly covered as it is light dependent for germination. I always plant in nursery flats for transplanting in 10 to 12 weeks. Cuttings do not readily root and are useful only if you want a few plants. Mature plants in the field will self sow readily if allowed to.

PLANTING Transplant in late spring/early summer with a transplanter or by hand. Spacing is 12 to 18 inches in the row with rows at 24 to 30 inches.

CULTIVATION Perennial, hardy to Zone 4. Grows in almost any soil, will produce in soils of marginal fertility though production will be higher in a fertile soil. Prefers full sun or partial shade. Can survive drought conditions but I irrigate it once a week in the west. Easy to cultivate as the stems are durable even when young. I've had no pest or disease problems with Feverfew. Deer will absolutely not touch it.

HARVESTING The tops are harvested just as the flowers are forming. Some companies prefer just the top leaves and flowers with little stem, but most of what is traded is whole herb including stem. It is sometimes possible to get two harvests in a year, a large early summer harvest and a smaller fall harvest. The first year you could get one small harvest but I wait until year two and get a very heavy harvest. Year three will yield a smaller harvest, and after this summer harvest it should be tilled under. Depending on your growing practices and whether you are harvesting just tops or whole herb, an acre will yield between 1,000 and 4,000.

PROCESSING AND DRYING The flowers dry easily in 4 to 6 days. If your customers want it stem free, you will have to garble it, or just harvest and dry the top 6 to 8 inches. It can easily be shipped fresh. Some of Feverfew's most important constituents break down rapidly. It should be sold and used within about 6 months of harvest. The tops are about 75% water.

SELLING IT The market for Feverfew is average and I don't anticipate any major jump in popularity in the near future. There seems to be somewhat of a glut of supply right now as it is an easy plant to cultivate and several growers over-planted thinking the market was going to expand. The dried herb sells for $7 to $12 per pound.

MISCELLANEOUS Feverfew is a good choice for the perennial flower garden, both for its leaves and its attractive flowers. It should be replaced after the second or third year. The flowers make excellent cut flowers for the florist or for your house. Feverfew has many medicinal uses but is best known for its ability to eliminate or diminish the symptoms of migraine headaches. You can use the leaves directly from the garden but be forewarned that some people will develop small sores in their mouths if they chew on the leaves. Also, Feverfew is one of the most bitter herbs around, in my humble opinion.

GARLIC

Allium sativum   *Liliaceae*

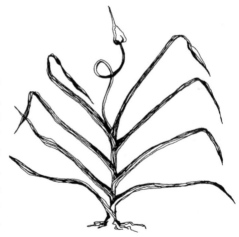

DESCRIPTION Grows up to 3 feet tall when in flower and spreads up to 6 inches. The leaves are flat, grasslike, and very pointed. The many small white flowers form in round clusters in early summer. Miniature bulbs, called bulbels, may form in the flower head. The underground bulbs contain 5 to 20 cloves encompassed in a paper like covering. Numerous varieties of garlic are grown in the U.S.

PROPAGATION By cloves or bulbels. Cloves are planted in the fall or spring directly into the field and are incredibly easy to grow. Bulbels are often started in nursery flats and then planted out with leaf growth already present. Nearly all garlic is planted from cloves.

PLANTING Cloves are field planted in the fall or spring with the fall being more common in warmer areas, and the spring in cold areas. One clove every 6 inches and row spacing of 24 inches. Plant them point up and about an inch deep.

CULTIVATION Perennial, hardy to Zone 4. Grows in full sun in a rich, well drained soil with a pH of 6.0 to 8.0. In warm areas where the ground doesn't freeze solid in winter the bulb is fall planted. Winter weeding is crucial; this usually means hand hoeing as the ground is too wet for equipment. Even in the west it needs little irrigation as it grows mainly during the wet season. Some irrigation may be necessary in late spring before the early summer harvest. Do not water within a couple of weeks of harvest time as you are trying to dry the plant up. I've had no major pest problems and disease-wise the biggest problem is root rot in poorly drained soils.

HARVESTING The bulbs are harvested in early summer in areas where it is fall planted, or in mid to late summer in areas where it is spring planted. The bulbs can be dug with a potato digger or a spade. Harvest is usually done as the tops start to die back.

PROCESSING AND DRYING Garlic can be dried in the shade in dry areas of the west or in the drying room. It is usually dried with the tops still in place. The tops are then cut and you have a finished product.

SELLING IT The market for garlic is gargantuan and growing. People are starting to use it as medicine now in a big way. It will continue to grow in popularity as people learn how wonderful it is. There are lots of garlic growers out there so make sure you have a market before planting it.

MISCELLANEOUS Garlic is an incredible food and medicine. It will definitely be with me on my travels throughout the galaxy. Most of the garlic in the U.S. is grown in California; the town of Gilroy advertises itself as "The garlic capital of the world." Mainly because of its use in cardiac disease, specifically high blood pressure, garlic has become one of the top selling medicinal herbs in the U.S. Ron L. Engeland wrote a wonderful book about garlic, *Growing Great Garlic*, which is available from Filaree Publications.

GINKGO

Ginkgo biloba Ginkgoaceae

DESCRIPTION Deciduous tree, up to 130 feet in height, with a spread of up to 60 feet; beautiful fan shaped leaves which turn yellow in the fall. Male and female flowers are borne on separate plants. The female produces nasty smelling small plum-like fruits. Ginkgo is considered the oldest living tree species on earth. Originally native to China, it is no longer found growing in the wild.

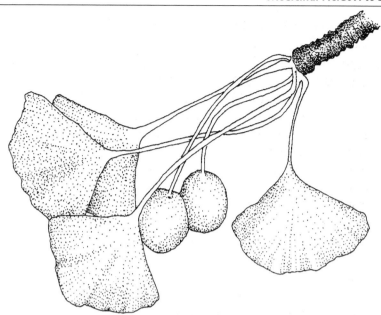

PROPAGATION Seed, cuttings, or grafting. Seeds are either sown in the fall after harvest or in spring after 4 to 6 weeks of stratification. Softwood cuttings done in spring are somewhat difficult but you can get male only plants that way. Female plants are considered undesirable because of the smelly fruit. Grafting is done on young seedlings the first winter to either insure male plants or to graft on a named variety.

PLANTING Small seedlings, 1 to 5 gallon specimens, or bigger can be purchased and planted any season of the year. Bare root plants are occasionally available in late winter/early spring. If you start your own plants pot them up in 1 to 5 gallon pots before planting them in the field. If you are going to grow it in rows and keep it pruned, put it on 10 to 20 foot centers. One large grower plants on 1 to 2 foot centers and never allows the plants to exceed 3 feet in height.

CULTIVATION Perennial tree, hardy to Zone 4. Ginkgo prefers a rich but reasonably well drained soil and full sun. It needs a regular deep watering to thrive but when mature it can withstand drought conditions. For production purposes it is best to prune it annually with your harvest and keep the trees almost shrub like. Ginkgo is incredibly resistant to pests and disease.

HARVESTING Ginkgo leaves are harvested in the fall after the tree has reached 6 to 8 feet in height and is healthy. The grower I previously mentioned harvests each year's annual growth once the trees have reached 3 feet in height. The leaves should just be turning yellow when you harvest. I use pruning shears, cut the branches, and then pull the leaves off. Over the years many people in areas where there are mature Ginkgo trees have harvested by waiting until the leaves fall from the tree. In cold areas this usually happens one clear night in the early fall when there is a very hard frost. Nearly all the leaves will fall off in one night and the harvesters just place large tarps under the trees and collect the leaves. They then sun dry them the next day, bag them up and sell them to a distributor. It is an easy way to harvest a lot of Ginkgo. The only problem is that by the time the leaves have fallen they have lost most of their medicinal potency.

PROCESSING AND DRYING After harvest either sell the leaves fresh or dry them. They dry easily in 4 to 7 days. They must be turned several times as they tend to mat together in the dryer. Ginkgo leaves vary from 60% to 75% water.

SELLING IT The market for Ginkgo is very large and growing. It is the number one selling herb in Europe by far and I believe it will soon be the number one selling herb in the U.S. Dry Ginkgo sells for $10 to $16 per pound while fresh leaves sell for $5 to $9 per pound.

MISCELLANEOUS Ginkgo is one of the most beautiful trees in the world. It is the most commonly planted tree in the U.S. due to both its beauty and its ability to withstand intense pollution and abuse. Drive through New York city and you will see Ginkgo trees everywhere. Medicinally Ginkgo is used to improve peripheral and cerebral blood flow, improve memory loss, tinnitus, and various stages of dementia among other things. As our population ages the baby boomers are going to embrace Ginkgo and it will be, in my very humble opinion, the number one selling herb for a long time.

GINSENG

Panax quinquefolius   Araliaceae

DESCRIPTION Grows one to two feet in height with a spread of one foot. The green leaves are divided into 3 to 7 toothed leaflets up to 6 inches long. The flowers are small, green-white, bloom in early summer, and are followed by bright red berries. The aromatic taproot is white and grows slowly. The older the root the bigger and deeper it grows. There are several species of Ginseng with the most important along with *P. quinquefolius* being *Panax ginseng* (also known as *P. pseudoginseng*) which is native to eastern Asia. *Panax quinquefolius* is native to the eastern half of North America, from southern Canada down through Minnesota,

Iowa, Oklahoma, Missouri, and across to Georgia and up to Quebec. American pickers often refer to it as "sang." Each year when the leaves drop they leave a circular scar, one scar per year. The age of a plant can be determined by the number of scars.

PROPAGATION From seed. Seed is either fall planted outdoors or stratified and then spring planted. Seed is slow to germinate but fall planted seed will usually germinate the following spring/summer. It is possible to buy pre-stratified seed. One or two year old roots are sold by several companies for fall or spring planting, but they are expensive.

PLANTING Seed is either planted in place in the field in the fall, or sown in flats and than transplanted in early spring, 18 months later. Seed is very expensive. Purchased seed often carries disease and it is best to treat it with a 10-1 water/bleach mix. Seeds or plants are placed 6 inches apart with a row spacing of 24 inches. Some growers plant in raised beds about 3 feet wide with plant spacing at 6 inches. This makes root harvest easier if you have a digger that will go 3 feet wide.

CULTIVATION Perennial, hardy to Zone 3. Ginseng requires approximately 75% shade. This can be accomplished either by growing under a forest canopy or by creating artificial shade. Most Ginseng in the U.S. is cultivated under artificial shade. Shade is created by using shade cloth which is supported by a variety of pole types and wire. I've used metal and wood posts, although I saw one Ginseng grower who used driftwood that had washed up on the beach near him. Wood lath was originally used before its price went sky high, and shade cloth is easier to put up. Shade cloth will usually last for 10 years or more. It costs between $8,000 and $15,000 to put up an acre of shade cloth.

Ginseng can be grown in the woods and "woods grown" Ginseng fetches a much higher price. The difficulties with growing it in the woods are numerous. It is difficult to clear the space so you can maximize your planting area. You can usually plant less than half as many plants in natural shade versus artificial shade. Other problems include deer, rodents, turkeys, and squirrels which love to harvest the berries. These pests will also "attack" a cultivated area; it's just that they are less likely to do so. Still, natural shade is a heck of a lot less expensive and you will get a higher price for your product.

Ginseng likes a humus-rich, loamy soil with good drainage. It loves slow release fertilizer and compost is ideal. It is hard to add too much organic matter to your Ginseng patch. Ginseng also loves mulch: leaves, grass, sawdust, or whatever is always beneficial. In dry areas, Ginseng must be irrigated once or twice a week with overhead sprinklers to help raise the humidity. Weeds are difficult to deal with because you do not want to damage the stems at all—so extra care must be taken. Mulch will help control weed problems. Ginseng is extremely susceptible to disease; commercial growers use a variety of toxic fungicides for control. I would venture to guess that Ginseng is the most heavily sprayed herb crop in the U.S. For organic cultivation the key is to not introduce disease and take extra care to insure good drainage. There are very few organic Ginseng growers at the moment though the numbers are growing.

HARVESTING Ginseng is harvested in the fall of the fourth year or later. The older the root the larger it is and the higher the price per pound. Many growers will harvest when disease is beginning to take over and threatens to destroy the entire crop. Roots can be harvested with a root digger or by hand. The seeds are harvested in the fall when the berry is ripe, and there are usually two seeds per berry.

PROCESSING AND DRYING Ginseng root is washed thoroughly after digging and then put out to dry. Traditionally it was, and still often is, dried outdoors over a long period of time. The important thing is to dry it slowly to keep the root from darkening. Low heat and dehumidifiers would be appropriate for a drying room. Ginseng roots are about 70% water.

SELLING IT The worldwide market for Ginseng is very large. About 90% of the American crop is sold to China. Most of the American supply is still grown in one county, Marathon County, in Wisconsin. Its dominance of the market is starting to fade though as Canada has taken a major role in Ginseng farming. Growers in other parts of the U.S. are also starting up, especially in the eastern woodlands and the Pacific northwest. The Chinese have also started to cultivate American Ginseng and prices are very low at the moment, with cultivated commercial Ginseng selling for between $20 and $60 per pound depending on the quality and the buyer. What little organic Ginseng there is may go for over $100 per pound and perhaps even much higher. Woods grown Ginseng, which may or may not be organic, will fetch more than commercial Ginseng on the Chinese market, as much as $200 per pound. Wildcrafted Ginseng is sometimes selling for up to $500 per pound though usually for less. If I had forested land in the eastern woodlands I would attempt to grow Ginseng. I would suggest starting small at first and then, once you have the knack for it, expanding. It has the potential to be a major cash crop but due to susceptibility to fungus it could also be a major cash losing crop.

MISCELLANEOUS Ginseng is on the Appendix 2 of the CITES (Convention on International Trade in Endangered Species) list. This discourages trade that might in any way be detrimental to its long term survival. Ginseng is also on the UpS primary list. My personal opinion is that we should no longer harvest or use wildcrafted ginseng. Since commercial Ginseng is heavily sprayed, the only alternative is certified organic. I think more and more growers will be attempting organic Ginseng cultivation in the next decade. Ginseng's medicinal actions mainly revolve around its "adaptogenic effect." It basically serves to enhance overall mental and physical health. It increases tolerance to stress, resistance to disease, increasing physical and mental performance, and has a mild stimulating effect. It is a wonderful herb, not a panacea for everything, but worthy of having around.

GOLDENSEAL

Hydrastis canadensis   Ranunculaceae

DESCRIPTION Grows up to 16 inches in height with a spread of 6 to 12 inches. Leaves are light green, palmate and deeply toothed. The late spring blooming flowers are small and hardly noticeable, with greenish-white stamens. The flowers are short lived—just a week or so—and are followed by a soft red berry containing 10 to 30 black seeds. The yellow rhizome is about one-half to three-quarters of an inch thick and about 2 inches long, covered with skinny fibrous rootlets. Goldenseal grows from southern Canada down through Minnesota to Arkansas, across to Georgia and back up to Quebec.

PROPAGATION Seeds, divisions, or by root buds. Seeds are difficult. The berry must be harvested as soon as it is ripe and then cleaned, to eliminate juice and separate out the seed. The berry usually ripens in mid-summer. The seed should be stratified immediately and not allowed to dry out. In the fall the seed can be planted into nursery flats outdoors. Then in early spring bring them into the greenhouse and hopefully they will germinate. By the next fall the tiny roots will be capable of being planted outdoors. The more common way to propagate Goldenseal is by root divisions in the fall or spring. A mature plant can produce 3 to 5 divisions. Some of the divisions will not produce leaf growth the first year but will the second year. Buds and plants will form on the fibrous roots that grow away from the main root. These small pieces can be planted separately and will also produce plants.

PLANTING Divisions are planted in the fall or spring at 6 inch spacing with rows at 12 inches or more. If I'm growing it under shade cloth I want to utilize every inch because of the cost of the shade and I might recommend 6 inch spacing all around. If I'm growing it under natural shade then I may space it farther apart.

CULTIVATION Perennial, hardy to Zone 4 and perhaps warmer parts of Zone 3. Goldenseal requires 75% shade which can be done either artificially or naturally. An artificial shade house was described earlier under Ginseng cultivation. There is another method of creating shade which I recently discovered. A friend of mine in Iowa, John Klosterboer, wanted to plant some Goldenseal so I went over to look at where he wanted to plant it. He had a number of young trees that had been planted in rows several years before. They were spaced at 6 foot centers and this allowed for easy planting of Goldenseal with little difficulty or waste of space. The trees only need to be 4 to 5 years old, especially if you are growing in Goldenseal's northern range where it seems to need less shade. This would be a simple and inexpensive way to get shade. Be aware as sometimes wildcrafters are a problem with cultivated woods-grown Goldenseal. Bev, in Virginia, was growing a number of Goldenseal plants in the woods on his property; the local wildcrafters found them and promptly dug them all up. Goldenseal will grow in similar conditions as Ginseng. Goldenseal likes a rich, humus filled soil with excellent drainage. I've seen growers lose whole crops to poor drainage. Lots of organic matter should be added to the soil; compost is ideal. Granular fertilizers that contain a broad array of nutrients, especially potassium and phosphorus, are beneficial. Regular watering in dry areas, or during drought, is important with overhead watering being preferred as it raises humidity. The pH should be between 5.5 and 6.5. Mulch is valuable for both the organic content and the ability to keep the soil moist and more weed free. Weed control is important; the first couple of years will be difficult and must be done by hand. Goldenseal does not have the same problem with fungus as Ginseng does, but it is somewhat susceptible and, like Ginseng, must have good drainage and airflow.

HARVESTING Rhizomes are harvested in the fall or early spring either by hand or with a root digger. Harvest starts after year 3, or 4 which is my preference, if growing from divisions or small bud/rootlets, and year 5 or 6 if grown from seed. There is a small market for the leaves which should be harvested in late spring/early summer. Data on yields varies so much and since I've only harvested small amounts I have no accurate numbers. I would estimate that a healthy crop grown under shade should yield 1,500 to 2,500 pounds of dry root per acre. Yields from woods grown patches will be less due to the difficulty in planting in consistent rows; normally harvests are less than half as much.

PROCESSING AND DRYING Goldenseal should be carefully washed before putting it into the dryer. Before washing put aside rhizomes that are for replanting. The root is about 70% water and should take about 2 weeks to dry. Turn the roots a little the first few days. Leaf should dry in about 7 days and should be turned regularly as they tend to mat together.

SELLING IT The market for Goldenseal is large and growing. Prices are rising as wildcrafted material becomes more difficult to secure, and as Goldenseal numbers diminish in the wild. Brokers or distributors will pay about $35 per pound dry for wildcrafted Goldenseal. The small amount of organic Goldenseal sells for nearly $50 per pound. This is a perfect time to plant Goldenseal. If I had forested land in Goldenseal's native habitat, I would definitely plant it now. Imagine spending $3,000 to $5,000 to plant an acre under trees; this would include root divisions, fertilizer, and some materials (chainsaw maintenance) to clear the acreage for planting. With some labor, which one person could easily handle, that acre in four years might yield 500 to 800 pounds of dry root. At $50 per pound that would be $25,000 to $40,000. Of course, lots of things could go wrong and prices might dip, but it still has lots of potential. Never forget though, that farming always has its share of unexpected disasters, so nothing is guaranteed.

MISCELLANEOUS Like Ginseng, Goldenseal is on the Appendix 2 CITES list and on the UpS primary list. We need to cultivate Goldenseal now. The longer we wait the more expensive the root will be and the more expensive for the grower to plant. Because of the cost of planting, and the need for more research, I believe that herb companies need to get more involved. Only a handful have: Eclectic, Gaia, and Herb Pharm have started to cultivate it; Herbs For Kids is promoting the use of Goldenseal substitutes and is encouraging organic cultivation. Frontier Herb Cooperative is doing an educational program, purchasing from organic growers. Frontier recently bought a farm in southern Ohio for research, that has lots of Goldenseal growing there. They are educating potential growers on how to grow it and running experiments on Goldenseal cultivation. Besides growing Goldenseal we can also educate the public on its appropriate use. A significant percentage of the Goldenseal sold in the U.S. is used by people who are about to take a drug test in the mistaken belief that it will help them pass the drug test. Goldenseal will not help you or anyone pass a drug test. What a sad waste of a good herb.

GOTU KOLA

Centella asiatica   Apiaceae

DESCRIPTION Creeping tropical plant growing 6 to 8 inches high and spreading forever. Leaves are kidney shaped, 2 inches across with serrated edges. The tiny pink flowers are hidden in the foliage and flower in summer. Native to parts of Africa, India, Sri Lanka, and Malaysia. Gotu Kola is sometimes called Brahmi. Another plant from India, *Bacopa monniera*, is also known as Brahmi and is used somewhat similarly. This is too confusing, so be careful when you hear the word Brahmi.

PROPAGATION Seed, cuttings, or divisions. Seeds germinate in 3 to 4 weeks at high temperatures, 70 to 90 degrees, and very moist conditions.

Best started in nursery flats. Cuttings are incredibly easy and can be done any time of the year. They are taken from the trailing stem and will include just 2 nodes. Cuttings root in 2 weeks and benefit from bottom heat and regular misting. Divisions can be accomplished at any time by simply pulling up rooted sections. Water heavily after dividing. I prefer to do cuttings as they are easy and you can get a transplantable plant in 4 to 6 weeks.

PLANTING Gotu Kola is tropical and will die in temperatures under about 30 degrees. I keep nursery stock in the greenhouse for propagation and harvesting but I also like to plant transplants out during the growing season for a bigger harvest. Seedlings can be transplanted out in 10 to 12 weeks either with a transplanter or by hand. Cuttings can be transplanted out directly from the cutting flats in 6 to 8 weeks, or if you pot them up then they can be hand planted in 8 weeks. Divisions should be planted as soon as you do them. You shouldn't plant outdoors until the soil and air temperature are warm in late spring or early summer. If you are planting in a greenhouse then plant as much as possible with as little pathway as necessary. Plant on 12 inch centers and you will fill up the greenhouse in 6 weeks or so. In the field I would suggest planting in rows 24 inches apart with plants 12 inches apart in the rows.

CULTIVATION Tropical perennial, hardy in Zone 10 and parts of Zone 9. Loves fertile rich soil with lots of water and high humidity. Fertilize regularly if you are repeatedly harvesting a patch. Water it every day with overhead irrigation to raise the humidity. Once established it is very good at smothering weeds but you will have to hand weed it several times. I grow it in full sun and it does very well. Some books recommend you use shade cloth, but with adequate moisture I don't think it is necessary. Other than slugs I've never had any pest problems other than the usual greenhouse pests like aphids and spider mites, and no disease problems.

HARVESTING Leaves are harvested several times a year in the greenhouse, while the outdoor planting will probably only yield one or maybe two cuttings. The roots can also be harvested when you do your last outdoor harvest. The leaves are harvested with pruning shears while the root/leaf combination is dug up and then cleaned.

PROCESSING AND DRYING The leaves are sold both fresh and dry. The leaves are about 90% water and are somewhat difficult to dry. The drying room temperature should be over 100 degrees; make sure the air flow is adequate and the dehumidifiers are going. It is best to dry it somewhat quickly or it might turn brown.

SELLING IT There is a large and growing market for Gotu Kola. It is used both fresh and dried. In southeast Asia it is eaten as a salad green and drunk as a juice. If the fresh market opens up in the U.S. we will need some local suppliers. The few companies that do buy it fresh are paying up to $8 per pound for quality herb. Most of the dry supply comes from India and it is one of the lowest quality herbs on the market. It is harvested in waste ditches there and often has a high bacterial level, ash level, and other impurities like (here I quote fellow herbalist, Richo Cech) "a Bengali cinema ticket or a battered hubcap." I personally would not touch commercial Gotu Kola. Unfortunately, the Indian material is cheap and it would be hard to compete against it. It sells for $3 to $4 per pound dry. I think several companies making medicinal products would be interested in organic Gotu Kola and paying a good price for it. If I lived in a warm area of the U.S. I would seriously look for buyers and then start growing it.

MISCELLANEOUS Gotu Kola has numerous medicinal uses including reducing inflammation, healing wounds, reducing scarring, balancing the nervous system, and improving memory. It is often used with Ginkgo in circulatory formulas to improve mental function. Gotu Kola is used in Ayurvedic medicine and if Ayurveda continues to become more popular then so will Gotu Kola.

GRAVEL ROOT, JOE PYE WEED

Eupatorium purpureum   *Asteraceae*

DESCRIPTION Grows up to 10 feet tall and spreads 2 to 3 feet. Leaves are finely toothed and grow in whorls, vanilla scented when crushed. The flowers are pink and stately and bloom in late summer. Rhizomes are thick, up to 1½ inches in diameter, hard and very bitter. Gravel Root is native to the eastern part of North America from Minnesota down to Georgia and up to New Hampshire. There are many other species of *Eupatorium* and one, *E. maculatum*, looks much like Gravel Root.

PROPAGATION Seeds, cuttings, or divisions. Seeds germinate in 3 to 4 weeks and are ready for transplanting in 12 weeks. Germination might be slightly enhanced by stratification but I don't consider it worth the effort. Cuttings root easily and are taken in late spring/early summer; they are ready for planting in about 8 to 12 weeks. Divisions are done in late fall/early spring by pulling or cutting apart the crown. This could be done when harvesting the rhizome.

PLANTING Seedlings can be transplanted into the field in late spring/early summer with a transplanter or by hand. Cuttings can be planted in late summer or held over in small pots for next spring's planting. Divisions should be planted as soon as they are divided. Spacing is 18 inches in the row and 24 to 30 inches between rows.

CULTIVATION Perennial, hardy to Zone 3. Prefers a rich fertile soil that holds moisture somewhat. It thrives on regular watering, as much as two or three times a week in the west, although it is capable of surviving for several weeks without water. Drip irrigation works well with Gravel Root. In its native environment it grows in very wet marshes or bog-like areas, but it adapts well to garden conditions. It needs full sun. It is fairly weed competitive when mature but young plants need regular weeding. The stem is very tough and you can cultivate close to it without worrying too much about damaging it. I've never had any disease or pest problems with it.

HARVESTING Rhizomes are harvested in the fall of the third year with a root digger or by hand. Due to the stems being so tall it is best to cut them before harvesting or they will be somewhat in the way.

PROCESSING AND DRYING The rhizome should be broken up and thoroughly washed. It should dry in 10 to 14 days.

SELLING IT The market is small but steady. All of the current supply comes from wildcrafted sources, so I think it would be an easy plant to sell to many companies. It sells for $7 to $8 per pound dry and companies would be willing to pay a higher price for certified organic. It is an easy and beautiful herb to grow and if you think you have a potential market for it then I would suggest growing a small crop.

MISCELLANEOUS This stately flower is perfect for the perennial flower garden and the cut flower is a beautiful addition to any flower arrangement. Medicinally it is used mainly for kidney and urinary disorders and as its common name suggests it is used for kidney stones, or gravel.

GRINDELIA

Grindelia robusta (and related species)
Asteraceae

DESCRIPTION Grows to 3 feet high and spreads up to 3 feet, looks somewhat bushy. Leaves are lanceolate, light green, and serrated on the edges. The mature plant is loaded with flowers which are yellow and are preceded by a gummy white resin which the flowers seem to grow out of. There are numerous species of Grindelia and I've harvested several but this is the only species I've cultivated.

PROPAGATION Seed or cuttings. Seed is best planted immediately after it matures in nursery flats. It grows slowly and should be transplanted the following spring by hand. Cuttings are difficult but they will root at a reasonable percentage. They should be taken in the late spring before flowering and will root in 6 to 8 weeks. They should be potted up but not planted until the following spring.

CULTIVATION Perennial, hardy to Zone 6 or maybe Zone 5. Needs excellent drainage but just average to poor fertility. Full sun and very little water, though in the dry west a watering every 2 weeks is necessary for it to thrive. Do not water near harvest time. Weed diligently when the plants are young but be careful as the stems are somewhat brittle. I've had no problems with disease or pests other than root rot associated with overwatering—although one species I've harvested grows in marshes in northern California.

HARVESTING A very fun herb to harvest. The flower buds are harvested when in the gummy resin stage in early summer. Picking is by hand and your fingers get really sticky.

PROCESSING AND DRYING It is very slow to dry even though it has little water content and is almost pure resin. Give it a couple of weeks. Do not stack in the dryer; leave it in thin layers.

SELLING IT The market for Grindelia is small for both fresh and dry. All the supply comes from wildcrafted sources, but I think if someone did grow it they could sell it to several companies who make medicinal products and are looking for organic herbs. The price is about $7 to $8 per pound dry.

MISCELLANEOUS This is one that few have grown but it makes an interesting addition to the herb garden, especially when in its gummy stage, which only lasts a couple of weeks.

HOREHOUND
Marrubium vulgare   Lamiaceae

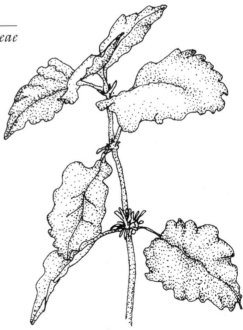

DESCRIPTION Grows up to 2 feet with a spread of 2 feet. Bush-like with numerous square, downy stems and downy gray-green opposite leaves with toothed margins. The small, white, hairy flowers bloom continuously throughout summer. It is native to western Asia, Europe, and North Africa, but has naturalized in many parts of North America.

PROPAGATION Seed, cuttings, and divisions. Seed germinates in 10 to 15 days and is ready for transplanting in 12 weeks. I find cuttings to be somewhat difficult which is unusual for a member of the mint family. They root slowly and at a low percentage. Divisions are done in early spring and are somewhat easy.

PLANTING Seedlings are transplanted by hand or transplanter, spring through fall. Cuttings are not recommended unless you just want a couple of plants. Divisions should be planted immediately after they are done. Plant at 12 inch spacing in the rows with row spacing at 24 to 30 inches.

CULTIVATION Perennial, hardy to Zone 4. Horehound can grow in the absolutely worst conditions, with poor soil and extended drought. It does require good drainage and full sun. Horehound might benefit from irrigation every 2 to 3 weeks in the west. Drip irrigation would be best as it reduces weeds and won't splash dirt on the plant. I have had no problem with pests or disease. Horehound is deer proof.

HARVESTING Harvest the above ground herb when it starts to flower which doesn't happen until the second year. Harvest with pruning shears. It should continue to produce through years 4 or 5 before it should be tilled in and replaced. Yields of dry herb should be about 2,000 pounds per acre. Do not water before harvesting.

PROCESSING AND DRYING It requires no cleaning and should dry easily in 5 to 10 days.

SELLING IT The market for Horehound is small and I don't anticipate any major changes. The dry herb sells for $8 to $10 per pound. Most of the present supply comes from wildcrafted sources so I believe it would be possible to sell to several companies who would prefer an organic supply.

MISCELLANEOUS An ideal herb for the drought tolerant landscape. It is used in thousands of medicinal lung preparations worldwide especially for treating coughs, chronic catarrh, and bronchitis.

HYSSOP

Hyssopus officinalis   *Lamiaceae*

DESCRIPTION Evergreen shrub up to 2 feet in height and spreading up to 2 or 3 feet. The leaves are opposite, shiny dark green, smooth edged, and lanceolate. The purple-blue, occasionally pink or white, flowers grow on dense spikes and bloom in summer. Hyssop is native to western Asia, central Europe, and the Mediterranean regions.

PROPAGATION Seed or cuttings. Seed germinates in 10 to 20 days and is ready to transplant into the field in 10 to 12 weeks. Cuttings are taken in late spring or late summer. They root easily and are ready for transplanting in 12 weeks, or they can be potted into larger pots and planted the following spring. Plants are spaced 24 inches in the rows, with the row spacing at 30 to 36 inches.

CULTIVATION Perennial, hardy to Zone 4. Hyssop is not sensitive to soil conditions and can grow in the worst soils with low fertility. Because it requires little water it can be grown on slopes where erosion might be a problem. As it is harvested over many years it is beneficial to improve the soil with cover crops before planting, and then add nitrogen annually in the amount of about 25 to 50 pounds per acre. It requires good drainage and full sun. In the dry west it might benefit from irrigation about once every 2 to 3 weeks, especially after harvesting. Drip irrigation would be ideal to reduce weeds and erosion if it is planted on a slope. Weeding is important the first year and second spring but after that Hyssop will be mature and fairly weed competitive and only occasional cultivation of the paths will be necessary. I've had no pest or disease problems with Hyssop and it is deer proof.

HARVESTING Harvesting starts in the second year (a small harvest is possible the first year if you get the plants out early) and will continue for up to 10 years before shrubs are tilled under and replanting is done. Peak production is from years 2 to 5. The top 6 to 10 inches of the flowering tops are picked in early summer and, if conditions are right, again in the late summer/early fall. Harvest is with pruning shears; you cut down to where the woody part of the stem starts. Harvest after the morning dew is dry and don't harvest after an overhead irrigation. Yields of 1,500 to 3,000 pounds per acre are possible with the amount depending on whether you can get a second harvest, your soil conditions, and how far down the stalk you harvest.

PROCESSING AND DRYING Hyssop is usually sold dry. The tops are 75% to 80% water and dry in 5 to 10 days. You should turn them once or twice to avoid matting together.

SELLING IT There is a good market for Hyssop and it is growing. Most of it is sold dry; the fresh market is small. The price is $9 to $12 per pound for certified organic though there is commercial Hyssop on the market that sells for much less. It is definitely worth growing and because it produces quickly you can start small and grow more if sales work out.

MISCELLANEOUS Hyssop is an exceptional herb for any landscape but especially for the drought tolerant landscape. Medicinally it has long been used for lung ailments like bronchitis and asthma though it is gaining popularity due to recent studies that show it has anti-viral activity.

LAVENDER

Lavendula angustifolia (formerly
L. vera and L. officinalis)
Lamiaceae

DESCRIPTION Small evergreen shrub growing up to 3 feet in height and spreading 3 feet. The leaves are grayish-green, linear, opposite, and up to 2½ inches in length. The tiny purple flowers appear on stalks up to 15 inches tall and bloom in summer. The water intake roots can penetrate down to 10 feet on a mature plant. There is much confusion due to popularity and long history of cultivation and breeding; consequently accurate identification is often difficult. Most of the lavender oil is harvested from Lavandin *(Lavendula x intermedia)*, a naturally occurring hybrid of *L. angustifolia* and *L. latifolia* (spike lavender).

PROPAGATION Seed or cuttings. Seed is slow and germinates poorly and unevenly. Seedlings take up to 6 months before they are ready for transplanting. Cuttings root readily especially if exposed to bottom heat and misting. Tip cuttings are done in late spring before flowering or in late summer. They will root in 4 to 8 weeks and be ready for transplanting in about 12 to 16 weeks.

PLANTING Plant seedlings or cuttings preferably in late spring/early summer, especially in Zones 4 and 5 where you want to get as much growth as possible before winter. Fall planting is okay in most zones, and even preferable in the dry warm parts of the west, where they will develop roots during the wet winter and spring, and be more drought tolerant by the next summer. Plants should be 24 to 36 inches apart in the row and rows should be 30 to 36 inches apart.

CULTIVATION Perennial, hardy to Zone 4. Tolerant of poor soils but needs good drainage. If you grow a good cover crop and add a little manure to the field before planting, you should not have to fertilize during the harvest life of the plant—which is about 10 years. Lavender likes a high pH, between 6.5 and 8.0, so many soils will have to be limed in order to raise the pH. Lavender requires full sun and very little water. Like Hyssop, it can be grown on slopes with drip irrigation to avoid erosion. Irrigate every 2 to 4 weeks in the dry west, especially after harvest or when taking cuttings. Weed carefully the first year as stems are somewhat brittle but after that you will probably only have to cultivate in spring and maybe again in summer. I've had no pest problems or disease with lavender. It is almost deer proof, although in a really dry year in California the deer did nibble on my Lavender, Thyme, and Peppermint.

HARVESTING Flowers are harvested starting in the second year. Harvest is done when the flowers are in full flower which lasts only about 10 days with *L. angustifolia*, but much longer with Lavandin cultivars. Harvest the flower stalk just under the first pair of leaves. Yields are about 150 to 250 pounds of dry flower per acre for *L. angustifolia* and 250 to 300 pounds per acre for Lavandin.

PROCESSING AND DRYING Lavender is dried and then crushed to separate out the flowers from the stalk, and then forced through a half-inch screen to further separate out the stalks. Lavender is 80% to 90% water and takes 7 to 14 days to dry.

SELLING IT The market for Lavender is large but dominated by the French, who use specialized machinery in the harvesting process. I would only suggest growing it if you have a buyer who is willing to pay top dollar for quality stuff. Prices are $10 to $15 per pound.

MISCELLANEOUS Lavender is a beautiful addition to the perennial garden especially a drought tolerant garden. The flowers are nice in any arrangement and a potpourri of Lavender is ideal in the bathroom. Medicinally Lavender is used mainly for headaches, general nervousness, and muscle spasms. The essential oil is one of the most popular herbal oils in aromatherapy.

LEMON BALM
Melissa officinalis   Labiaceae

DESCRIPTION Grows up to 3 feet and spreads to 2 feet. Lemon scented leaves are ovate, and toothed around the edges. Flowers are small, white to pale yellow, and bloom in summer. Lemon balm is native to Europe, western Asia, and northern Africa. Melissa is the Greek word for honeybee, referring to its origin as being cultivated for bees.

PROPAGATION Seed, cuttings, or divisions. Seeds grow easily and germinate in 10 to 20 days and are ready for transplanting in 12 weeks. If allowed to they will self sow and dominate your garden. Cuttings in late spring or late summer root easily and are ready for transplanting in 12 weeks. Divisions can be done in fall or spring and should be planted immediately.

PLANTING Seedlings should be planted in late spring/early summer ideally but can be planted until late fall. Cuttings can be planted at the same times. Divisions should be planted when they are done. Spacing is 12 to 18 inches in the rows and 24 to 30 between rows.

CULTIVATION Perennial, hardy to Zone 3. Lemon Balm produces best in a fertile soil with a pH of 5.0 to 7.0. Because the whole herb is harvested regularly for years, it must be fertilized annually—especially with nitrogen. Though Lemon Balm can grow in drought situations, it produces best with regular watering; once a week is adequate, and it can tolerate a fairly moist soil. Overhead watering is best I think because the plants seem to like a more humid environment. It can be grown in full sun or partial shade. In partial shade, it seems to be a bit more succulent, but with regular watering it does very well in full sun. It is somewhat difficult to weed when it starts to spread, so cultivate intensely the first year and try to eliminate as many weeds as possible. After that, it will still need regular weeding. Weeds don't hamper its growth much, but they do make harvesting more difficult—because you have to sift out the weeds. I've had no pest or disease problems with Lemon Balm.

HARVESTING The entire above ground herb is harvested when it is starting to bloom in early summer and then again in late summer/early fall before the first frost. Harvest is by hand and should be done after the dew is gone; irrigation should be avoided before harvest. Lemon Balm should continue to produce for 5 to 10 years in one location and then should be tilled under. Yields of dry herb are 1,500 to 2,500 pounds per acre.

PROCESSING AND DRYING Lemon Balm should be dried immediately with effort made to avoid bruising. If it is bruised or heats up in the field it could turn brown pretty fast. The leaf dries quickly in 4 to 7 days and is approximately 80% water. Some companies want it fresh, in which case it should be harvested in the morning and shipped before it gets hot. Don't pack it too tight, because you still want to avoid bruising. Some companies want leaf only, in which case you'll need to garble the leaf from the stem.

SELLING IT The market for it is average, but it could grow. The price is $7 to $10 per pound for certified organic, though there is some commercial stuff selling for a little less. It is an easy crop to grow. With a little marketing it is possible to sell some—but don't plant too much.

MISCELLANEOUS Lemon Balm is a nice addition to the perennial herb garden both for its smell and its hardiness. It will also do well in gardens that are not necessarily dry gardens but seldom watered. Given a chance it will take over as it reseeds prolifically. Medicinally it is used as an antispasmodic and tranquilizer, especially in children's formulas.

LICORICE

Glycyrrhiza glabra and G. uralensis   Apiaceae

DESCRIPTION *G. glabra* grows up to 5 feet in height and spreads eventually to the ends of the earth. The root is a large and deep taproot from which stolons spread as far as 20 feet if given the time. The pinnately compound pea-like leaves have 9 to 17 leaflets. The flowers are blue-violet, pea-like and borne in loose spikes, followed by oblong pods which contain 3 to 5 large seeds. *G. glabra* is native to southwest Asia and the Mediterranean region. There are several varieties including *typica*, *glandulifera*, and *beta-violacea*.

G. uralensis is native to central Asia, China, and Japan. It grows up to 3 feet in height with a 12 to 24 inch spread. Leaves are similar to *glabra* but shorter with the leaflets slightly more rounded. The violet flowers bloom in denser spikes, and the root system is not as extensive.

PROPAGATION Seed, root division, or stolon cuttings. Seed germinates in 7 to 14 days and is ready for transplanting in 12 to 16 weeks. *Glabra* seeds are very expensive at this time. Root division is done at harvest and means breaking up or cutting the main root system. Stolon cuttings are the best way to plant it. Dig up the stolons of mature plants in the fall and

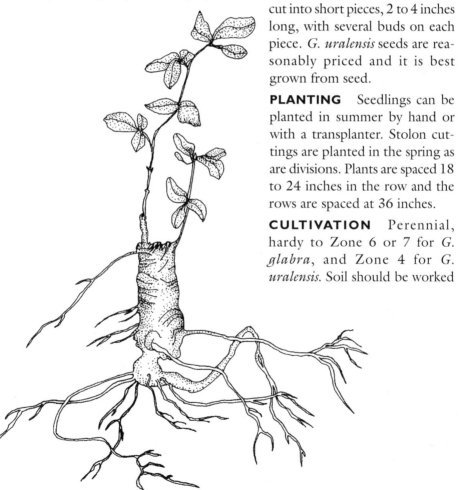

cut into short pieces, 2 to 4 inches long, with several buds on each piece. *G. uralensis* seeds are reasonably priced and it is best grown from seed.

PLANTING Seedlings can be planted in summer by hand or with a transplanter. Stolon cuttings are planted in the spring as are divisions. Plants are spaced 18 to 24 inches in the row and the rows are spaced at 36 inches.

CULTIVATION Perennial, hardy to Zone 6 or 7 for *G. glabra*, and Zone 4 for *G. uralensis*. Soil should be worked deeply and manured and cover cropped the year before planting. Good drainage is essential and watering should be somewhat minimal. I once walked a farm I was working on with Hu Shu Lin, a famous Chinese pharmacognosist, and an expert on cultivation of Chinese herbs. After telling me that my Astragalus was in soil that was too rich (he said the same to Richo Cech at his farm) we then walked past some Licorice. Once more he shook his head and soon thereafter we walked near some rocky poor soil and he lifted his head and said, "good soil for Licorice." I guess the key with Licorice is to have relatively dry, well drained soil that isn't too fertile. It likes a high pH of 6.5 to 8.0. It requires full sun. Weed diligently in the first two years but, by the third year, it will crowd out most weeds. I've never had any problem with pests or disease. Growth is slow the first year or two but after that watch out. The stalks should be cut down each fall.

HARVESTING The roots and stolons are harvested in the fall after 3 to 5 years. Do not let the plants flower at any time before harvest as it will negatively affect the quality of the root. The roots will have to be dug by hand due to the depth. Licorice is like Comfrey in that once you plant it you will always have it, unless you remove every single root and stolon piece. Most likely it will come back and you will have a harvest in another 3 to 5 years. Dry root yields can be as high as 5,000 pounds per acre.

PROCESSING AND DRYING Thoroughly wash the roots and stolons. The roots will need to be cut vertically in order to facilitate drying. Drying time is slow, 10 to 20 days or more, depending on temperatures in the dryer.

SELLING IT The market for Licorice is very large and growing. Most of the American supply of *G. glabra* comes from Europe; the Chinese Licorice comes from China. Organic Licorice from Europe sells here for $10 to $15 per pound. Commercial Licorice sells for $4 to $6 per pound. There is potential for growing and selling it here. Though somewhat easy to grow don't forget that once you commit some land to Licorice it might always stay in Licorice.

MISCELLANEOUS For many years growers were buying seeds and plants that they thought were Licorice but were actually Goat's Rue (*Galega officinalis*). I purchased such a plant in 1980 and I'll bet there is more Goat's Rue in the U.S. than Licorice today. One Licorice species native to the U.S., *G. lepidota*, is used by some American herbalists. However, my experience with it is that it lacks the sweetness of *G. glabra* and *G. uralensis*, and thus contains little *glycyrrhizin*. Licorice has many medicinal uses including being a cough suppressant and anti-inflammatory for ulcers. It stimulates the adrenals, and is used for numerous things in Chinese Medicine—where it is the most used herb after Ginseng. Licorice can have side effects if taken regularly, including raising blood pressure so read more about it before taking large doses daily.

LOBELIA
Lobelia inflata   Lobeliaceae

DESCRIPTION Grows up to 24 inches in height with a spread of 6 to 12 inches. Hairy herb with ovate, toothed leaves. Flowers are light blue to white, very small, bloom in summer and are followed by inflated seed pods. Lobelia is native to central and eastern North America. There are over 360 species worldwide, many of which have been used medicinally.

PROPAGATION By seed; tiny seeds germinate in 2 to 3 weeks. They are light dependent, so they must not be covered too deeply or they won't germinate. Seeds must be kept wet but not flooded; water flats gently so as not to wash away the seeds. Seedlings should be thinned out while in the nursery flats: one plant per cell. Seedlings are ready for transplanting in 8 to 12 weeks.

PLANTING Seedlings are transplanted in late spring with a transplanter or by hand. Water immediately after planting. Plant on 9 to 12 inch spacing in rows, with rows at 24 inches.

CULTIVATION Annual herb can be planted anywhere. Prefers a rich loamy soil and full sun or partial shade. A good manure spreading followed by a year of healthy cover crops should prepare the soil adequately. Irrigate often if necessary, twice a week in the west, preferably from an overhead source to raise the humidity. Weed constantly, especially when the plants are small. Plants will definitely produce more if weeded. I've had no pest problems or disease in my Lobelia plantings.

HARVESTING The entire above ground portion is harvested after some seed capsules have developed. It is important to allow it to develop green seeds due to the high concentration of an important constituent, lobeline, contained in the seeds. Plants are harvested with pruning shears and lots of caution. Lobelia is somewhat toxic and can be absorbed through the skin or by breathing it. When harvesting or processing wear a mask or respirator, gloves, long pants, long sleeves, and eye protection. Lobelia is called pukeweed for a good reason and believe me, you do not want to get sick from it. Yields of dry herb are 1,000 to 1,500 pounds per acre.

PROCESSING AND DRYING Herb dries easily in 5 to 7 days. Once again care should be taken when handling it. The herb is approximately 75% water.

SELLING IT There is a fairly good market for Lobelia. The price for dry herb is $12 to $20 per pound. Much of what is sold on the market is from wildcrafted sources which has been shown to be of inferior medicinal quality (Krochmal, Wilken, and Chien 1972). This is a good herb to grow and try to sell. The price is reasonable and a good grower could compete easily with high quality. Start out small and grow more if you can sell it.

MISCELLANEOUS Medicinally, Lobelia is mainly used as an antispasmodic—especially for bronchial spasms. It is also used to reduce the symptoms of tobacco withdrawal, because of lobeline's similarity to nicotine. Only small doses should be used. Large doses are toxic and can cause a variety of problems. Lobelia *inflata* is not a candidate for the flower garden, but many other species of Lobelia are, including *L. cardinalis* and *L. syphilitica*.

LOVAGE

Levisticum officinale   Apiaceae

DESCRIPTION Grows up to 6 feet in height with a spread of up to 3 feet. The leaves are large, dark green, and celery like. The stem is hollow and the flowers, which bloom in summer, are small, greenish-yellow in an umbel 2 to 3 inches across on the top of the plant. The seeds are large and elliptical with 3 prominent wings. The roots are white and fleshy. The whole plant is aromatic.

PROPAGATION Seeds or divisions. The seeds lose their viability within a few months so plant them in the summer or fall after harvesting them, or stratify them in the refrigerator until spring and plant them then. Fall planted seed will germinate in the greenhouse but if planted outdoors they probably won't germinate until spring. Seeds will germinate in 2 to 3 weeks and will be ready for transplanting in about 10 to 12 weeks. Divisions are done in the fall or early spring and are planted immediately.

PLANTING Seedlings are transplanted in late spring/early summer. Divisions are planted in the fall or early spring. Spacing is 18 inches in the rows and the rows are 24 to 30 inches apart.

CULTIVATION Perennial, hardy to Zone 4. Likes a rich, deep soil though it will grow in nearly any soil. Needs good drainage; I've had several plants rot from poor drainage. Irrigate once a week in the dry parts of the country. A pH of 5.5 to 7.5 should be adequate. If you harvest the leaves annually you will need to fertilize annually with a balanced fertilizer and extra nitrogen. I've never had any major pest or disease problems with Lovage as long as it has good drainage. The plant should be replaced after 4 years as production starts to diminish.

HARVESTING Leaves are harvested starting the second year in late spring, before the flower stalk appears, and then again in the late summer/early fall. Harvest with pruning shears. The root is harvested in the fall of the third or fourth year. It can be dug by hand or with a root digger. Yields of dried leaf are close to 1,000 pounds per acre per year. Root yields are 1,000 to 1,300 pounds of dry root per acre.

PROCESSING AND DRYING   Leaves should be carefully handled and dried immediately. The water content of the leaves is between 80% and 90%. The root should be thoroughly washed and then vertically and horizontally cut into smaller pieces to facilitate drying. Drying time should be 5 to 15 days. Roots are about 80% water.

SELLING IT   The market in the U.S. for Lovage is small. In this country, we just haven't realized its potential. In Europe, it is much more popular. The root sells for about $7 to $8 per pound. I would not recommend planting it until the market for it grows.

MISCELLANEOUS   Personally I think Lovage is a great herb. The root is an excellent diuretic and diaphoretic. For me it works a lot like Osha root. Also, due to the fact that Osha is proving nearly impossible to cultivate, and is perhaps being over-picked, I think Lovage is a good substitute for Osha. The leaves make a fine addition to salads and salad dressing, soups, and even stir fried veggies. The leaves seem to enhance the flavors of whatever they are mixed with.

MARSHMALLOW
Althaea officinalis   Malvaceae

DESCRIPTION   Grows up to 4 feet in height and spreads up to 3 feet. Leaves are ovate, toothed, grayish-green, and velvety-hairy. Flowers are white to pale pink and bloom in summer. The root is fast growing, dark outside and white inside. Marshmallow is native to the European continent.

PROPAGATION   Seed or divisions. Seed germinates in 3 to 5 weeks and is ready for transplanting in about 10 to 12 weeks. The root crown can be divided when harvesting in the fall.

PLANTING   Seedlings can be transplanted in late spring/early summer with a transplanter or by hand. Divisions can be planted in the fall or stored in sawdust over winter and then planted in spring. Spacing is 18 inches in the rows and 24 to 30 inches between the rows.

CULTIVATION   Perennial, hardy to Zone 4. Likes a deep fertile soil. Likes water and can grow in areas of poor drainage but does better with at least adequate drainage. A well manured field followed by a good cover crop the year before planting should provide all the nutrients needed. Needs to be irrigated deeply at least once a week in the west. Marshmallow needs full sun. Young plants should be intensely weeded the first year. Though somewhat weed competitive the crop will need to be cultivated several times to reduce the competition. The roots tend to get pithy and rotten in spots after a couple of years. I've had no major pest or disease problems with Marshmallow.

HARVESTING Roots are harvested in the fall of the second year. Roots harvested in the fall seem to have a higher mucilage content than those harvested in winter or spring (Cech, 1995). They can be dug with a root digger or by hand. The expected yield is 1,000 to 1,500 pounds of dry root per acre.

PROCESSING AND DRYING The roots should be washed and then cut vertically and horizontally to facilitate drying. They are about 80% water and dry in 5 to 10 days. They reabsorb water easily so take extra care to store them in a dry spot.

SELLING IT There is an average market for Marshmallow. The going price is $6 to $9 per pound for certified organic. It is an easy plant to grow and I think it is worth taking the risk of finding a buyer. It would fill the niche if you had some wet ground that needed a crop.

MISCELLANEOUS Marshmallow is a nice plant for the perennial flower bed. A few flowers are a colorful addition to a salad. The plant is very mucilaginous; the chewed leaves make a soothing oral poultice and are soothing to irritated tissue internally as well as externally. It is wonderful for soothing irritated urinary tracts caused by infections and for any prostate irritations. Marshmallow also has a slight immune enhancing action. Contrary to popular belief, Marshmallow does not produce white, soft, mushy fruits.

MEADOWSWEET

Filipendula ulmaria   Rosaceae

DESCRIPTION Grows up to 6 feet in height with a spread of 18 to 24 inches. The compound leaves have 2 to 5 pairs of leaflets with finely serrated edges and are green above and white and downy below. The flowers are creamy white, almond scented, absolutely beautiful, and bloom in summer. Meadowsweet (*F. ulmaria*) is native to Europe but there is a species, *F. rubra*, which is native to the midwest.

PROPAGATION Seed or divisions. Seeds germinate in 2 to 4 weeks and are ready for transplanting in about 12 weeks. Divisions can be taken from mature plants in the fall or spring.

PLANTING Seedlings can be transplanted into the field in late spring/early summer with a transplanter or by hand. Divisions are planted when they are done. Spacing is 18 inches in the row and 24 to 30 inches between rows.

CULTIVATION Perennial, hardy to Zone 3. Likes a fertile soil. Fertilize with manure or compost before planting and then fertilize annually with a balanced fertilizer and extra nitrogen. Thrives on lots of water and can stand a poorly drained soil much like Marshmallow. Must be irrigated often in the west and even in the wet summer areas if there is an extended drought. Irrigate at least twice a week in the west from overhead sources. Likes full sun but will grow in partial shade in hot areas. I've had zero pest trouble, and the only disease was when I tried to grow it in full shade which it did not like. It can remain in the ground and remain productive for a long time though it might be beneficial to divide it after a few years.

HARVESTING The leaf and flowers are harvested in early summer as the flowers start to open. Usually a second cutting can be had in late summer/early fall in areas with a long growing season. The harvesting is done with pruning shears. The first year you might get a small late harvest but starting in year 2 you will be at full production. Yields are about 1,000 pounds of dry leaf and flower per acre.

PROCESSING AND DRYING It dries quickly in about 3 to 5 days and it should be turned the first couple of days. The leaf and flower are about 70% water. The flowers are somewhat fine so you might want to put something under the screens (if you use screens) to catch the flowers that have sifted through.

SELLING IT Meadowsweet sells for between $9 and $14 per pound. Most of it comes from wildcrafted or organic sources in Europe. It would be easy to market certified organic Meadowsweet grown in the good old U.S.A. I would recommend this as a small scale crop; it is somewhat easy to grow and harvest, and I think the price is okay and the market is available.

MISCELLANEOUS This is perhaps my favorite herb. This is often the focus of my perennial flower garden and also my herb garden. The flowers are absolutely mesmerizing to me and make excellent cut flowers. Medicinally it was from Meadowsweet that salicylic acid was first isolated and aspirin was named after it. *Filipendula* used to be *spirea* and from *a spirea* we got aspirin. The herb is used for the same illnesses that aspirin is but, unlike aspirin, it is used for irritations or ulcerations of the gastrointestinal tract, due to its own natural buffering agents.

MILK THISTLE

Silybum marianum   *Asteraceae*

DESCRIPTION Grows up to 4 feet in height and spreads up to 2 feet. The large leaves have spiny margins with milky white variegated veins. The purple flowers are up to 2 inches across, and are followed by large black seeds each bearing white hairs, similar to Dandelion. Native to the Mediterranean, Milk Thistle has naturalized on the west coast of the U.S.

PROPAGATION Milk Thistle is propagated from seeds which germinate in 10 to 14 days. The large seeds need to be sown ½ inch deep either in nursery flats or outdoors.

PLANTING Seeds can be direct sown in the field in the summer to early fall or in early spring. Nursery seedlings that are spring planted should be put out as soon as weather permits. For fall planting from nursery starts, sow the seeds in mid to late summer. If sowing directly into the field plant seeds every 4 to 6 inches and then thin to 18 to 24 inches. Transplants should also be on 18 to 24 inch spacing in the rows. The rows should be spaced at 4 feet to allow access for harvest. This implies harvesting by hand. If harvesting with a combine, the rows can be on 24 inch spacing.

CULTIVATION Annual or biennial, can be grown anywhere with a growing season of at least 150 days. In areas with warm winters it can be grown as a biennial, allowing for more growth and a larger harvest. Milk Thistle can grow in the absolute worst soils and can survive and even thrive in dry conditions. Still, I had a plant come up in a compost pile a few years ago that was over 6 feet in width and had dozens of flower stalks. I think it is okay to grow it on poor soils but a little manure on the field won't hurt. It does require good drainage and full sun. If summer or fall planted, irrigate until the winter rains come. If spring planted, in the dry west, irrigate regularly until it is established, and then once every 2 weeks should do. Cultivate when the plants are young; once they have grown a bit they will smother most of the weeds. I've never had any pest or disease problems with Milk Thistle.

HARVESTING The seeds of the Milk Thistle are harvested. They are somewhat difficult to harvest due to the uneven flowering of the various plants in the field. When hand harvesting cut the flower head off when the white pappus tuft starts to develop just after the flower dries up. You will have to harvest every few days for a couple of weeks. Be careful when harvesting, as the spines on Milk Thistle are sharp and can penetrate a tank. Wear stout gloves, glasses, long pants and shirt, and thick boots. Yields from hand harvesting will average about one quarter pound of seed per plant (Cech, 1995). If harvesting with a combine the seeds are harvested when the first plants have matured, and are probably ready to drop, but most of the field is near ready. Seeds do continue to ripen after they are harvested. Yields of up to 2,000 pounds per acre can be expected.

PROCESSING AND DRYING Cut flower heads are placed in a burlap bag and allowed to dry for 5 to 7 days. The flower heads are then run through a hammermill with a one inch screen. The material can then be run through a seed cleaner, winnowed in the open air on a windy day, or you can supply wind with a fan. The seeds are then ready.

SELLING IT Milk Thistle is one of the biggest selling herbs in the world. The price is $10 to $14 per pound for certified organic and a few dollars less per pound for wildcrafted. Most of the Milk Thistle today comes from South America and Europe. I think that soon more growers will attempt to grow Milk Thistle on a commercial scale in the U.S. It can grow on fairly marginal soils, so it might just find a niche on some over-grazed land along the California or Oregon coast. On a small scale it might still be practical if you can get the absolute top dollar for the best quality seed available. There's no doubt that hand harvesting produces a more uniform quality because all of the seeds are harvested when they are just ripe.

MISCELLANEOUS It is an interesting plant for the herb garden but don't let it go to seed. In some areas, milk thistle planting can actually be restricted. Medicinally Milk Thistle has the wondrous ability to protect the liver from damage and also to heal the liver after it has been damaged.

MOTHERWORT

Leonurus cardiaca   *Lamiaceae*

DESCRIPTION Grows up to 5 feet in height with a spread of 24 inches. The leaves are lobed, toothed, and hairy. The flowers are pinkish-white and grow in numerous many-flowered whorls, blooming in summer. Native to Europe, it has naturalized in many parts of the U.S.

PROPAGATION Motherwort is propagated from seeds, which germinate in 2 to 3 weeks. Nursery starts are ready for transplanting in 8 to 12 weeks.

PLANTING Nursery seedlings are ready for transplanting in late spring/early summer; it can be done using a transplanter or by hand. Plants are spaced 12 to 15 inches in the row, with row spacing at 24 to 30 inches.

CULTIVATION Perennial, hardy to Zone 3. Grows in almost any soil but production will increase if you give it a relatively rich soil. Manuring followed by a cover crop the year before planting should be sufficient—or a manure spreading several weeks before planting. Motherwort does require adequate drainage; it can grow in full sun or partial shade. Though it is somewhat drought tolerant when mature, it does like water, and should be irrigated once a week in the drier parts of the country during the growing season. Either drip or overhead irrigation would be okay. Weed it often because, even though it is somewhat weed competitive, the weeds will make harvesting more difficult. I've had no pest or disease problems with Motherwort.

HARVESTING   The above ground herb is harvested when the plant is in flower. There is usually a small crop the first year and then two cuttings a year after that for several years. At some point productivity will diminish and the crop should be turned under. Harvest by hand. Yields of 1,200 to 2,500 pounds per acre can be expected. Yield depends on whether the whole herb is sold or just the leaf and tops.

PROCESSING AND DRYING   If selling fresh, be careful when handling it, as it does heat up quickly. If selling dried leaf and tops, you can garble fresh leaf by cutting off the top 10 inches or so and stripping the leaves from the stem before putting them into the dryer. This will save dryer space. Motherwort dries easily in 3 to 5 days, though it should be turned the first couple of days. The leaves and tops are about 80% water; with the stem added, it is less than 75% water.

SELLING IT   The market for Motherwort is fairly substantial. The price for dry Motherwort is $9 to $11 per pound. This is a worthwhile crop if you can find a market for it. Make sure you are clear with the buyer on the amount of stem to be included.

MISCELLANEOUS   Motherwort makes an interesting addition to the flower garden mainly because of its attractive leaves which look somewhat like marijuana leaves but have very different medicinal actions. Motherwort, as its species name cardiaca implies, is used for heart conditions—specifically tachycardia. Very little research on Motherwort has been done, but it has a long history of safe and effective medicinal use.

MUGWORT

Artemisia vulgaris; Artemisia douglasiana
Asteraceae

DESCRIPTION   Grows up to 6 feet in height and spreads to 3 feet; continues to spread via underground rhizomes. Very aromatic with purple stem and dark, deeply toothed leaves, green on top with gray underneath. The flowers are tiny, red-brown, and bloom in summer. *A. douglasiana* has grayer leaves and longer and more significant flowers. *A. vulgaris* is native to Asia and has naturalized in the eastern U.S. *A. douglasiana* is native to the western U.S.

PROPAGATION Seeds or divisions. Seeds germinate in 2 to 4 weeks and are ready for transplanting in 10 to 12 weeks. Divisions are done in spring or fall. A two year old plant will yield close to 100 divisions. It is probably possible to propagate from cuttings but I haven't tried it yet; I've gotten all the plants I need from divisions.

PLANTING Seedlings are transplanted in late spring/early summer and divisions are transplanted in fall or early summer. Plants are spaced 24 inches in the row and rows are spaced at 36 inches.

CULTIVATION Perennial, hardy to Zone 3. Likes a fairly rich soil with good drainage. It grows best in full sun and should be watered, in the dry parts of the country, every 10 days. Mugwort is an aggressive grower; it will fill in a large area in a short time. Be wary where you plant it as it is difficult to control. If you are aggressively harvesting it then it should be fertilized annually with a balanced fertilizer and some additional nitrogen. Weed it after planting, but soon thereafter it will probably be the weed. I've had no pest problems with Mugwort nor any disease. If you have problems keeping plants alive, grow Mugwort; it would probably survive a nuclear holocaust.

HARVESTING Above ground herb is harvested as it starts to flower. Pick it with pruning shears. It is possible to get two cuttings a year. Yields of dry herb will be several thousand pounds per acre but I can't say exactly as I've harvested very little.

PROCESSING AND DRYING Most buyers would prefer leaf and tops only though I've seen cut-and-sifted Mugwort with stem for sale. Mugwort dries easily but it should be turned regularly as it tends to mat together.

SELLING IT The market is small for its medicinal value, but there is a small market for its potpourri value. The price for dry herb is $8 to $10 per pound. If I knew I could sell it I would not hesitate to grow it but the market is small and hard to locate.

MISCELLANEOUS When I lived in northern California we used to harvest Mugwort when we were camping and then put it around and under our sleeping bags to facilitate dreaming. Dream pillows made out of Mugwort are quite common. Of the two species I prefer *A. douglasiana* which I think has an incredible smell, one of my favorites. I used to harvest it as a cut flower and sold quite a bit. *A. vulgaris* is the herb used to make "moxa" which is used in acupuncture. Mugwort is a popular herb in Chinese medicine.

MULLEIN

Verbascum thapsus; Verbascum olympicum
Scrophulariaceae

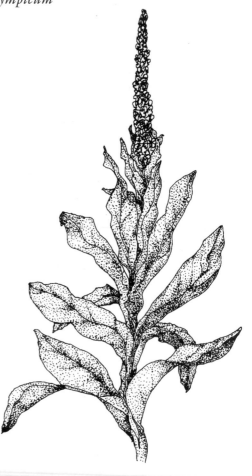

DESCRIPTION Both species grow up to 8 feet with a spread of 3 feet. Leaves are gray-green, large, woolly, oval to lanceolate, and grow in a rosette the first year. The second year smaller leaves grow on the flower stalk. Flowers are yellow, and grow in a dense spike-like cluster and bloom during summer. One big difference between the two species is that *thapsus* has flowers that cling tightly to the stalk and bloom slowly over several months. *Olympicum* tends to bloom over a shorter period and the flowers are more open and showy. Both are native to Europe and Asia; *V. thapsus* has naturalized throughout North America.

PROPAGATION Mullein is propagated from seed which germinates in 10 to 20 days. Started in the greenhouse they are ready for transplanting in 8 to 12 weeks.

PLANTING Seedlings are transplanted into the field in late spring/early summer with a transplanter or by hand. Plants are spaced at 24 inches in the row, 30 to 36 inches between rows.

CULTIVATION Biennial, hardy to Zone 3. Mullein is capable of growing in pavement. It doesn't require a rich soil but it does produce best when the soil is fertilized somewhat. It prefers full sun and good drainage, though I've seen it survive in poorly drained areas. It needs very little irrigation. In the dry west, water until the plants are established, and then after that once every 2 weeks or more should do. It can survive without any water for up to 6 months in parts of the west. I've never had any pest or disease problems with Mullein.

HARVESTING Leaf is harvested in the spring of the second year before a flower stalk appears. Cut the whole plant at the base with pruning shears and throw out any bad leaves. Flowers are harvested in the late morning as they open. *V. thapsus* flowers only last one day, and in my humble opinion are too difficult to harvest, so I only harvest flowers from *V. olympicum*. *V. olympicum* flowers can be stripped off the stalk with your hands quite easily.

PROCESSING AND DRYING The leaves dry slowly due to the thickness of the midrib and can take up to 2 weeks. They must be turned regularly. The flowers are generally sold fresh. They can be dried easily but either way be careful not to let them heat up as you harvest them. When harvesting the flowers you often have to compete with the bees. Both the flowers and leaves are about 75% water.

SELLING IT There is a steady market for Mullein but not large. The flowers are highly sought after by companies making ear oil with it. The leaf price is $5 to $9 per pound dry and the flower price is $15 to $18 per pound for fresh. *V. olympicum* is worth growing as a fresh flower if you are anywhere near a company who makes ear oil. Mullein leaf is so common that it probably isn't worth growing unless you have it pre-sold.

MISCELLANEOUS *V. olympicum* and another species, *V. bombyciferum*, are absolutely gorgeous in the garden. They are perhaps the showiest flower in the herb garden. Even the leaves are attractive, especially *V. bombyciferum's*. Mullein can reseed prolifically so be prepared for it.

NETTLE

Urtica dioica   Urticaceae

DESCRIPTION Grows up to 6 feet with a spread of 2 to 3 feet or forever. Leaves are dark green, deeply toothed, and covered with stinging hairs. Flowers bloom in summer and are tiny, green, and grow on hanging clusters. Roots are forever creeping and yellow. Nettle is native to Europe and Asia but has naturalized throughout North America. There are over 50 species of nettles that grow worldwide, many of which are harvested for food or medicine.

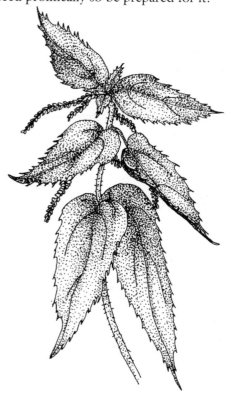

PROPAGATION Seed, cuttings, or divisions. Seeds germinate in 10 to 15 days and are ready for transplanting in 8 to 12 weeks. Cuttings can be taken in late spring or late summer and even though they root okay it is my least favorite way to propagate it. Divisions are easy and are done off mature plants in fall or early spring.

PLANTING Seedlings are transplanted in late spring/early summer or if started in summer can be fall planted. Divisions should be planted after they are done in fall or spring. Plants are spaced 12 to 18 inches in the row; the rows are 24 to 30 inches apart.

CULTIVATION Perennial, hardy to Zone 2. Nettles grow best in a rich, fertile soil. Soil should be high in organic matter and rich in nitrogen with a pH of 6.0 to 7.5. After harvesting each year fertilize with a balanced fertilizer and extra nitrogen. Nettle can grow in full sun or partial shade; however, if it is in full sun in a hot area it will need lots of moisture. In the dry west irrigate once or twice a week from overhead sprinklers. Nettles like a lot of water but not a bog-like situation. Weed thoroughly the first year and continue to cultivate as needed but it will out compete most weeds. Nettle can grow in the same spot indefinitely. I've had no disease problems with nettle. Certain caterpillars will eat Nettle leaves but if you harvest them often the caterpillars don't have a chance to become established. If you let the plants flower they will be attacked but they won't cause enough damage to undermine seed production. As the leaves age they develop oxalate crystals so for culinary use harvest early.

HARVESTING Leaves are harvested before the flowers start the first year. From year two on you should be able to harvest 2, 3, or even 4 times a year depending on the fertility of your soil and the length of your growing season. When harvesting just cut the plant to the ground, taking care not to sting yourself too badly. The roots are harvested in the fall of the second year either by hand or with a root digger. The seeds are harvested when they ripen.

PROCESSING AND DRYING Nettle leaf is easy to dry and should take about 3 to 5 days. The roots should be washed and then dried. The roots are 75% to 80% water while the herb is about 85% water.

SELLING IT The market for Nettle is fairly large and could get much bigger due to its many uses. The going price is $7 to $11 per pound for organic, dry leaf. The root is seldom sold but is catching on. Some companies are purchasing fresh Nettle. I think it is a good crop because most of it still comes from wildcrafted sources, it is easy to grow, and it is gaining in popularity. I wouldn't plant much unless I had it pre-sold though.

MISCELLANEOUS My friend David Hoffman said at a recent conference, "If you don't know what herb to take, take Nettle. It's good for everything." You really can't take too much Nettle. Medicinally it is used for allergies, excessive internal bleeding, arthritis, skin conditions, and much more. The roots are being used for enlarged prostates and one extensive study showed conclusively how well it can work (Belaiche and Lievoux, 1991). Nettle is a wonderful food when steamed or pickled, one of the most nutrient rich foods there is. Nettle definitely goes with me on my journeys around the galaxy.

OATS

Avena sativa   Graminaceae

DESCRIPTION Do I have to describe Oats? Everyone must know them. Oats grow up to 6 feet high and spread 6 to 9 inches. The leaves are green; the flowers bloom in late spring to summer.

PROPAGATION Oats are grown from seed which is sown in the field and germinates in 7 to 10 days.

PLANTING The seeds are sown directly in the field in either the fall or spring. The seeds are either broadcast or drilled in. If broadcast they are lightly worked into the soil.

CULTIVATION Annual, capable of being grown anywhere. Produces best in a fertile soil with adequate moisture and reasonable drainage. Spring planted Oats need irrigation in the dry west. Oats require full sun. The biggest pests I've had with Oats, literally, are the deer that like to graze on it.

HARVESTING Oat seeds are harvested while in the milky stage. This stage only lasts for about a week so you will need to monitor the plants almost daily as they start to flower. The green seed is harvested by hand. If harvesting the entire "straw" you pick during the milk stage but harvest to the ground.

PROCESSING AND DRYING Milky Oats are mainly sold fresh. Drying them is easy, taking 4 to 7 days.

SELLING IT There is a small but steady market for fresh Oats. If you live near a company that makes medicinal products and uses Oats then you might have a market. The price is $4 to $8 for fresh Oats, and dry milky seeds go for $10 to $14 per pound. Dry Oat straw sells for $3 to $4 per pound.

MISCELLANEOUS Though mainly known for their food value, Oats have long been used for medicine. Oats soothe the nervous system and studies show that they work well with withdrawal symptoms. With so many people trying to get away from cigarettes and coffee, Oats will always have a market.

PASSIONFLOWER
Passiflora incarnata   Passifloraceae

DESCRIPTION Deciduous vine capable of growing up to 30 feet in one season. The deeply lobed green leaves grow 4 to 6 inches. The fragrant lavender to white flowers are 2 to 3 inches across and amongst the most beautiful of flowers. They bloom in summer, followed by 2 inch long yellow fruits which are called Maypops and are quite edible. This is one of the hardiest of over 500 species worldwide. It is native to the southeastern U.S. from Florida to Virginia, across to Ohio and down to Texas.

PROPAGATION Seed, cuttings, divisions, or layering. Seeds germinate in 3 to 5 weeks and benefit from high heat. Cuttings root in 3 to 6 weeks and benefit from misting and bottom heat. Divisions need to have some of the main tuber attached; otherwise they are just like a cutting. I made that mistake several times when I first started growing it thinking I had a ready-to-go plant. Layering is fairly easy but only nets a few plants. My preference is cuttings which are best taken in the late summer/early fall.

PLANTING Plant outdoors in late spring after it has warmed up. Passionflower prefers to grow up something, so when possible plant near fences, trellises, or whatever. It can be just allowed to spread on the surface also. Plant on 18 to 24 inch centers. Make sure your plants are well rooted before planting them.

CULTIVATION Perennial, hardy to Zone 6 and maybe down to Zone 4 with heavy mulching. Passionflower grows in relatively poor sandy and acidic soils but does a little better with some fertilizer. Apply a small amount of slow release fertilizer like cottonseed meal when you plant. It does require good drainage, and will need to be irrigated in the dry west. I water weekly with overhead sprinklers though drip would work fine also. I've had no pest or disease problems with Passionflower but I haven't grown very much of it.

HARVESTING The above ground parts of the plant are harvested when it is in flower. I use pruning shears and usually gawk at the flowers for a long time before I finally get anything picked. You get one harvest a year and each plant will produce indefinitely. The plants multiply and spread as they age so the older the patch the greater the harvest.

PROCESSING AND DRYING Passionflower is sold both fresh and dry. It starts to decompose quickly so handle it with care and get it into the drying room as soon as possible. If shipping fresh pick it early and pack it before it gets hot. Passionflower is about 80% water.

SELLING IT The market for Passionflower is average. Most of the supply is wildcrafted. The average price is $7 to $9 per pound for dry herb. It is a difficult herb to grow because it prefers something to climb on. I would not recommend growing it except on a small scale for a good customer, or just for the sheer joy of it.

MISCELLANEOUS Passionflowers are truly an aphrodisiac. Try looking at one and not getting a warm fuzzy feeling. The fruits are edible; John Muir considered them to be the best tasting fruit he'd ever eaten. Of course it was when he was young, walking across the country and nearly starving.

PLANTAIN

Plantago lanceolata; Plantago major
Plantaginaceae

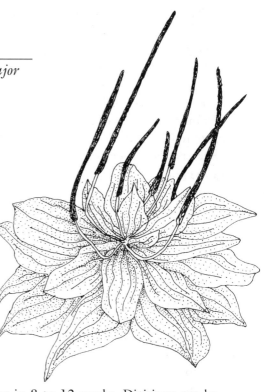

DESCRIPTION Grows up to 16 inches tall and spreads up to 16 inches. Leaves grow in a basal rosette and are ovate to lanceolate, 6 to 9 inches long. The flowers are produced on thin stalks, are tiny, yellow-green, and bloom in summer. There are many species of Plantain used medicinally. Plantain has naturalized throughout the universe. In the western U.S. we have mainly *P. lanceolata* whereas in the eastern U.S. we have mainly *P. major*.

PROPAGATION Seed or divisions. Seed germinates in 1 to 2 weeks and is ready for transplanting in 8 to 12 weeks. Divisions can be done any time of the year and are very easy to do.

PLANTING Plant seedlings or divisions any time from spring through fall. Spacing should be 12 inches in the row and the rows spaced at 24 to 30 inches.

CULTIVATION Perennial, hardy to Zone 2. Plantain will grow in any soil but produces best in a soil of average fertility and drainage. If you continue to harvest it for several years it should be fertilized annually with nitrogen. Plantain will grow in full sun or partial shade and will produce best if watered once a week in the dry west. Weed heavily when young and continue to cultivate when needed. I've never had any pest problems or disease. Plantain is the hardiest plant in the universe.

HARVESTING Leaves are harvested before flowering. Two to four harvests are possible annually starting in the second year. Cut the leaves with pruning shears. You can continue to harvest the same patch for several years but at some point it should be tilled in and replanted elsewhere. A yield of 2,000 pounds of dry herb per acre is possible.

PROCESSING AND DRYING Plantain turns brown easily so dry it immediately. It dries easily in 3 to 7 days. Plantain leaves are about 85% water.

SELLING IT Though it is a weed there is a lot of Plantain sold. It sells for $8 to $11 per pound dry. Nearly all of the supply is from wildcrafting.

Until recently I don't think anyone was concerned about our Plantain supply. In mid-1997 though a batch of Foxglove was sold as Plantain, resulting in several people being poisoned and hospitalized. The Foxglove/Plantain came from Europe and was sold to an American herb company. That company sold it to other companies as "domestic wildcrafted Plantain." Claiming it was "domestic wildcrafted Plantain" was an out and out lie. Since then many people have been more concerned about where their Plantain originated. If I had had more organic Plantain last year I could have sold it all very easily. I think for the next few years memories will linger and anyone with certified organic Plantain will be able to sell it.

MISCELLANEOUS Plantain is used mainly in formulas to facilitate healing of wounds. The first poultice I ever used was chewing some Plantain leaf in my mouth and then putting it on a bee sting. It of course relieved the pain instantly and reduced the inflammation.

POKEROOT

Phytolacca americana   *Phytolaccaceae*

DESCRIPTION Grows up to 12 feet tall and 3 to 5 feet wide. Very imposing plant with a thick hollow stem which divides in two just above the ground. The leaves are alternate, lanceolate, and grow to 12 inches. The flowers have a white calyx but no petals and are followed by intensely purple berries hanging in long clusters. The root is very thick and long with many sideshoots. It is native to eastern North America.

PROPAGATION Seeds or divisions. Seeds are either fall planted outdoors, or stratified and spring sown in flats or direct. Divisions are done in late fall or early spring and require cutting the crown with leaf buds attached.

PLANTING Seedlings started in the nursery are transplanted into the field in late spring/early summer. Seeds that are directly sown in the fall or early spring will not germinate until the soil warms up. Divisions can be done at harvest time in the fall and stored in sawdust until spring and planted then. Space plants 18 inches in the rows with the rows spaced at 24 to 30 inches.

CULTIVATION Perennial, hardy to Zone 3. Pokeroot likes a deep and fertile soil. It grows best in full sun and likes reasonable drainage. It likes it moist so in the west it will need irrigation once a week from overhead or drip. If planting seed or divisions directly into the field it will need a severe weeding that first spring, and cultivating when needed after that. As long as weeds can be controlled I think Pokeroot grows quickest from direct sowing; it grows even quicker from divisions. This is probably due to the taproot getting somewhat stunted in the nursery flats. I have also grown it for years from flats just fine. I've had no pest or disease problems with Pokeroot.

HARVESTING Though a perennial, the roots are harvested in the fall of the second year—in some cases, if you really need some, in the fall of the first year. After that they start getting woody. The roots can go deep and wide so harvest carefully to get them all. A root digger can be employed and it will probably cut off the bottom of the root which will try to regrow and sometimes succeed. It is not like Comfrey though; you can cultivate it away. I've never done an accurate measurement but I would guess a yield of well over 1,500 pounds of dry root should be possible in an acre.

PROCESSING AND DRYING The root is thoroughly washed and then cut vertically and horizontally to facilitate drying. It will dry in 7 to 10 days and is 75% to 80% water.

SELLING IT The market for Pokeroot is small due to the fact that it is extremely toxic. The going price is $7 to $10 per pound dry. Most of the supply comes from wildcrafters but I think many companies would buy organic Poke. The market is small though. There is also a small fresh market.

MISCELLANEOUS Pokeroot is a striking plant that is ideal for the background of a perennial bed. The young leaves in early spring have long been eaten in this country. Care should be taken though as they and the whole plant are toxic. They should be boiled twice in fresh water before eating. I had a student who ate some leaves after boiling them. He got extremely ill, with diarrhea, vomiting blood, and severe cramping and fever. I personally do not recommend eating the leaves no matter how long they are boiled. The herb should only be used medicinally by someone who knows what they are doing as too high a dose can kill.

RED CLOVER

Trifolium pratense   Apiaceae

DESCRIPTION Grows up to 24 inches and spreads until you stop it. The leaves are, well, clover-like, with long stalks divided into 3 obovate leaflets. The flowers are purple-pink and are borne on roundish heads from spring through fall. Red Clover has naturalized in much of the U.S.

PROPAGATION Seed or divisions. Seed germinates easily in 7 to 14 days and is directly sown into the field. Divisions can be done from mature plants, but why bother when the seed is so easy to grow?

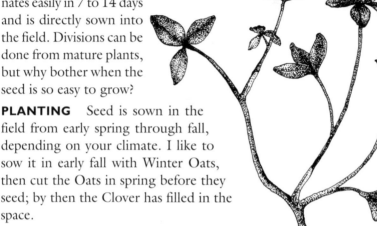

PLANTING   Seed is sown in the field from early spring through fall, depending on your climate. I like to sow it in early fall with Winter Oats, then cut the Oats in spring before they seed; by then the Clover has filled in the space.

CULTIVATION Perennial, hardy to Zone 3. Clover will grow in nearly any soil but prefers a reasonably fertile soil with adequate drainage. If you are starting with poor soil add several tons of manure per acre and your Red Clover will love you for it. Red Clover needs regular watering, about once a week in the dry west, from overhead sprinklers. Red Clover, like all legumes, fixes atmospheric nitrogen into solid nitrogen through little bacteria that cling to its roots. It really isn't possible to weed Red Clover once it is planted but it usually smothers most weeds. Try to till under weeds before planting. I've had no pest problems with Clover. I have had just a little powdery mildew on the leaves and flowers in the late summer or early fall as the harvest is winding down.

HARVESTING The flowers are hand picked when they are open. I usually pick the first leaf with it as well, as it makes it easier to pick. Some farmers combine leaf, stem and flower and then dry it but the flower is what is generally considered the most medicinal and only hand picked Red Clover is of superior quality. Each patch needs to be picked two to three times each week to stay on top of the flowers. The picking season goes on from late spring through early fall but it seems like forever. A fast picker can pick about one pound of dried flowers an hour if the field is healthy, but the average picker picks one-half to three-quarters of a pound per hour. A field is usually picked for two years and then turned under.

PROCESSING AND DRYING   Red Clover dries easily in 4 to 7 days. Turn the flowers the first couple of days. When dry the flowers should maintain the same color as when they were fresh. The flowers are 75% to 80% water.

SELLING IT   There is a large market for Red Clover blossoms. The price for just blossoms is $10 to $30 per pound dry. The $10 price is way too low and I was surprised to see a company selling it for that. Thirty a pound is more reasonable. The whole herb sells for $5 to $7 per pound. This is a good crop for the small grower but it requires a lot of difficult hand labor. I wouldn't harvest it until I was pretty sure I had it sold.

MISCELLANEOUS   Red Clover, somewhat like Nettle, is good for almost everything. It is used mainly for skin complaints, cancers, and many chronic diseases.

ROSEMARY

Rosmarinus officinalis
Lamiaceae

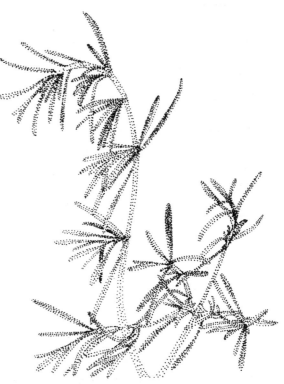

DESCRIPTION   Evergreen shrub growing up to 6 feet and with a spread of 4 to 6 feet. Very stately plant with upright branches and tough needle-like leaves. Flowers are blue to white, and appear in whorls from early spring (even winter in really warm areas) through early summer. The entire plant is wonderfully aromatic. It is native to the Mediterranean. There are numerous cultivars of Rosmarinus including Prostratus, a trailing plant; Alba, with white flowers; Sudbury Blue, a somewhat hardier variety; and Arp, the hardiest variety capable of surviving temperatures down to -10 degrees. Though Arp is hardy I found it one of the least aromatic of the cultivars and only recommend growing it in Zone 6 where it is all you have.

PROPAGATION Seed or cuttings. Seeds are difficult and I simply don't recommend them. Cuttings are easy and root in 4 to 6 weeks and are ready for transplanting in about 10 to 12 weeks. Cuttings benefit from bottom heat. They should be from succulent growth and can be cut nearly any time of the year but the dead of winter.

PLANTING Rosemary is best planted in spring or early summer. Transplanting is done by hand; I prefer to do it from established plants into a 4 inch pot or larger. I generally take late summer cuttings which are ready for transplanting in spring. Plants are spaced 24 to 36 inches in the row; rows are spaced at 36 to 42 inches.

CULTIVATION Perennial, hardy to Zone 8 or with some varieties Zones 7 and even 6. Most cultivars are only hardy to Zone 8 but Prostratus will survive in Zone 7 as will Sudbury Blue and both are excellent for harvesting. Arp is hardy to Zone 6 but I don't recommend it for harvesting except for personal use. Rosemary is incredibly drought tolerant and can survive without water for as long as 6 months in the hot parts of California. I like to water it about once a month in summer, after it is established. Young plants will need more water. Drip irrigation is ideal. Rosemary needs full sun; in the shade it gets straggly and weak. Rosemary needs exceptional drainage; when it dies prematurely it is nearly always from overwatering. Soil can be of low fertility but it might help just a bit to cover crop or manure the field once before planting if the soil is pathetic. The soil pH should be 5 to 8. You can grow it on slopes, especially Prostratus; it will reduce erosion and allow you to harvest a crop on marginal soil. Weed intensely when it is young because eventually it becomes difficult to get machinery between the rows. I've never had any pest problems and the only diseases I've had resulted from too much water or shade. If you live in Zone 5 or colder you can still grow it in a large pot. You can put it out during the warm season and then bring it in during the winter. The most important factor in growing it in pots is give it full sun—and do not, I repeat do not, overwater it.

HARVESTING The succulent tops are harvested starting in the second year continuing for many years. Pick with pruning shears after the dew has dried. Eventually the plants tend to get too woody for maximum production and they are replaced. In long growing seasons two crops a year is normal. Don't cut into the woody stem, just the succulent growth. The first cutting is usually in late spring. For essential oil production the plant is picked when in flower. Production of Rosemary will be best in Zone 9 and then Zone 8. I would not try a commercial operation in Zone 7 though I've had much success in the warmer part of that zone. Yields can be as high as 1,500 pounds per acre of dry herb per year in good situations.

PROCESSING AND DRYING Rosemary dries easily in 4 to 7 days. Its water content is about 60%. There is a small medicinal market for fresh Rosemary. If shipping fresh it must be harvested after moisture from the dew is gone. It can be harvested the evening before and then packaged the next day as it wilts incredibly slowly.

SELLING IT There is a fairly large market for Rosemary but much of it is from commercial sources. The average price is $7 to $10 per pound dry for certified organic, but the commercial price is less than half that. In Zones 8 or 9 Rosemary is a good crop to grow especially if you have some sloped or marginal soil. I think more companies will be purchasing organic in the near future. There is a good sized market for fresh culinary Rosemary; this is worth looking into in your region.

MISCELLANEOUS I have probably harvested more Rosemary by hand than any other hand harvested crop. I've been growing and selling it for 20 years and when I have fond thoughts of harvesting, it is usually when I'm thinking of picking Rosemary. It is an exceptional herb for drought tolerant landscaping. Trailing Rosemary is absolutely beautiful as it trails down over rock terraces. You can grow bonsai Rosemary with a little effort. My friends Jim and Dottie Becker from Goodwin Creek Nursery, in Williams, Oregon (a great place to buy mail order plants), have a beautiful bonsai which gave Heather the idea of trying her own. We now have a circular growing bonsai Rosemary which I think is just so cool. Rosemary is an alternate on my top 5 list of plants that will travel with me across the galaxy, due to the fact that on many planets it won't be quite cold hardy enough.

RUE

Ruta graveolens   Rutaceae

DESCRIPTION Evergreen shrub growing to 3 feet in height with a spread of 2 to 3 feet wide. Leaves are pinnately compound, somewhat lacy, deeply divided, and grayish-green or almost bluish-gray. Flowers are yellow and bloom in early summer. The fruit is a globular capsule, somewhat resembling a citrus fruit which it is related to. The entire plant is strongly aromatic. It is native to southern and southeastern Europe.

PROPAGATION Seed or cuttings. Seeds germinate in 10 to 20 days and are ready for transplanting in 10 to 12 weeks. They grow slowly at first so field sowing is absolutely not advised. Cuttings do not root really well. I usually do cuttings when I only need a few plants.

PLANTING Seedlings are best planted in late spring/early summer with either a transplanter or by hand. Spacing is 18 inches in the row and 24 to 30 inches between rows.

CULTIVATION Perennial, hardy to Zone 4. Rue grows best in a rich, well drained soil. It will grow in poor soils where nothing else thrives but production is dramatically increased by fertilization. Rue should be fertilized annually if you are harvesting it. Fertilize with a balanced fertilizer with some extra nitrogen. Before planting definitely improve the soil with cover crops and manure or compost. Rue requires full sun and should be irrigated once every two weeks or so. Drip irrigation is ideal for Rue and due to its low water requirements it can be planted on slopes. Cultivate intensely the first year and when needed after that. Rue will continue to produce at a high level for 5 to 7 years, at which point it should be tilled under and replaced. I can't imagine any pests attacking Rue and deer won't touch it. Other than root rot I've never had any disease problems with Rue.

HARVESTING The non-woody tops are picked when the plant is in flower. Harvest with pruning shears down to the woody stem. The first year you might get a small harvest, but in areas with a reasonably long growing season you can get two harvests a year from year two. The leaves can cause contact dermatitis especially on hot sunny days so be a little careful about rubbing in it too much. Wear gloves for sure and maybe long pants and sleeves. Yields can be as high as 2,000 to 3,000 pounds of dry herb per acre. There is a small market for the fresh herb with some companies wanting just the very succulent tips when the plant is starting to fruit.

PROCESSING AND DRYING Rue dries easily in 4 to 7 days. If you have a buyer who wants it stem free then garble it in the open air and wear a mask. It is very strong smelling and somewhat irritating. The herb is 75% to 80% water. Rue can be shipped fresh fairly easily.

SELLING IT The market for Rue is fairly small in the U.S. Most of what is sold is commercial from Europe. The price for commercial is $5 to $7 per pound for dry herb. I think there is a small market for organic Rue and worth trying on a very small scale.

MISCELLANEOUS Rue is an attractive plant that should be in the perennial garden. Though not as drought tolerant as Rosemary, Rue is fairly drought tolerant and can be planted in western gardens that get little summer water. Rue's main medicinal use is as an antispasmodic; it is also used in many eyewash formulas as well as a multitude of other uses. A number of plants do not like to grow near Rue. One of the first things you learn in companion planting is not to plant Basil near Rue.

SAGE

Salvia officinalis   Lamiaceae

DESCRIPTION Evergreen shrub with many branched stems growing up to 3 feet in height and spreading to 3 feet. The leaves are grayish-green and hairy. The flowers are spikes of purple that bloom in early summer. The root penetrates deeply into the soil in search of water. There are numerous cultivars of *S. officinalis*. Sage is native to the northern Mediterranean.

PROPAGATION Seed or cuttings. Seeds germinate readily in 2 to 3 weeks and are ready for transplanting in 10 to 12 weeks. Cuttings root fairly easily in about 4 to 6 weeks and are ready for planting into the field in about 12 weeks. Cuttings can be done in late spring or late summer/early fall.

PLANTING Seedlings are best transplanted in late spring or early summer. Cuttings can be planted when ready but I like to take cuttings in early fall and plant them out the next spring. Spacing is 18 inches in the row and 24 to 30 inches between the rows.

CULTIVATION Perennial, hardy to Zone 4. Though many books say it isn't very winter hardy I've over-wintered it in Zone 4 without problems. It might be advisable to mulch it in the fall. I won't recommend growing it commercially, however, in either Zone 4 or 5. Though Sage will grow in poor soils it produces best in a fertile but reasonably drained soil. The soil should be well fertilized before planting, preferably with manure and cover cropping. Fertilize annually after the first harvest with a well balanced fertilizer high in nitrogen. Sage should be irrigated every 7 to 14 days in the drier parts of the country with drip irrigation being ideal. It requires full sun and a pH of 6.0 to 6.5. I've had no pest or disease problems with Sage.

HARVESTING Pick the herb before it flowers. There is sometimes a small harvest the first year, but usually the first harvest is in the late spring of the second year. It is important to cut the plant down to 4 inches at this point to facilitate branching out. A second harvest will occur in late summer/early fall and 2 or 3 harvests a year is the norm through years 4 or 5. Essential oil content reaches its peak in the middle of the day so pick then. After year 5 it is best to till it under and replant elsewhere. Don't forget that whenever you are going to till a crop under you need to have replacement plants already in the ground somewhere else. Large commercial growers of Sage will harvest with mowers but I've always used my trusty pruning shears. Yields of 1,000 to 2,000 pounds of dry herb are possible.

PROCESSING AND DRYING Sage leaves dry readily in 2 to 4 days. Do not harvest when the leaves are wet. Sage leaves are approximately 80% water. There is a market for fresh Sage but if shipping fresh make sure the leaves are dry before packing.

SELLING IT The market for medicinal Sage is small whereas the culinary market is quite large. Certified organic sells for $6 to $8 per pound dry. The market for fresh culinary Sage is good especially around Thanksgiving. I've sold a lot of fresh Sage that went into turkeys. I wouldn't recommend Sage unless you have a dependable market already set up.

MISCELLANEOUS A good herb for the perennial landscape. Many of the cultivars are especially attractive. Sage has a longtime use as a gargle for laryngitis, tonsillitis, and sore throats. When Bill Clinton was running for president he seemed to constantly get laryngitis and sore throats. Every time I heard or saw him on television (I don't watch often) I wondered if he had tried Sage gargles, or an Echinacea-Propolis throat spray.

ST. JOHN'S WORT

Hypericum perforatum   *Hypericaceae*

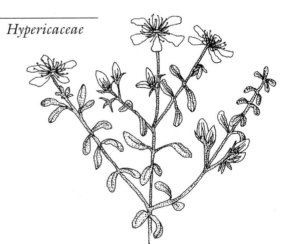

DESCRIPTION Much branched plant grows 2 to 3 feet tall and spreads up to a foot. The pale green leaves are opposite, linear-ovate, and about an inch long. The flowers are bright yellow, 5 petaled, about ¾ of an inch across, and bloom in summer. Spreads from underground rhizomes. Species name *perforatum* comes from the fact that leaves have translucent dots which appear to be holes when they are put up to the light. There are about 370 species of *Hypericum* but *H. perforatum* is easy to identify. It is native to Europe and Asia but has naturalized in North America amongst other places.

PROPAGATION Seeds, cuttings, or divisions. Very easy from seed which is light dependent and should be very lightly covered. Seed is small and germinates in 3 to 4 weeks; it should be thinned at about 6 weeks. Seedlings are ready to plant in about 12 weeks. Seed viability is maintained for many years. Cuttings have never rooted very well for me so I don't use them any longer. Divisions can be done in late fall or early spring.

PLANTING Seedlings should be transplanted into the field in late spring or early summer. Divisions should be planted when they are done in the fall or early spring. I do all my propagation for row crops from seed. Spacing is 12 inches in the row and 24 to 30 inches between rows.

CULTIVATION Perennial, hardy to Zone 3. Will grow in pathetically poor soils but produces best in a field of at least average fertility. Cover cropping and manuring before planting should do it. Prefers a well drained field but I've grown thousands of plants in pretty wet fields. It needs full sun. It grows slowly the first year and needs extensive weeding. In the subsequent years cultivate when necessary. St. John's Wort is drought tolerant but does best when irrigated somewhat. The first year water weekly, but in year two every 2 to 3 weeks will do.

It has several pests but the worst by far is the Klamath Beetle (*Chrysolina spp.*). The Klamath Beetle was introduced into California by the USDA in 1944 to control the spread of St. John's Wort which can have a toxic effect on cattle when they graze on large quantities of it. The beetle adapted well and is now found seemingly everywhere that St. John's Wort grows in the west. I have not seen the beetle east of the Rockies. Most of the damage to the plant is caused by the larvae which hatch in winter or early spring. They feed all spring before maturing into adult beetles. The adult beetle continues to feed for a while before going dormant in the soil during the hot summer months. They come alive in the early fall, mate, and lay eggs on the lower parts of the plant. The larvae hatch and the cycle is repeated. Control might be possible by using Bt, *Bacillus thuringenensis* (Colorado Potato Beetle variety), which is applied to the larvae. I've not had any disease problems with St. John's Wort.

HARVESTING The flowering tops are harvested when part of the inflorescence is open and the rest is in bud. Flowering will start in the second year; you will get a harvest the third year at which point it should be tilled under. Year 2 will be the most productive year, with year 3 slightly less. Most companies prefer cuttings 6 to 12 inches down from the top but more and more is being picked lower or completely down to the ground. Picking the top 6 to 8 inches will yield ½ to ¾ of a pound of fresh flowers in a healthy plant. This could give you a yield of as much as 13,000 pounds of fresh flower tops per acre. Of course, some plants may die in the field and many will have diminished production due to pests or other environmental factors. All things considered a yield of at least 5,000 pounds of fresh flower per acre should be expected the second year. Yields vary greatly depending upon the spacing and how much of each plant you harvest.

PROCESSING AND DRYING   I've always used and sold St. John's Wort fresh and that is mainly how it has been used in the U.S. in the past 20 years. Recent data seems to indicate that the freshly dried herb might be as effective. The fresh herb bruises readily and it starts to decompose almost immediately. When shipping fresh flowers take steps to keep the harvested material cool at all times and ship a.s.a.p. after harvest. I've seen several examples of St. John's Wort that were shipped second day air; upon opening the box the smell of decomposing plant matter overwhelmed my senses. St. John's Wort is approximately 75% water. It dries in 3 to 7 days.

SELLING IT   The market for St. John's Wort is gargantuan. After an episode on the *20/20* television show which portrayed it in a positive light St. John's Wort sales shot up several hundred percent virtually overnight. Any grower who had certified organic flowers last year could have sold them by standing on a street corner. The average price for fresh tops is $4 to $8 per pound and for dry it is $10 to $14 per pound. Virtually all of the American supply is wildcrafted in California and Oregon. Many companies would love to have organic St. John's Wort and now is the time to grow it. In the future there might be a glut but for the next few years I think it will be an easy sell.

MISCELLANEOUS   There have been a few cases of shipments of harvested St. John's wort being held up in states where it is considered an undesirable invasive weed. Be sure to check with your buyer and make sure that couldn't happen to your crop. St. John's Wort is used for so many things medicinally but most of the focus at the moment is on its antidepressant action. It seems to be very effective for mild to medium cases of depression and has no significant side effects. It is also an incredible emollient capable of healing wounds internally and externally. The flowers are so uplifting to look at and to harvest. I think I'll have to include it in my list of plants I shall carry with me as I cross the galaxy in search of new herbs.

SHEPHERD'S PURSE
Capsella bursa pastoris   Cruciferae

DESCRIPTION Grows up to 20 inches and spreads 2 to 6 inches. Leaves form in a basal rosette; they vary quite a bit from deeply toothed to smooth edged and are much smaller on the slender stem that holds the flower. The flowers are small and white and bloom slowly up the stalk. They can be found blooming almost any time of the year but most bloom in spring to early summer. The triangular seed pods give rise to its name because they look like little purses. Shepherd's Purse has a slender taproot. It is native to Europe but has naturalized in many areas including North America.

PROPAGATION Shepherd's Purse is propagated from seed sown in early spring or in the fall. It needs to be sown direct. When I've grown it in flats it wants to bolt and go to flower too quickly. It seems to germinate best when fall planted and allowed to stratify naturally; then it comes up in spring.

PLANTING Plant the seed in rows or beds in the fall or spring. If you plant it in rows thin it to 3 inches. Plant rows close together as you won't be able to cultivate with machinery. It's best to grow it in an area that doesn't have too much weed growth as weeding is difficult.

CULTIVATION Annual or biennial, can be grown anywhere. Will grow in full sun or partial shade, definitely grows best when grown in a fertile soil. Irrigate often if necessary. Fall sown seed should reach maturity in late spring the following year in warm winter areas. Spring sown will mature in early summer.

HARVESTING The whole above ground herb as it is flowering. Use pruning shears and cut to the ground. I sometimes yank it out of the ground which makes it easier to cut. Some companies using fresh herb want the root also.

PROCESSING AND DRYING Most companies want it fresh but it is also commonly sold dry. It dries easily in 3 to 5 days. It is 80% to 90% water. It ships fresh easily and should be picked early in the day while still slightly moist and cool. It seems to lose much of its medicinal action within about a year so it should be sold as soon as possible, and old herb should be tossed.

SELLING IT The market is small but because Shepherd's Purse is so effective it is commonly sold. The dried herb sells for $4.50 to $8 per pound. The fresh herb sells for around $3.50 per pound. It is so easy to grow sometimes and so difficult at others. I haven't quite figured it out yet. I think once you get it started it is best to simply let it reseed itself. I'm not sure if it is worth growing but everywhere I've been people have asked me if I had some.

MISCELLANEOUS Medicinally it is used internally and externally to stop bleeding. I've used it for someone who had profuse vaginal bleeding that the hospital emergency room could do nothing for, but the Shepherd's Purse stopped the bleeding in about 10 minutes. The exact mechanism of its action is unknown but who cares, it works.

SKULLCAP
Scutellaria lateriflora   Lamiaceae

DESCRIPTION Grows up to 3 feet in height and spreads until you stop it. The leaves are ovate to lanceolate, toothed, and almost pointed at the end. The flowers are blue and bloom on just one side of the stalk; they bloom in summer. Native to North America it is one of about 300 species of *Scutellaria*. Another popular medicinal species is *S. baicalensis*, which is used in Chinese medicine.

PROPAGATION Seeds, cuttings, or divisions. Seeds germinate easily in 2 to 4 weeks and are ready to transplant in 10 to 12 weeks. Cuttings are somewhat difficult due to the plants being so soft and succulent. I don't do cuttings any longer. Divisions are easy and can be done in spring or late fall.

PLANTING Seedlings should be transplanted in late spring or early summer. Divisions should be planted right after they are done in spring or late fall. Spacing is about 12 inches per plant and they can either be planted in rows or in 3 foot wide beds. They will spread quickly and fill in the rows, so it might be best to just plant them in 3 foot wide beds and try to contain them in the beds. Water immediately after planting.

CULTIVATION Perennial, hardy to Zone 4. Likes a fertile soil. If you are harvesting it, then you will need to fertilize it once or twice annually with a balanced fertilizer and extra nitrogen. Skullcap loves water and should be irrigated twice a week in the west, and even in areas of summer rain it will need extra moisture if rainfall lacks for any given period of time. Overhead irrigation is best. It can grow in full sun or partial shade. Several people over the years have tried to tell me that it can't be grown in full sun and yet I've grown it in full sun more often than not. The key is water. If you can't give it much then plant it in partial shade. Weeding of Skullcap is very difficult because it grows in a thick clump, so even hoes are useless, making hand weeding the preferred method. It is best, before you put in your permanent patch, to eliminate weeds as much as possible via smothering cover crops and intensive cultivation. I've had no pest or disease problems with Skullcap.

HARVESTING Above ground herb is harvested when it starts to flower. First year you might get a small crop but starting in year 2 and forever after you will get two cuttings a year. Use pruning shears and don't allow it to heat up as you are picking. Keep it in the shade in thin piles or take it to the drying room immediately. Yields of over 2,000 pounds of dry material per acre are possible.

PROCESSING AND DRYING Skullcap dries easily in 3 to 5 days but should be turned often. The herb is about 80% water. Fresh Skullcap is fairly easy to ship, but harvest and ship it early while it is still cool.

SELLING IT There is a fairly substantial market for Skullcap in the U.S. It is used both fresh and dried. The dry price is $12 to $15 per pound, while the fresh price is $6 to $9 per pound. The potential monetary yield for Skullcap is good if you can sell it. The main reason for not growing it is the intense labor it takes to weed it and also the moisture requirement.

MISCELLANEOUS Skullcap is used medicinally mainly for its action on the nervous system. It is used in numerous nervine or sedative formulas. In the perennial garden it is an interesting addition but be wary of its ability to spread.

SPILANTHES

Spilanthes spp. *Asteraceae*

DESCRIPTION Grows up to 2 feet and spreads 3 feet or so the first year if conditions are right. The stems and leaves are green to purple. The flowers are yellow-gold with dark red eyes in the middle, and about one-half inch across. It is very striking. Spilanthes is native to the tropics.

PROPAGATION Seeds or cuttings. Seeds germinate in 2 to 3 weeks and are ready for transplanting in 8 to 12 weeks. The seeds need hot conditions to germinate. Cuttings can be done any time during the growing season. Take a 3 to 4 inch tip and trim off most leaves. Keep it moist and use bottom heat if possible. Cuttings will root in 3 to 4 weeks.

PLANTING Seedlings should be planted in early summer when the soil has warmed up. Cuttings are generally over-wintered in pots and then planted out in late spring/early summer. Spacing is 12 to 18 inches in the row and 24 to 30 inches between the rows. Water immediately after planting.

CULTIVATION Tropical perennial, hardy in Zone 10. Spilanthes can be grown as an annual anywhere. It thrives on very rich fertile soil high in nitrogen. It needs frequent watering, 3 times a week in dry areas during summer. Even in areas of summer rain it might need irrigation during extended dry spells. If it looks wilted, water it. Overhead watering is definitely the way to go. It will grow in full sun or partial shade. Like Skullcap the key is water. I've had no pest or disease problems with Spilanthes.

HARVESTING The entire plant, root and all, is harvested before the first frost. Don't cut it close, one frost will kill it all. Dig the plants with a fork or spade taking care not to damage the tops. The plants will all be grown together when you harvest and you almost feel like you are in a jungle. A healthy plant will weigh between 3 and 10 pounds.

PROCESSING AND DRYING The plants are carefully washed and then shipped either fresh or dried. The plant is 85% to 90% water and dries in 3 to 7 days. Spilanthes will put a lot of moisture in the air in the drying room so dehumidifiers should be on for sure.

SELLING IT The market for Spilanthes is very small. Most people have never heard of it. Had you before you read this? What little sells goes for $4 to $6 per pound fresh, and $13 to $16 per pound dry. I would not recommend growing it unless you have a buyer already picked out. I do think this plant has the potential to become a major selling herb though.

MISCELLANEOUS Spilanthes is an incredible medicinal plant. It is an immune stimulant, antiparasitic, antibacterial, and it makes a great mouthwash (Cech, 1997). My first introduction to this plant was in 1982 when I got some seed. I planted it not knowing anything about it other than that it was called toothache plant. When it flowered I picked one and starting chewing. Wow. You will salivate like you've never salivated before. It stimulates blood flow also, and makes a good mouthwash and gargle. I have high hopes that this plant will become popular because it has so many good uses.

STONEROOT

Collinsonia canadensis   *Lamiaceae*

DESCRIPTION Grows up to 4 feet and spreads up to 4 feet. Bushy growth with very straight and rigid stems. Leaves are opposite, ovate, slightly serrated on the edges, and up to 8 inches long. The flowers are pale yellow and appear in summer. Both the leaves and the flowers are somewhat lemon scented when crushed. The rhizome is thick and as hard as a stone, thus its name Stoneroot. Stoneroot is native to the woodlands of the eastern U.S.

PROPAGATION Seeds, cuttings, or divisions. Seeds require stratification for 4 to 8 weeks. Seeds can also be planted outdoors in the fall and stratified naturally. They will reseed themselves. The best success I've had with seeds so far is just letting the plants drop their seeds in the rows and then going out in spring and digging up the seedlings. For whatever reason I haven't been able to duplicate that success in the nursery. Cuttings are taken before flowering and root slowly but okay in 4 to 6 weeks. Misting and bottom heat will help. Cuttings are ready for transplanting in 10 to 12 weeks. The main problem with doing cuttings is that the nodes are so far apart that it is difficult sometimes to get 2 nodes close enough to make an easy cutting. The cuttings will almost always be tip cuttings because the nodes are closer together at the tip. Divisions from mature plants can be done in late fall or early spring when you harvest. You will have to use pruning shears, as the roots are so hard that they don't separate easily, and the pruning shears will provide much needed assistance.

PLANTING Seedlings are planted out in late spring/early summer. Cuttings can be planted in the late summer or early fall but I prefer to over-winter them in 4 inch pots and plant them out in spring. Divisions are best planted in early spring. If you harvest in the fall over-winter the rhizomes in sawdust. Spring planting is easier due to easier weed control. Plants should be watered after planting. Spacing is 18 inches in the row and 24 to 30 inches between the rows.

CULTIVATION Perennial, hardy to Zone 3. Grows best in rich, somewhat moist soil. Fertilize before planting; liberal additions of organic matter are beneficial. Water needs are high; in the west irrigate twice a week with overhead sprinklers. *Collinsonia* grows best in partial shade in the dry and hot areas of the country but it will grow in full sun if you aren't in too hot an area and give it lots of water. Like Skullcap, water is the key. Weed often when it is young. The plants get bushy in mid-summer so mechanical cultivation can only be easily done before then each year. I've had no disease or pest problems with *Collinsonia*.

HARVESTING The rhizomes are harvested in the fall after 4 to 5 years. If you are growing it from seedlings or cuttings wait at least 4 years but preferably longer. The first 2 years it grows slowly. If growing it from root divisions you might be able to harvest after 3 years. The rhizomes can be dug by hand or with a root digger.

PROCESSING AND DRYING Clean the roots and separate them before drying them. There is a small market for fresh *Collinsonia* and it ships very easily. The roots are about 60% water and dry easily in 3 to 10 days.

SELLING IT The market for Stoneroot is small but growing. The price is $5 to $9 per pound for dry root. All of the world's supply comes from wildcrafting, so if it were grown certified organically it would be easy to sell. The key question is whether the companies would be willing to pay quite a bit more. I think many would.

MISCELLANEOUS Stoneroot is on the UpS secondary list and if it ever became popular then it would be on the primary list. I have it on my list of priority herbs to grow because I've grown it successfully and I know others can grow it also. If the price went up enough it would be worth growing. It is an interesting plant for the perennial garden; the flowers aren't showy but the whole plant is somewhat attractive. Medicinally it is used mainly for hemorrhoids and other conditions with weak or swollen veins.

THYME

Thymus vulgaris
Lamiaceae

DESCRIPTION Low growing and spreading herb up to a foot in height and spreading one to two feet. The leaves are gray-green and small. The flowers are white to lilac and bloom in early summer. There is much confusion in the genus as to how many species there are and what the correct botanical names are. I won't attempt to shed any light on the subject. There are many cultivars of which my favorite for growing and harvesting is *Thymus vulgaris*, or English Broadleaf. I also like Silver Thyme (*T. vulgaris Argenteus*). These names may be incorrect but that is how I purchased them so I'll stand by them until someone says I'm wrong, which will probably be soon.

PROPAGATION Seed or cuttings. Seeds germinate easily in 14 to 20 days and are ready for transplanting in about 12 weeks. If growing cultivars you will have to propagate from cuttings, which root easily and can be done nearly any time of the year except the dead of winter. I like to root my Thyme cuttings in sand as it has worked better for me than perlite or any mixes of perlite, vermiculite, and sand. Cuttings root in 3 to 5 weeks and are ready for planting in about 12 weeks.

PLANTING Seedlings are planted in late spring/early summer. Cuttings are planted in when they are ready, but like most cuttings I like to plant them in spring from large healthy plants. Spacing is 12 inches in the row and 24 to 30 between rows.

CULTIVATION Perennial, hardy to Zone 4. In colder climates it is best to mulch it in winter especially if you have one of those cold winters with little snow to insulate the plants. I've over-wintered it in Zone 4 though with zero mulch, so don't worry too much. Thyme can survive in poor soils, but production is greatly increased by having a fertile soil and fertilizing annually. It likes a pH of 6.0 to 8.0 and demands good drainage. Full sun is critical. It requires minimal irrigation; in the dry west I've irrigated it every 2 weeks. Thyme produces less essential oil in humid areas so quality is diminished. The best Thyme comes from areas with climates similar to the Mediterranean, like California and much of the west. Weed control is important before planting and cultivation should continue throughout the life of the crop. Weeds make harvesting much more difficult. I've had no pest or disease problems with Thyme. Thyme gets woody after a few years and production decreases so replace it at that point.

HARVESTING The herb is harvested once the first year as it starts to flower in late summer, and then twice a year after that. The first harvest is when it is in full flower and the second is in the fall. Cut the plant down to 4 to 6 inches or so but do not cut into any woody growth. Yields of 1,000 to 1,500 pounds of dry herb per acre are possible.

PROCESSING AND DRYING Thyme dries easily in 3 to 5 days. The herb is about 70% water.

SELLING IT The market for medicinal Thyme is small though the culinary market is huge. Overseas there is a large market for the herb to be converted into essential oil. The price here is $9 to $12 per pound for dried certified organic Thyme. The commercial price is much lower, $2.50 to $4 per pound. Thyme is worth growing at $10 per pound or higher, but not at $4 per pound. I would only suggest growing it if you have a buyer in mind and you live in the dry parts of the west.

MISCELLANEOUS Everyone should grow Thyme in their garden. There are so many cultivars available from many species that are incredibly beautiful. Thyme does well in the drought tolerant garden also. Medicinally Thyme has many uses and one of its main constituents, thymol, is the key ingredient in many mouthwashes.

UVA-URSI, BEARBERRY
Arctostaphylus uva-ursi   Ericaceae

DESCRIPTION Prostrate evergreen shrub with dark green leaves. The flowers are white to pink and appear in spring, and are followed by glossy red fruits. Uva-ursi is native throughout the northern hemisphere and common in western North America. There are many cultivars available.

PROPAGATION Seed, cuttings, or divisions. Seeds are difficult and not worth trying in my humble opinion. Cuttings are not easy but practical. Cuttings benefit from bottom heat and misting. When I was in college I

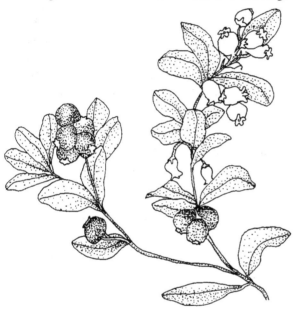

did an experiment with Uva-ursi trying various techniques for propagating it. I found that cuttings root far better when using hormones at relatively high concentrations. It is the only herb I would recommend using hormones for that I've mentioned in this book. Check with your certifier to determine what is okay to use. Cuttings root very slowly, 6 to 12 weeks and aren't ready to transplant for 6 months. I suggest doing late spring cuttings one year and planting them into the field the next year. Divisions are a pain and I only suggest it if you want only a plant or two.

PLANTING Plant the healthy plants in spring to mid-summer. Spacing is 2 to 3 feet between plants and rows at 3 feet. Eventually they will grow together in a mat.

CULTIVATION Perennial, hardy to Zone 2. Uva-ursi will grow in virtually any soil though it needs a little drainage. If you are cutting it heavily you will have to fertilize it regularly. It likes full sun and a pH of 6.0 or less. It requires very little water but occasional irrigation in the dry west is beneficial, maybe every 2 to 3 weeks. The first year or two it will require more water. It is an ideal herb to grow on slopes and when it fills in, after

3 years or so, it will provide excellent erosion control. I've never had any problem with pests or disease with Uva-ursi.

HARVESTING The leaves are harvested starting in the second or third year. They can be cut pretty low to the ground; since they will be garbled it is okay to cut into woody stems. I've never measured yields but I would estimate between 500 and 1,000 pounds of dry leaf per acre.

PROCESSING AND DRYING Uva-ursi dries easily in 3 to 7 days but should be turned regularly at first. Garbling is done after drying with the goal of nearly total elimination of the stems.

SELLING IT The market for Uva-ursi is medium but not growing much. Other herbs have started to replace it and its reputation is diminishing somewhat. Of course with the herb market growing so much I'm sure the total sales of Uva-ursi are growing at least a wee bit. The price is $8 to $10 per pound for certified organic dry leaf and the wildcrafted price is about half of that. I wouldn't recommend growing Uva-ursi as a crop unless you have a buyer in mind.

MISCELLANEOUS Uva-ursi makes an excellent landscape plant especially for drought tolerant landscapes. It grows well on slopes; many hillsides in California are planted in Uva-ursi. Medicinally it is used mainly as a urinary tract antiseptic. It can irritate the stomach so don't drink too much and avoid it if you have stomach problems. The berries taste like Vitamin C, and are quite tasty when crushed in water. The seeds inside are quite hard though so don't bite down. Bears feed copiously on the leaves and especially the fruit, hence its name, Bearberry.

VALERIAN
Valeriana officinalis   Valerianaceae

DESCRIPTION Grows 4 to 8 feet in height with a spread of 1 to 2 feet. The leaves are highly variable but generally deeply divided into 7 to 10 segments. The stems are hollow. The flowers are umbel-like clusters of white to pink and appear in summer. The root is made up of a bunch of spindle-like fibrous roots that are dark on the outside and white inside. There are 150 to 250 species of Valerian worldwide; many are used medicinally on smaller scales, but *V. officinalis* dominates the American market. It is native to Europe and northern Asia.

PROPAGATION Seeds or divisions. Seeds germinate easily in 2 to 3 weeks and are ready for transplanting in 8 to 12 weeks. Divisions are easy and are usually done when harvesting in the fall or early spring.

PLANTING Seedlings should be transplanted into the field in late spring/ early summer either by transplanter or hand. Divisions are best done with the fall harvest and held over the winter and planted in spring. Spacing is 12 to 15 inches in the row and the rows are spaced at 24 to 30 inches. Water immediately after planting if it is hot and dry.

CULTIVATION Perennial, hardy to Zone 4. Valerian grows best in a rich and moist soil. Prepare fields ahead of time with manure and a nice cover crop. Extra nitrogen and especially phosphorus should be added to the soil before planting. Water is essential. In the dry west irrigate once or twice a week by drip or overhead. Valerian can grow in soils too wet for many other plants. For root production it is best to cut the flower stalks off before flowering; however, I've always had a hard time with that because a field of Valerian flowers is one of the prettiest sights. Valerian grows in full sun or partial shade and likes a pH of 6 to 7. Weed intensely when young and cultivate when necessary until harvest. I've had no pest or disease problems with Valerian.

HARVESTING The roots are dug in the fall of the second year. They can be dug by hand or root digger. It is best to cut the stalks first. Yields of 1,500 to 2,500 pounds of dry root are possible.

PROCESSING AND DRYING Valerian is sold both fresh and dry. Fresh roots ship easily. Roots need to be thoroughly cleaned before drying or shipping though. They are one of the most difficult roots to clean as the many fibers hold soil and rocks really well. Companies hate to have little rocks in their hammermills so clean until there are no rocks left. Valerian is about 75% to 85% water.

SELLING IT There is a large and growing market for Valerian root. The price is $10 to $12 per pound for certified organic dried root while commercial root goes for less than half of that. Fresh root sells for $6 to $8 per pound. This is still a good herb to grow even though there are several large growers growing it. It is easy to grow and the price for organic is reasonable.

MISCELLANEOUS *Valeriana officinalis* makes up nearly all of the American market but a small amount of the western North American native *V. sitchensis* is entering the market. I feel very strongly that we should not be harvesting this native species. We already have good quality Valerian available from organic growers. Valerian is a beautiful flower for the perennial flower garden. Medicinally it is used mainly for its sedative properties though it has a multitude of uses besides that. Yes, it does smell bad. Most say it smells like dirty socks. I have to strongly disagree. I was once traveling with a friend in our car and we thought we smelled dog poop. We stopped the car and looked at our shoes and around the car and found nothing. Later after arriving at our destination we found a small bag of

Valerian under the seat that I had been showing to a class. At no point did we say, "Smells like dirty socks in here." We said, "All right, who stepped in the dog s—t."

WOOD BETONY

Stachys officinalis   Lamiaceae

DESCRIPTION Grows up to 24 inches tall with a spread of 12 to 18 inches. Stems are hairy and square. Leaves grow in a rosette and are deep green, hairy, about 4 to 5 inches in length, and have serrated edges. Flowers are spikes of blue and bloom in summer. Wood Betony is native to Europe.

PROPAGATION Seed or divisions. Seed germinates easily in 2 to 3 weeks and is ready for transplanting in 10 to 12 weeks. Divisions are easy and are done in the fall or spring.

PLANTING Seedlings are transplanted in late spring/early summer with a transplanter or by hand. Divisions can be planted in fall or spring. Spacing is 12 inches in the row and 24 to 30 inches between the rows.

CULTIVATION Perennial, hardy to Zone 4. Grows best in a rich, somewhat moist soil. A cover crop and manuring ahead of time will supply the necessary nutrients for a few years. If you continue to cut it for many years it will need to be fertilized. Irrigate once a week in the dry west. Grows in full sun or partial shade. Weed early and cultivate when necessary. Wood Betony is pretty hardy and weed competitive as it bulks out quickly and the leaves somewhat smother the weeds. I've had no major pest or disease problems with it.

HARVESTING The above ground herb is harvested twice a year starting in year 2. Harvest when it is just starting to flower and cut close to the ground. A second harvest occurs in late summer whether it starts to flower again or not. I've never kept accurate data on yields but I would estimate 1,500 pounds of dry herb per acre per year.

PROCESSING AND DRYING Wood Betony dries easily in 3 to 7 days. When you harvest it be sure to cull out any leaves that are starting to rot. The herb is about 85% water.

SELLING IT The market for Wood Betony is small but has potential to grow. The going price is around $10 per pound. I enjoy growing it but I would not recommend it as a crop due to the small market, unless you have a buyer. The market could grow as it is a very effective medicinal herb.

MISCELLANEOUS A nice addition to the perennial garden with attractive foliage and subtle but showy flowers. Medicinally it is used as a nervine and is excellent at eliminating tension headaches.

WORMWOOD

Artemesia absinthium   *Asteraceae*

DESCRIPTION Bushy shrub growing to 4 feet and spreading 3 to 4 feet. Leaves are gray, deeply cut, with silky hairs on both sides. The flowers are yellow, very small, and bloom in summer. The plant has a soft almost lacy appearance. Wormwood is native to Europe.

PROPAGATION Seeds, cuttings, or divisions. Seeds are somewhat difficult and slow growing. They germinate in 2 to 4 weeks. Softwood cuttings root easily in 4 to 6 weeks and are ready for transplanting in 12 weeks. Cuttings are best taken in late spring or late summer/early fall. Divisions are done in fall or spring from mature plants but don't yield a lot of plants. Cuttings are my preferred method for propagating Wormwood. I like to take fall cuttings and leave them in the greenhouse all winter.

PLANTING Seedlings can be planted in late spring/early summer. Cuttings are best planted in the late spring, though they can also be fall planted. Divisions are best done in spring and planted immediately. Spacing is 24 to 36 inches in the row and the rows are spaced at 36 to 48 inches.

CULTIVATION Perennial, hardy to Zone 4. Wormwood will grow on almost any soil as long as there is adequate drainage. If your soil is totally infertile you will want to manure it and plant a cover crop first; otherwise don't bother to fertilize. Wormwood likes a pH of 5.5 to 7.5 and grows best in full sun. Its water needs are minimal, and even in the dry west it only needs water every 2 to 4 weeks, though it should be deeply irrigated after the first harvest each year. Weed thoroughly the first year. After the first year it is pretty weed competitive especially in poorer soils where it outgrows them. Cultivate when necessary after the first year. Plants will produce at their peak for 6 to 8 years and then should be replaced. I've had no pest or disease problems with Wormwood.

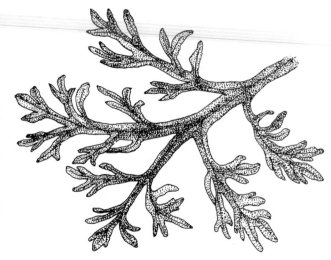

HARVESTING First harvest is in the summer of the second year when it is in full flower. Cut with pruning shears down to 6 to 12 inches. Every cutting after that will be down to the woody growth. Second harvest each year will be in the late summer/early fall. A yield of 2,000 pounds of dry herb per acre per year can be expected.

PROCESSING AND DRYING Wormwood dries relatively easily. Most companies would prefer just leaf so garbling of the lower portion of each stalk is usually necessary. You can garble it fresh to save dryer space or garble it dry which goes quicker. When garbling care should be taken not to inhale or rub against the herb. I recommend gloves, eyeglasses, and a mask. Some don't react like I do but I get sick if I garble it too long without a respirator. Wormwood is 65% to 70% water.

SELLING IT The market for Wormwood is fairly substantial especially since someone wrote a book about parasites and health and named Wormwood as the herb of the millennium. The average price is $9 to $13 per pound for certified organic, and $5 to $7 for commercial. It is a good herb to grow at the moment, as long as it can be sold for $10 per pound or more.

MISCELLANEOUS Wormwood is an excellent plant for the perennial garden. For the drought tolerant landscape it is one of the best. Medicinally Wormwood is used mainly to eliminate worms and to stimulate gastric secretions.

YARROW
Achillea millefolium   Asteraceae

DESCRIPTION Grows up to 3 feet in height with a spread of 1 to 2 feet. Yarrow will continue to spread. The leaves are feathery and up to 6 to 9 inches long. The white flowers are clustered in beautiful umbels and bloom in summer. There are numerous cultivars of *A. millefolium* but only the pure species is desired in commerce.

PROPAGATION Seeds or divisions. Seeds germinate in 10 to 20 days and are ready for transplanting in 8 to 12 weeks. Divisions are done in early spring or late fall. Divisions are easy to do but somewhat time consuming to plant. I do most of my Yarrow from seed.

PLANTING Seedlings are planted out in late spring or early summer. Divisions are planted when they are done in fall or early spring. Spacing is 12 to 18 inches in the rows and the rows are 24 to 30 inches apart.

CULTIVATION Perennial, hardy to Zone 2. Yarrow can grow in almost any soil with adequate drainage. If your soil is really poor then fertilize with manure first. Yarrow is very drought tolerant and in the west only needs to be irrigated every 2 to 3 weeks; drip irrigation works great.

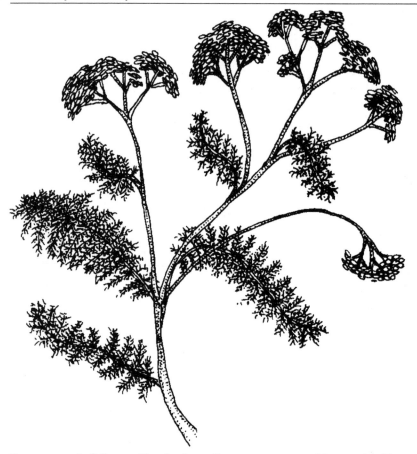

Yarrow needs full sun. I've had no disease or pest problems with Yarrow. It doesn't get much easier than Yarrow.

HARVESTING The flowers are harvested as they start to bloom in summer. The flowers will continue to bloom for several weeks. Pick the flowers with the old fingers.

PROCESSING AND DRYING Yarrow flowers dry readily in 3 to 5 days. They are 65% to 70% water.

SELLING IT The market for Yarrow is a little bigger than small. Most of the supply comes from wildcrafters, but I know companies would buy certified organic. Wildcrafted Yarrow sells for $6 to $10 per pound dry.

MISCELLANEOUS Yarrow is a nice addition to the perennial bed. Some of the cultivars come in other colors and are quite pretty. Yarrow is perfect for the drought tolerant landscape. Medicinally Yarrow is used for a wide variety of things including easing diarrhea, reducing bleeding internally and externally, and as a diaphoretic.

YERBA MANSA

Anemopsis californica Saururaceae

DESCRIPTION Creeping perennial with basal leaves 3 to 6 inches long, green until winter when the whole plant turns red. The white flowers come in conical spikes and are, to me anyway, really neat looking. The plant spreads and spreads and spreads above ground and roots at the nodes. The entire plant is aromatic. It is native to the desert southwest but unlike most desert plants it thrives on water.

PROPAGATION Seeds, cuttings, or divisions. I had no success growing it from seed until I applied bottom heat at which point it germinated in 4 weeks. Seedlings are ready for transplanting in 12 weeks or more. Cuttings root easily in 2 to 3 weeks. The main difficulty is that the nodes are far apart and many cuttings are 6 to 8 inches long. Divisions are easy and are done in early spring.

PLANTING Seedlings are planted in early summer by hand or transplanter. Cuttings are best planted the spring after they are taken. Divisions are planted in early spring right after they are done. Spacing is 12 to 18 inches in the row and the rows are spaced at 24 to 30 inches.

CULTIVATION Perennial, hardy to Zone 4. In colder areas it should be heavily mulched to insure that it gets through the winter, though I've over-wintered it in Zone 4 without mulch. It likes a high pH, 6.5 to 8.0 or even higher. It will grow in an average soil with lots of water. It will grow in seasonal standing water. I irrigate it twice weekly in an average draining soil in the west and it does fine. It needs full sun. Weed heavily the first year and cultivate when needed. The runners start to spread quickly so either train them along the row, or let it fill in the space between the rows. I've had single runners over 4 feet long. I've had no pest or disease problems with Yerba Mansa.

HARVESTING The roots are harvested in the fall by hand. You can harvest the most mature plants and leave younger plants in the ground. Roots are harvested after the third or fourth year.

PROCESSING AND DRYING The roots are washed and then dried. They will dry in 5 to 10 days.

SELLING IT The market for Yerba Mansa is small at the moment but it has a lot of potential due to its potent medicinal action. Many are touting it as a substitute for Goldenseal though their actions are somewhat different. The price is about $12 per pound for dry herb. I would not recommend growing it at this time because the market is tiny, but right now the entire supply comes from wildcrafters and it is on the UpS secondary list.

Also, desert wet areas are often where agricultural runoff ends up. Much of the Yerba Mansa that is picked is probably not too "pure." I definitely would not want wildcrafted Yerba Mansa from the Imperial Valley in California.

MISCELLANEOUS Yerba Mansa has always been used by the people who live in the southwest, from the ancient Native American peoples to the present Native American people and now the Hispanic culture. I think it might someday be a somewhat popular herb. Medicinally it is used as an anti-inflammatory, a diuretic, antibacterial, antifungal, and especially to reduce inflammation of the mucous membranes similar to what Goldenseal does.

Resources

Contents

RESOURCES FOR GROWERS
Recommended Books on Medicinal Herb Growing
The following small publications, all written by Richo Cech, are available from Horizon Herbs, PO Box 69, Williams, OR 97544. They cost only three or four dollars each.

Milk Thistle—Spiny Friend
Growing Chinese Herbs Organically
Forest Roots: Black Cohosh, Ginseng, Goldenseal and Wild Yam
Echinacea—Native American Tonic Roots
Middle Earth Cultivation of Medicinals from the English Tradition
Growing Tropical Perennials in the Temperate North
Herb of the Sun, St. John's Wort

Growing Great Garlic, by Ron Engeland, 1991. Filaree Productions, Rt. 1, Box 162, Okanogan, WA 98840. 220 pp.

Herbal Renaissance: Growing, Using and Understanding Herbs in the Modern World, by Steven Foster, 1993. Gibbs Smith, Publisher, Layton, UT.

Herbal Remedies in Pots: Growing and Making Herbal Remedies for Common Ailments, by Effie Romain & Sue Hawley. Available from Northwind Publications, 439 Ponderosa Way, Jemez Springs, NM 87025-8036.

Encyclopedia of Herbs and Herbalism, edited by Malcolm Stuart. Orbis Publishers, London. Now out of print but a very good and useful book to look for in used book stores.

Magic and Medicine of Plants, 1986. Reader's Digest Books, NY. 464 pp.

Cultivation and Processing of Medicinal Plants, 1992. Budapest, Hungary. Akademiai Kiado.

Herbs, An Illustrated Encyclopedia, by Kathi Keville, 1994. Friedman, Fairfax, NY.

Encyclopedia of Herbs and Their Uses, 1995. Dorling Kindersley Ltd., London.

The Random House Book of Herbs, by R. Phillips and N. Foy, 1990. Random House, NY.

Recommended Books on Market Gardening
Backyard Market Gardening: The Entrepreneur's Guide to Selling What you Grow, by Andrew Lee, 1993. Good Earth Publications. 350 pp.

Metrofarm: Guide to Growing for Big Profit on a Small Parcel of Land, by Michael Olson, 1994. T. S. Books. 498 pp.

The New Organic Grower, A Master's Manual of Tools and Techniques for the Home and Market Gardener, by Eliott Coleman, 1989. Chelsea Green. 269 pp.

Sell What you Sow: Growers Guide to Successful Produce Marketing, by Eric Gibson, 1994. New World Publishing. 302 pp.

The Small Commercial Garden, by Dan Haakenson, 1995. PC Services, PO Box 7294, Bismarck, ND 58507. 208 pp.

No need to buy any of these fine books until you've had a look at them. All were available through my library.

Other Grower Resources
Dr. Branka Barl will send list of 50 crops that can be grown in Saskatchewan. Most are perennials. Will send them to any who get in touch with her. Also has names of brokers for wild medicinal plants from the prairies. University of Saskatchewan, 51 Campus Dr., Saskatoon SK S7N 5A8.

ATTRA: Appropriate Technology Transfer for Rural Areas Resource Center, PO Box 3657, Fayetteville, AR 75702. Contact them for packet of herb growing information and organic certification information.

U.S Department of Agriculture
Office for Small-Scale Agriculture
Ag Box 2244
Washington DC 20250-2244
202-720-5245. Fax 202-205-2448
Ask for newsletters and publications on medicinal herbs.

Resources for Herb Drying
Gen MacManiman
Living Foods Dehydrators
3023 362nd S.E., Fall City, WA 98024
425-222-5587

Supplies both dehydrators and plans, plus detailed directions, even recipes. Popular with herb people in my area.

Freeze Dry Co.
Highway 371 South
PO Box 570
Nisswa, MN 56468
218-963-2100. Fax 218-963-0761

Expensive machines, but freeze dried herbs are used by a few large medicinal herb companies because of the quality results. Also available to rent.

Plans for 4'x4'x8' cabinet dryer are available from Bert Van Dalfsen, Mechanization Engineer, B.C. Ministry of Agriculture, Fisheries & Food, Abbotsford, BC V3J 2M3.

Recommended Medicinal Plant, Seed & Root Sources

There are many plant and seed companies to choose from these days. These are only a few of the recommended ones that carry at least some medicinal herbs. I have put in the current catalog charges plus e-mail and web sites when available.

For even more herb seed catalogs, I recommend, as always, Gardening by Mail, by Barbara J. Barton, published by Mariner Books. In her current edition, Barton lists 85 reputable sources for herb seeds and plants. Your library should have a reference section copy; if not, perhaps you'll want to suggest it.

Borealis Botanicals: Box 91, Cochrane, Alberta TOL OWO. **S** $3

Companion Plants: 7247 N. Coolville Ridge Rd., Athens, OH 45701. **SP** $3. 614-593-3092. www.frognet.net/companion-plants/; e-mail: complants@frognet.net

Dabney Herbs: PO Box 22061, Louisville, KY 40252-0061. **SP** $2 502-893-5198. www.dabneyherbs.com; e-mail: davydabney@aye.net

Desert Woman Botanicals: PO Box 263, Gila, NM 88038. **SP** 505-535-2860. Fax 505-535-2252

Elixir Farm Botanicals: General Delivery, Brixey, MO 65618. **SP** $2. 417-261-2355. efb@aristotle.net. Specialize in Chinese medicinal herbs.

Goodwin Creek Gardens: PO Box 83, Williams, OR 97544. **SP** $1. 541-846-7357

Herb Farm: 323 Parleeville Rd., Norton, New Brunswick E0G 2N0. **S** $2 US$3

Herbs-Liscious: 1702 So. 6th St., Marshalltown, IA 50158. **SP** $2. 515-752-4976. herbs@marshallnet.com

Horizon Herbs: PO Box 69, Williams, OR 97544-0069. **PSR** $1. 541-846-6233. www.chatlink.com/herbseed; e-mail: herbseed@chatlink.com Specialize in medicinals.

Inside Passage: Forest Shomer, PO Box 639, Port Townsend, WA 98368. **S**

Johnny's Seeds: Rt. 1, Box 2580, Foss Hill Rd., Albion, ME. **S** n/c. 207-437-9294. www.johnnyseeds.com; e-mail: commercial@johnnyseeds.com

Native Seed Foundation: Star Rt., Moyie Springs, ID 83845. **S**

Northwoods Nursery: 27635 S. Oglesby Rd, Canby, OR 97013. **P** $3. 503-266-5432. e-mail: 102742.3327@compuserve.com

One Green World: Box 1080, Molalla, OR 97038. **P**. 503-651-3005. Specialize in fruits and herbs from the former Soviet Union and Eastern Europe.

Ontario Seed Co.: Box 7, Waterloo, ON N2J 3Z6. **S** 519-886-0557

Pan American Seed Co: 728 Tonn Rd., West Chicago, IL 60185. **S.** 708-231-1400

Piroche Plants, Inc.: 20542 Mc Neil Road, Pitts Meadows, BC V3Y 1Z1. **P.** 604-465-7101

Redwood City Seed Co: PO Box 361, Redwood City, CA 94064. **S** $1. 415-325-7333. www.batnet.com/rwc-seed/

Richter's Herbs: Goodwood, ON L0C 1A0, Canada. **PSR** n/c. 905-640-6677. www.richters.com; e-mail: catalog@richters.com

Ron's Rare Plants and Seeds: 415 Chappel, Calumet City, IL 60409-2122. **PS** $3.

Seeds of Diversity: Box 36, Station Q, Toronto, ON M4T 2L7. **S.** Seeds free, membership $25. Includes newsletter.

Terra Flora Botanicals: 16775 60th Ave., Cloverdale, BC V3S 1S8. **SP** $2.

Western Biologicals: Box 283, Aldergrove, BC V4W 2T8. **SP** $3.

Wild Botanicals: PO Box 2264, Corvallis, OR 97339. **PS.** 503-929-4753

If you are especially interested in growing native medicinal plants, please see the note on native seed sources in the wildcrafting resource section.

Herbs of Economic Importance to the Canadian Prairies

List prepared by Dr. Branka Barl, Saskatoon Herb Research Centre, Univ. of Saskatoon, 51 Campus Dr., Saskatchewan, SK S7N 5A8. Fax 306-966-8106; e-mail: barlb@duke.usask.ca

Bearberry/Kinnickkinnick	*Arctostaphylos uva ursi*
Chickweed	*Stellaria media*
Dandelion	*Taraxacum officinale*
Echinacea	*Echinacea angustifolia, E. Purpurea, E. Pallida*
Elecampane	*Inula helenium*
Evening primrose	*Oenothera biennis L.*
German chamomile	*Matricaria chamomilla*
Ginseng, Oriental	*Panax ginseng*
Ginseng, American	*Panax quinquefolium*
Ginseng, Siberian	*Eleutherococcus senticosus*
Goldenseal	*Hydrastis canadensis*
Horsetail	*Equisetum arvense L.*
Licorice root	*Glycyrrhiza glabra*
Plantain	*Plantago spp*
Sarsaparilla	*Aralia nudicaulis*
Seneca root	*Polygala senega*
Stinging nettle	*Urtica dioica*

Valerian root	*Valeriana officinalis*
Yarrow	*Achillea millefolium*
Feverfew	*Tanacetum parthenium*

Possible Alternative Herb Crops for Western Canada

List prepared by Al Oliver, Provincial Ginseng Specialist, BC Ministry of Agriculture, Fisheries & Food, 162 Oriole Rd., Kamloops, BC V2C 4N7

Arnica	*A. montana*
Barberry	*Berberis vulgaris*
Bearberry	*Arctostaphylos uva ursi*
Billberry	*Vaccinium myrtillus*
Bloodroot	*Sanguinaria canadensis*
Burdock	*Arctium lappa*
Chinese Boxthorn	*Lycium chinense*
Chicory	*Cichorium intybus*
Comfrey	*Symphytum officinale*
Dandelion	*Taraxacum officinale*
Devils Club	*Oplopanax horridus*
Dock	*Rumex crispis*
Echinacea	*Echinacea spp.*
Elderberry (Black)	*Sambucus canadensis*
Feverfew	*Tanacetum parthenium*
Foxglove	*Digitalis purpurea*
Garlic	*Allium sativum*
Ginkgo	*Ginkgo biloba*
Ginseng	*Panax spp.*
Goldenseal	*Hydrastis canadensis*
Hawthorn	*Crataegus spp.*
Horsetail	*Equisetum arvense*
Juniper	*Juniperus commumis*
Linden	*Tillia spp.*
Milk Thistle	*Silybum marianum*
Mullein	*Verbscum thapsus*
Nettles	*Urtica dioica*
Oregon Grape	*Mahonia aquifolium*
Chinese Rhubarb	*Rheum officinale*
Rose Hips	*Rosa spp.*
Sea Buckthorn	*Hippephae rhamnoides*
Seneca	*Polygala senega*
Siberian Ginseng	*Eleutherococcus senticosis*

St. John's Wort	*Hypericum perforatum*
Witch Wormwood	*Artemisia absinthium*
Yarrow	*Achillea millefolium*

Medicinal Plants Now Grown for Commerce in Canada

List prepared by Conrad Richter, Richters Herbs, Goodwood, Ontario L0C 1A0

Ginseng–3 species	Echinacea–3 species	Borage
Evening Primrose	Feverfew	Goldenseal
Catnip	St John's Wort	Valerian
Milk Thistle	Foxglove	Chamomile
Angelica	Sheep Sorrel	Burdock
Comfrey	Nettle	

Promising Medicinal Plants for the Praries

List prepared by D. V. C. Awang, MediPlant Natural Products Consulting Services, Box 8693, Ottawa, ON K1G 3J1

American Ginseng	*Panax quinquefolium*
Feverfew	*Tanacetum parthenium*
Goldenseal	*Hydrastis canadensis*
Siberian Ginseng	*Eleutherococcus senticosus*
Angelica	*Angelica archangelica, A. sinensis - Dong Quai*
Bilberry	*Vaccinium myrtillus*
Chamomile	*Matricaria recutita*
Hawthorn	*Crataegus spp.*
Horsechestnut	*Aeculus hippocastanum*
Lemon Balm	*Melissa officinalis*
Licorice	*Glycyrrhiza glabra, G. uralensis*
Nettle	*Urtica dioica*
St. John's Wort	*Hypericum perforatum*

Resources for Ginseng Growers

Northwest Ginseng Growers Association: Don Hoogesteger, Pacific Rim Ginseng, 1504 N.E. 234th St., Ridgefield, WA 98642

Ginseng Growers Association of Canada: 395 Queensway West, 2nd Floor, Simcoe, ON N3Y 2N4. 519-426-7046. Fax 519-426-9087. Publishes bi-monthly newsletter.

Canadian Ginseng Research Foundation: Dr. Tom Francis, 150 College St., Toronto, ON M5S 1A8

Albert Ginseng Assoc: 105.150 Crowfoot Cres. N.W. #706, Calgary, AB T3G 3T2

Ginseng Canadian Agriphone: 519-426-6047. Weekly reports on crop conditions, etc.

Jan Schooley, Prov. Ginseng & Medicinal Herb Specialist, Ontario Ministry of Agriculture, Food and Rural Affairs, Box 587, Simcoe, ON N3Y 4N5

Ginseng Enterprise Budget, by Charles A Brun, WSU Cooperative Extension, & Don Hoogesteger, Pacific Rim Ginseng. Available from: Bldg. C, Ste. 100, 11104 N.E. 149th St., Brush Prairie, WA 98606

Illinois Ginseng Grower Assoc: 3201 South Prospect, Champaign, IL 61821. 217-351-8858

White Crane Trading Co: 447 Tenth Ave, New York, NY 10001. 212-736-1467. Buys from organic (only) growers.

Recommended Reading on Ginseng

Ginseng Industry Directory & Suppliers Guide
Available from Al Oliver, 162 Oriole Road, Kamloops, BC V2C 4N7

Diseases of Cultivated Ginseng, by J. L. Parke and K. M. Shotwell
Available from Ag. Extension Service, Wisconsin State University, Ad Bulletins, Rm. 245, 30 N. Murray St., Madison, WI 53715

Ginseng Production Guide for Commercial Growers, 1996 edition
Available from B. C. Ministry of Agriculture, Fisheries and Food, 162 Oriole Rd, Kamloops, BC V2C 4N7

Ginseng, by Kathi Keville, Keats, New Canaan, NY. Medicinal information on ginseng.

American Ginseng–Green Gold, by W. Scott Persons, Bright Mountain Books, 138 Springside Rd., Ashville, NC 28803. $15.95 ppd.

Methods to Utilize Tobacco Kilns for Curing (drying) and/or Storage of Alternate Crops, by D. L. VanHooren and S. J. Ratavicius. Available from Ag Energy Centre, Guelph Ag Centre, PO Box 1030, Guelph, ON N1H 6N1

Effects of Conditioning and Drying Ginseng Roots, by D. L. VanHooren and H. R. Lester. Available from Ontario Ministry of Ag, Food and Rural Affairs, Ag & Agri-Food Research Station, Delhi, ON N4B 2W9

Ginseng Market Opportunities in the Asia Pacific Region for the B.C. Ginseng Industry. Available from Ministry of Economic Development, Small Business & Trade, Ste. 629, 999 Canada Pl., Vancouver, BC V6C 3E1

Facts About Ginseng, Elixir of Life, by Florence Lee. Available from Hollym International Corp., 18 Donald Pl., Elizabeth, NJ 07208

Close Up Look at the Chinese Ginseng Industry, by Andy Hankins. Published in several issues of Business of Herbs, 439 Ponderosa Way, Jemez Springs, NM 87025-8036

The Ginsengs…A User's Guide, Christopher Hobbs, 1998. Interweave Press, CO

Computer Related Ginseng Resources
(from Dr. Chas. A Brun)

Panax Discussion Group. Several hundred ginseng growers exchange information through a Listserve:

To subscribe, send an e-mail message to:
    mailserv@cariboo.bc.ca
In the body of the message, type the one line command:
    subscribe panax   your first name   last name

There are color pictures of ginseng diseases and cultivation practices on this web site from the Pest Management Center at Delhi, Ontario: http//res.agr.ca/london/pmrc/pmrchome.html

B.C. Ministry of Ag, Fish and Food has a web site on major crops including ginseng:
    http://www.agf.gov.bc.ca

American Ginseng Society has their newsletter on the web:
    http://earthwks.com/earthwrks/AGSI

Don Hoogesteger, Pacific Rim Ginseng has an interesting web page:
    http://www.e-z.net/~ginseng

Sources for Ginseng Seed & Roots

Ginseng America Inc: Bridge St., Box 246, Roxbury, NY 12474

Barney's Ginseng Patch: Rt 2, Box 43, Montgomery City, MO 63361

Nature's Cathedral: Rt 1, Box 120, Blairstown, IA 52209-9721. (Also buys ginseng & goldenseal from other growers.)

Mama's Ginseng Garden: 370 14th St. West., Simco, ON N3Y 4K6

Wild Wonderful Farm, Inc: PO Box 256, Franklin, WV 26268. 212-736-1467. Toll free order 1-800-977-4372

Ginseng Gardens: Rt 2, Box 261, Pittsfield, IL 62363. 217-285-6022

Scott Persons Ginseng Co: 138 Springside Rd., Asheville, NC 28803

Resources for Mushroom Growing
Recommended Books

Growing Gourmet and Medicinal Mushrooms, by Paul Stemets, Ten Speed Press, Berkeley, 1993. 550 pp. Enthusiasm & information. Many kinds of mushrooms. Covers all aspects of mushroom growing; accent on indoor growing on sterilized sawdust. Bibliography, glossary, resource directory.

Medicinal Mushrooms, by Christopher Hobbs, Botanica Press, Santa Cruz, CA. 2nd Edition, 1995. 250 pp. Medicinal studies associated with more than 30 varieties of mushrooms. Information on nutrition included. Hobbs offers his own 20 years of experience with and use of medicinal mushrooms, plus a wealth of information from Europe and Asia.

Medicinal Mushrooms You Can Grow for Health, Pleasure and Profit, by Hajo Hadeler, Cariago Publishing House, Box 1428, Sechelt, BC V0N 3A0, Canada. 200 pp.
Offers an understanding of mushrooms and their complex, fascinating place in the world. Contains information on growing and using medicinal mushrooms, including making tonics.

Shiitake: The Healing Mushroom, by Kenneth Jones, Healing Arts Press, 1995. For cooking, eating, and appreciating the medicinal properties of the shiitake.

Growing Shiitake Mushrooms in a Continental Climate, by Mary Ellen Kozak and Joe Krawczyk, 2nd Edition 100+ pp.
Field & Forest Products: N3296 Kozuzek Road, Peshtigo, WI 54157 Production techniques for log culture of shiitake.

Shiitake Growers Handbook, by Paul Przbylowicz and John Donoghue, 1988. Kendall Hunt Publ. 215 pp.
Considered the definitive source book on both log and substrate shiitake cultivation.

Spawn & Equipment Suppliers

Allied Mushroom Products: PO Box 490, Tontitown, AR 72770. 501-361-5938

Western Biologicals, Ltd.: PO Box 283, Aldergrove, BC V4W 2T8. 604-856-3339

Fungi Perfecti: PO Box 7634, Olympia, WA 98507. 206-426-9292. Fax 206-426-9377. Seminars on Cultivation. Book Suppliers. Commercial catalog.

Mushroom People: Box 220, Summertown, TN 38483. 612-964-2200

Northwest Mycological Consultants: 702 NW 4th, Corvallis, OR 97330. 541-753-8198

Mushroom Grower Associations

Alabama Shiitake Grower's Assoc.: c/o Hosea Nall, Cooperative Extension Service, Alabama A&M University, 819 Cooke Ave., Normal, AL 35762. 205-532-1697

American Mushroom Institute: 907 East Baltimore Pike, Kennett Square, PA 19348. 215-388-7806

Appalachian Mushroom Growers Assoc.: c/o Margery Cook, Rt 1 Box BYY, Haywood, VA 22722

Canadian Mushroom Growers Assoc.: 310-1101 Prince of Wales Rd., Ottawa, ON K2C 3W7

Carolina Exotic Mushroom Assoc.: c/o Ellie Litts, PO Box 356, Hodges, SC 29653

Florida Mushroom Growers Assoc.: c/o Charlie Tarjan, 3426 SW 75th St., Gainesville, FL 32607

Northwest Shiitake Growers Assoc.: PO Box 207, Salem, OR 97308. 800-577-5515

Shiitake Growers Assoc. of Wisconsin: PO Box 99, Birchwood, WI 54817

Mushroom Grower Newsletters

Mushroom Growers Newsletter: c/o Mushroom Co., 464 Fulton St., Klamath Falls, OR 97601

Cultivated Mushroom Report: University of Toronto, Mississauga, ON, Canada

Mushroom Journal: Box 3156, Moscow, ID 83843

Shiitake News: Forest Resource Center, Rt. 2, Box 156A, Lanesboro, MN 55949

The Mycophile: No. American Mycological Assoc., 3556 Oakwood, Ann Arbor, MI 48104

Growers Interviewed for
Medicinal Herbs in the Garden, Field and Marketplace

Mark & Marggy Wheeler
Pacific Botanicals
4350 Fish Hatchery Road
Grants Pass, OR 97527

Jim Lawrence
Thirsty Goose Farm
Friday Harbor, WA 98250

Mike and Lynn Monroe
Fungus Among Us
PO Box 352
Snohomish, WA 98291
360-568-3403
www.premier1.net/~shrooms/

Elaine & John McLeod
Meadowbrook Corner
Box B24
Bowen Island, BC V0n 1C0
604-947-9988
Fax 604-947-0858

Jim Macpherson
Snow Peak Mushroom Co.
34962 Bond Rd.
Lebanon, OR 97355
541-258-2626
Fax 541-259-4434

Phil Schulz
Friday Harbor, WA 98250

Herb Apprenticeships

Don't mix these too closely in your mind with herb schools, although both can contribute greatly to your herb education. Herb apprenticeships can often be very hard physical work with relatively poor working conditions. Be certain you understand all the conditions (and costs) before you enroll. Write and ask for details on their programs.

Susan Weed, Wise Woman Center
PO Box 64
Woodstock, NY 12498

Dry Creek Herb Farm &
Learning Center
13935 Dry Creek Road
Auburn, CA 95602

Frontier Botanical Preserve
Apprentice Program
Tim Blakley, Heather McNeill
33560 Beechwood Grove Rd.
Rutland, OH 45775
740-742-4401
Fax: 740-742-4401

Kathi Keville
Oak Valley Herb Farm
PO Box 2482
Nevada City, CA 95959

Ryan Drum, Ph.D.
Island Herbs

Waldron Island, WA 98297
EagleSong/Ravencroft
PO Box 229
Startup, WA 98293

Wise Woman Herbals
Sharol Tilgner, N.D.
PO Box 279
Creswell, OR 97426-0279

Michael Pilarsky
Friends of the Trees
PO Box 4469
Bellingham, WA 98227
360-738-4972

CAEP, Communicating for Agriculture Exchange Program.
Places young people on farms, ranches, and businesses around the world.
112 E. Lincoln, Fergus Falls, MN 56537. Fax 218-739-3832

Organic Growing Information Resources

To learn about and/or comment on national organic standards, contact:

Eileen S. Stommes, Deputy Administrator, Agriculture Marketing
Services, USDA, Room 4007, Ag Stop 0275, PO Box 96456, Washington, DC 20090-6456. Fax 202-690-4632.

Or call 202-512-1800 for a copy of the National Organic Proposed Rules.
You can buy a copy with an $8 credit card purchase.

The rules are posted on the following web site:

http://www.ams.usda.gov/nop

North American Organic Resource Directory. Offers free listings for certified organic growers. Put out by Organic Trade Association, PO Box 1078, Greenfield, MA 01302

To locate a private certifier near you, speak with your County Agent or call a local organic grower.

Resources for Wildcrafters
Recommended Books

Medicinal Plants of the Pacific West
Medicinal Plants of the Mountain West
Medicinal Plants of the Desert and Canyon West

All are written by Michael Moore, respected (almost legendary) herbalist who heads the Southwest School of Botanical Medicine, PO Box 4565, Bisbee, AZ 85603.

All are published by Red Crane Books, 2008 Rosina St., Ste B, Santa Fe, NM 87505.

A Peterson Field Guide of Medicinal Plants: Eastern & Central North America, by James Duke and Steven Foster. Houghton Mifflin, Boston, 1990.

Forest Pharmacy: Medicinal Plants in American Forests, by Steven Foster. 1995. Published by Forest History Society, 701 Vickers Ave., Durham, NC 27701.

The EcoHerbalist's Fieldbook, Wildcrafting in the Mountain West, by Gregory L. Tilford. 1993. Mountain Weed Publishing Co., HC 33 Box 17, Conner, MT 59827. 300 pp.

Domestication of Wild Medicinal Plants, by Richo Cech. 1995. Available from Horizon Herbs, PO Box 69, Williams, OR 97544. 12 pp.

Medicine From the Mountains, by Kimball Chatfield, Box 2000153, S. Lake Tahoe, CA 96150. Details medicinal plants of the Sierra Nevadas.

Ginseng: How to Find, Grow and Use America's Forest Gold, by K. D. Pritts.

A Plant Lover's Guide to Wildcrafting: How to Preserve Wild Places and Harvest Medicinal Herbs, by Krista Thie, 1549 W. Jewett Blvd., White Salmon, WA 98672

Videos

Medicinal Plants in the Field with Michael Moore, Vol. 1, The Rio Grande Gorge, available from Plant Planet Films, PO Box 727, Silver City NM 88061.

Four Hour Ethnobotanical Herb & Plant Walk Video with Ryan Drum. Available from Dominion Herbal College, 7527 Kingsway, Burnaby, BC V3N 3C1.

Wildcrafting herbal videos also available from:
Debra Nuzzi, 997 Dixon Rd, Boulder, CO 80302
The Seeker Press, PO Box 2899, Lafayette, IN 47906

Other Wildcrafting Resources

Friends of the Trees Society
Michael Pilarski
PO Box 4469
Bellingham, WA 98227
360-738-4972. Fax 360-671-9668
tern@geocities.net
www.geocities.com/rainforest/4663

Rocky Mountain Herbalist Coalition
412 Boulder St.
Gold Hill
Boulder, CO 80302
303-786-9667

Northwest Special Forest Products Assoc.
Gail Hampton
PO Box 7803
Brooking, OR 97415

For a long listing of plant nurseries that specialize in native medicinal plants, send a SASE and a small donation to:
United Plant Savers, PO Box 420, East Barre VT 05649. Better yet, join up and they will send you the nursery listing free.

A partial list of these nurseries can be had for free on the UpS web site:
    http://www.plantsavers.org

If you are interested in keeping up with USDA Forest Service work with wildcrafters, contact Tammi Hartung, 1270 Fields Ave., Canon City, CO 81212.

British Columbia Ministry of Forests; Forest Practices Code:
    http://www.for.gov.bc.ca

Chinese Medicinals Resources
Recommended Books

The Web That Has No Weaver, by Ted J. Kapchuck. Congdon and Weeds, 1983. 402pp.

Between Heaven and Earth: A Guide to Chinese Medicine, by Harriet Beinfield. Ballantine, 1991. 432 pp.

Herbal Emmissaries: Bringing Chinese Herbs to the West. Steven Foster and Yue Chongxi, 1992. Healing Arts Press, Rochester VT.
Detailed instructions for growing nearly 50 important Chinese medicinal plants in American gardens. Includes cultivation, harvesting, processing, and the medicinal uses.

Growing Chinese Herbs Organically, by Richo Cech. 1995. Horizon Herbs, PO Box 69, Williams, OR 97544. 12 pp.

Other Information

Lyle Craker, of University of Massachusetts Dept. of Plant & Soil Sciences, Stockbridge Hall, Amherst, MA 01003. An Evaluation of Chinese Medicinal Herbs as Field Crops in the Northeastern U.S. Contact for report.

A recent listing in the American Herb Assoc. Newsletter:

Rare Chinese Seeds. 200 native plants. $1 per packet (no import permit needed.) Seed List: $2. Quingpu Paradise Hort. Co. Ltd., PO Box 031-116, 1337 Middle Huai Rd., Shanghai, People's Republic of China.

For brief, interesting overview of Market Report on Traditional Chinese Medicines, see HerbalGram #38, Fall '96, excerpted from long (243 pp.), expensive ($1500) report from London.

See also the seed and plant resource listing

HERB EDUCATION & INFORMATION
Medicinal Herb Organizations & Associations

These are all important herb associations—with at least some medicinal herb focus. You may not want to join any of them, but I would suggest you do consider becoming a member of one or more as you get more involved in growing and marketing herbs. I also suggest you write, first of all, for the free descriptive brochure from each organization. From that, you should be able to tell which group might fit your interests.

American Assoc. of Naturopathic Physicians
2366 Eastlake Ave., Ste. 322
Seattle, WA 98102
206-323-7610

American Herb Association
PO Box 1673
Nevada City, CA 95959
530-274-3140
Quarterly newsletter
See also their resource listing in Education

American Herbalists Guild
Box 746555
Arvada, CO. Fax 303-423-8828
http://www.healthy.net/herbalists

British Columbia Herb Growers Assoc.
PO Box 1415
Aldergrove, BC V4W 2V1

Canadian Association of Herbal Practitioners
1745 West 4th Ave
Vancouver, BC V6J 1M2

Canadian Herb Society
5251 Oak Street
Vancouver, BC V6M 4H1
http://www.herbsociety.ca

Citizens for Health
PO Box 2260
Boulder CO 80306
Works on legislative issues concerning herbs.
www.healthfreedom.com

Herb Research Foundation
1007 Pearl Street, Ste. 200
Boulder, CO 80302
www.herbs.org

International Herb Assoc.
PO Box 317
Mundelein, IL 60060-0317
847-949-4372. Fax 847-949-5896
www.herb-pros.com

National Certification Commission for
Acupuncture & Oriental Medicine
202-232-1404
www.nccaom.org

National Nutritional Foods Assoc.
3931 MacArthur Blvd., Ste. 101
Newport Beach, CA 92660
714-622-6272. Fax 714-622-6266
nnfa@aol.com

Ontario Herbalists Assoc.
11 Winthrop Pl.
Stoney Creek, ON L8G 3M3
416-536-1509

United Plant Savers
PO Box 420
East Barre, VT 05649
802-479-9825. Fax 802-476-3722

Educating Yourself About Herbs

There are so many ways to learn about herbs: by reading and studying on
your own; by learning in a field or classroom setting from more experienced and educated herbalists and botanists; by correspondence classes;
or by attending a school with more formal programs.

To learn about your local plants, check the programs offered at your
local colleges—especially at the community or junior college level. Often
local plant specialists will share their knowledge in inexpensive classes intended for nearby residents. Even if the teachers don't talk much about
the medicinal uses of the local plants, the ability to identify the plants and
learn about their habitats is very important to any would-be herbalist.

Perhaps you live in an area where Native North Americans still live.
You could be lucky and find one who would teach you about their local
plants and plant medicine traditions.

Almost all herb farms and herb nurseries around the country offer
herb classes each year, many of them about medicinal herbs. So do many
food co-ops and health food stores. To learn about the herb businesses
close to your own home, you can consult the yellow pages under herbs,

health food stores, or nurseries. Often that first phone call will lead to other, more specialized people. As I've said before, the herb networks are being woven in every location of the country as I write this book. They may not have reached your neighborhood yet, but they are definitely taking shape in your area.

There are also two national guides to herb businesses in the U.S. with another one being produced at this time for Canada. Many of the businesses listed in these directories offer classes. Here are the contacts for those publications:

1. *The Herbal Green Pages,* published by the Herb Growing and Marketing Network. (See their listing on page 278.)
2. *The Herb Resource Directory,* published by Northwind Publications. (See their listing on page 278.)
3. Contact the Canadian Herb Society (their listing is on page 272) for a copy of their new directory of herb businesses.

If you learn what is being offered and taught in your own area first, it will then be easier to decide how much more time and expense you will want to expend in educating yourself about herbs. Learning from experienced hands at the local level first means you will learn and know the important medicinal plants in your own area. Our tendencies are often to seek out the rare and the exotic—whether we are talking about bird watching or medicinal plants. We shun the sparrow and our local "weeds" in search of the threatened species. I can't explain that. I just know it's foolish. And probably dangerous, both to us and the planet. How happy I would be to learn that this book caused some of you to look down when you step out of your front door tomorrow and say to yourself: "These could be important medicinal plants growing here beside this sidewalk; I need to learn about them."

When it comes to the more formal and well known schools for teaching about herbs, I've chosen to list only those that have been recommended to me by herbalists, or those that are primarily run by, or associated with, well known herb professionals. But please get recommendations about these schools from many other people, too, as there are no national standards for herb schools, and there is lots of hype out there these days about all things *natural* and *herbal.* Schools can change over time, getting better or becoming less well focused. I would always make an effort to find recent graduates of any of these programs in order to learn more about their true value to their students. I suggest you start by getting a brochure from any of these school programs that interest you. Some offer correspondence courses.

Australasian College of Herbal Studies: PO Box 57, Lake Oswego OR 97034

Avena Institute: 20 Mill St., Rockland, ME 04841

Bastyr University: 14500 Juanita Dr., N.E., Bothell, WA

Blazing Star Herbal School: PO Box 6, Shelbourne Falls, MA 01370

Blue Sky School of Herbal Studies: N5821 Fairway Dr., Fredonia, WI 53021

California School of Herbal Medicine: Box 39, Forestville, CA 95436

East West Herb Course: Michael Tierra, Box 712, Santa Cruz, CA 95061

Frontier Botanical Preserve Program: Tim Blakley, 33560 Bechwood Grove Rd., Rutland, OH 45775

Institute of Medical Herbalism: PO Box 1149, Calistoga, CA 94515

Jeanne Rose Herbal Studies Course: 219 Carl St., San Francisco, CA 94117-3804

Mountain Weed Company: HC 33 Box 17, Conner, MT 59827

National College of Naturopathic Medicine: 049 S.W. Porter, Portland, OR 97201

National College of Phytotherapy: 120 Aliso S.E., Albuquerque, NM 87108

Ojai College of Phytotherapy: PO Box 66, Ojai, CA 93024

Rocky Mountain Center for Botanical Studies: PO Box 19254, Boulder, CO 80308

Rocky Mountain Herbal Institute: PO Box 579, Hot Springs, MT 59845

Sage Mountain Herbs: PO Box 420, E. Barre, VT 05649

School of Herbal Medicine: PO Box 168K, Suquamish, WA 98392

School of Natural Healing: PO Box 412, Springville, UT 84663

Southwest College of Naturopathic Medicine & Health Sciences: 2140 East Broadway Road, Tempe, AZ 85282

Southwest School of Botanical Medicine: PO Box 4565, Bisbee, AZ 85603

Therapeutic Herbalism: 2068 Ludwig Ave, Santa Rosa, CA 95407

Wise Woman Center: PO Box 64, Woodstock, NY 12498

The American Herb Association offers a *Directory of Herbal Education* for $3.50 which lists over 50 herb schools, correspondence courses, etc. Available from AHA, PO Box 1673, Nevada City, CA 95959

Canadian Schools

Canadian College of Naturopathic Medicine: PO Box 2431, Toronto, ON M4P 1E4

Dominion Herbal College: 7527 Kingsway, Burnaby, BC V3N 3C1

Douglas College: PO Box 2503, New Westminister, BC V3L 5B2

University of Saskatchewan Herb Research Program: 51 Campus Dr., Saskatoon, SK S7N 5A8

West Coast College of Complementary Health Care: 6th Fl., Spencer Bldg., Harbour Center, 555 West Hastings St., Vancouver BC V6B 4N6

Wild Rose College: 302 1220 Kensington Rd N.W., Calgary, AB T2N 3P5

Olds College, 4500 50 Street, Olds, AB T4H 1R6
403-556-4684. FAX 556-4711
Sometimes offers classes in commercial herb production.

Oriental Medicine Schools
American College of Trad. Chinese Medicine: 455 Arkansas St., Ste. 302, San Francisco, CA 94107

Canadian College for Chinese Studies: 853-859 Cormorant St., Victoria BC V8W 1R2

Emperor's College of Trad. Oriental Medicine: 1801 Wilshire Blvd, Santa Monica, CA 90403

Institute of Chinese Herbology: 1533 Shattuck Ave, Oakland, CA 94709

International Institute of Chinese Medicine: PO Box 4991, Santa Fe, NM 87502

Pacific College of Oriental Medicine: 702 W. Washington St., San Diego, CA 92103

Seattle Institute of Oriental Medicine: 916 NE 65th, Ste. B, Seattle, WA 98115

Toronto School of Trad. Chinese Medicine: 2010 Eglington Ave. W., Ste. 302, Toronto, ON M6E 2K3

Other Educational Opportunities
American Institute of Vedic Studies: PO Box 8357, Santa Fe, NM 87504

Ayurvedic Institute: PO Box 23445, Albuquerque, NM 87192-1445

New Mexico Academy of Massage and Advanced Healing Arts: PO Box 932, Santa Fe, NM 87504

Contact James E. Simon, Department of Horticulture, Purdue University, 1165 Hort. Bldg., West LaFayette, IN 47907-1165. 317-494-1328. Fax 317-494-0391 for a list of classes now offered in medicinal plants and essential oils.

In 1997, the Rocky Mountain Center for Botanical Studies in Boulder, Colorado, created an educational program entitled Herbal Supplements Retail Training Program. Designed to help salespeople in retail stores deal with issues in the areas of herbs and herbal products, including reading and evaluating labels, and guidelines for legal discussion of health concerns with customers. The program is coordinated by well known herbalist Feather Jones. For more information, 303-442-6861. HerbalGram #40.

Other Sources for Herb Information
Herb Book Sources
Following are several book companies that feature medicinal herb books. You might want to send for their book brochures.

American Botanical Council
PO Box 201660
Austin, TX 78720-1660
One of the most complete medicinal herb book collections available. Plus special reports, videos, software, etc.

Food Products Press
Haworth Press, Inc.
10 Alice St.
Binghampton, NY 13905-1580
Agriculture and horticulture books, plus many on food production.

Interweave Press
201 East Fourth St.
Loveland, CO 80537
www.Interweave.com
Many herb books from the publishers of *Herb Companion* and *Herbs For Health* magazines.

Churchill Livingstone
PO Box 3188
Secaucus, NJ 07096-9927
Specializes in complementary medicine, Chinese medicine, etc.

Audio Tapes, Proceedings, etc.
Tree Farm Communications, Inc.
23703 N.E. 4th Street
Redmond, WA 98053-3612

Herb conference proceedings are often available from:

Herb Growing and Marketing Network, PO Box 245, Silver Springs, MD 17575-0245

The Business of Herbs, 439 Ponderosa Way, Jemez Springs, NM 87025

Computer Herb Databases
GlobalHerb: Steve Blake, 1613 Elm Ave., Richmond, CA 94805

American Herbal Pharmacopoeia
Box 5159
Santa Cruz, CA 95063
408-461-6317
herbal@got.net
www.herbal-ahp.org
Herb monographs.

Newsletters

Medical Herbalism: A Clinical Newsletter for the Herbal Practitioner,
Paul Bergner, PO Box 33080, Portland, OR 97283

Herb Growing & Marketing Network
Maureen Rogers, PO Box 245, Silver Springs, MD 17575-0245
http://www.herbnet.com
The Herbal Connection is the newsletter;
The Herbal Green Pages is a huge annual directory listing most of the
herb businesses in the U.S. A primary herb business link.

The Business of Herbs
Northwind Publications
Paula & David Oliver
439 Ponderosa Way
Jemez Springs, NM 87025-8036
Great and long time source for herb information: all the conferences; all
the events; all the organization news.

Growing For Market
PO Box 3747
Lawrence, KS 66046
Not often about herbs, but always good info for market growers.

Magazines

Herbs for Health
Bi-monthly from Herb Companion Press
741 Corporate Circle, Ste. A, Box 4101
Golden, CO 80401
www.interweave.com
Produced for medicinal herb consumers with solid input from American
herb pros.

HerbalGram
Quarterly Journal of the American Botanical Council &
Herb Research Foundation
PO Box 201660
Austin, TX 78720
A primary publication linking herbalists to the world of herbal prod-
ucts, the regulatory environment, and the world of plant research.
Indispensable.

Small Farm Today
*The Original How-To Magazine of Alternative and Traditional Crops,
Livestock, and Direct Marketing.*
3903 W. Ridge Trail Rd.
Clark, MO 65243-9525
Always good articles on market farming with occasional articles on herb
crops.

Herb Companion
Bi-monthly from Interweave Press
PO Box 55295
Boulder CO 80322
Now carries a section on medicinal herbs.

Herb & Whole Food Retailer Magazines

Natural Foods Merchandiser
1301 Spruce St.
Boulder, CO 80302
303-939-8440. Fax 303-939-9559

Whole Foods
3000 Hadley Rd.
So. Plainfield, NJ 07080-1117
908-769-1160. Fax 908-769-1171

Internet Resources for Medicinal Herb Enthusiasts

This category grows by the day. I'll list just a few important stops that can then link you to enough other medicinal herb information to keep you desk-bound for a whole growing season. Take care. Enjoy.

http://www.rt66.com/hrbmoore/HOMEPAGE/HomePage.html

http://www.herbnet.com

http://www.herb.com

http://countrylife.net/ethnobotany/

http://sunsite.unc.edu/herbmed/

http://www.richters.com

http://www.ars-grin.gov/~ngrlsb/   Complete herb chemical database

http://www.nal.usda.gov/   U.S. Dept. of Ag. Library

Usenet newsgroup:
alt.folklore.herbs

ListServe on herb use:
LISTSERV@TREARNPC.EGE.EDU.TR
message should be: SUBSCRIBE HERBS your name

On Line Herb Newsletters

Conrad Richter, of Richter's Herbs in Canada, puts out an always interesting, informative newsletter.

To subscribe:
majordomo@richters.com

Message should be:
SUBSCRIBE RICHTERS-L [your e-mail your name]
Don't use brackets.
For archive issues, see www.richters.com

Resources for Product People

Books on Product Making
The Herbal Medicine-Maker's Handbook, by James Green, 1990. WildLife & Green Publications, Box 39, Forestville, CA 95436.

Handmade Medicine, by Christopher Hobbs. Interweave Press, Loveland, CO, 1998.

The Herbal Medicine Cabinet, by Debra St. Claire, Celestial Arts Publishing, Berkeley, 1997.

Profitable Dream Pillows, by Jim Long. $12.95 postpaid from Long Creek Herbs, Rt. 4 Box 730, Oak Grove, AR 72660.

Herb Formulas for Clinic and Home, by Michael Moore, Southwest School of Botanical Medicine, PO Box 4565, Bisbee, AZ 85603.

Medicines From the Earth, Thomson, W., ed., 1978. Gage Publishing, Vancouver, BC.

Backyard Medicine Chest, by Douglas Schar, 1995. Elliott and Clark. 160 pp.

The Medicinal Garden: How to Grow and Use Your Own Medicinal Herbs, by Anne McIntire. Henry Holt, 1997. 150 pp.

Special Report on Tea Products
U.S Tea is 'Hot' Report

Available from:

Sage Group, 1712 Warren Ave. No., Seattle, WA 98109. 206-282-1789; Fax 206-282-2594

Videos on Making Herbal Products
Herbal Medicine Videos available from:
Debra Nuzzi, 997 Dixon Rd., Boulder, CO 80302
The Seeker Press, PO Box 2899, Lafayette, IN 47906

Making Your Own Herbal Salves, video available through Dominion Herbal College, 7527 Kingsway, Burnaby, BC V3N 3C1

Small Herbal Tincture Presses
Longevity Herbs
Tincture Presses
Krista Thie
1549 West Jewett Blvd.
White Salmon, WA 948672
509-493-2626
Also produce PNW Herb Directory.

Mathres Presses
486 Rich Gulch Road
Mokkelumne Hill, CA 95245
209-286-1232. Fax 209-286-1368. http://www.mathrespresses.com
They are also starting to make larger hyrdraulic presses.

Distillation Equipment for making essential oils.

BENZALCO
Purdue Business & Technology Center
1291 Cumberland Ave., West Lafayette, IN 47906-1385
765-497-1313; Fax 765-463-7004

Hammermills
Most small product people use heavy duty blenders for grinding herbs.
One source is:

Vitamix
8615 Usher Road
Cleveland, OH 44128
1-800-848-2649. Fax 216-235-3726

For FDA labeling information, check out the following Internet site:
http://vm.cfsan.fda.gov/~ams/fig-1.html

Product People Interviewed
for *Medicinal Herbs in the Garden, Field & Marketplace*

Kelly Van Allen
Wind Dancer Llama & Herb Farm
PO Box 86
Bow, WA 98232
winddanc@cnw.com
www.cnw.com/~winddanc/

Robyn Martin
O-LALA Farms
PO Box 75
North San Juan, CA 95960

Wonderland Teas, Herbs & Spices
Linda Quintana, Owner
1305 Railroad Ave.
Bellingham, WA 98225
360-733-0517

Tierney Salter
The Herbalist
2106 N.E. 65th
Seattle, WA 98115
the herbalist@the herbalist.com
www.theherbalist.com

Other Product Supply Information

For suppliers of bottles, packaging, labels etc., I suggest you check in the latest editions of *The Business of Herbs* or the *Herb Growing Marketing and Network* newsletters, or their herb business directories.

Recommended Sources for Bulk Herbs

* means they may also be interested in purchasing organically grown herbs

*Frontier Cooperative Herbs
3021 78th St.
PO Box 299
Norway, IA 52318
www.frontierherb.com

*Pacific Botanicals
4350 Fish Hatchery Rd.
Grants Pass, OR 97527
541-479-7777, Fax 541-479-5271

*Global Botanical
RR 8
545 Welham Rd
Barrie, ON L4M 6E7
705-733-2117, Fax 705-733-2391

*Blessed Herbs
109 Barre Plains Road
Oakham, MA 01068

Trinity Herbs
Bodega, CA

Montana Arnica
PO Box 350057
Grantsdale, MT 59835

*Nature's Cathedral
1995 78th St.
Blairstown, IA 52209-9721
319-454-6959

*Star West Botanicals
11253 Trade Centre Dr.
Rancho Cordova, CA 95742
916-638-8100
Fax 916-638-8100

*Trout Lake Farms
149 Little Mountain Road
PO Box 181
Trout Lake, WA 98650
509-395-2025, Fax 395-2645

*Desert Woman Botanicals
Monica Rude
PO Box 263
Gila, NM 88038
desertwoman@wnmc.net

Regulatory Information

U.S. Food and Drug Administration

Their main offices are located at:

U.S. Food & Drug Administration (HFE-88)
Rockville, MD 20857
1-800-532-4440, Fax 301-443-9676
e-mail: execsec@oc.fda.gov

FDA on Internet: http://www.fda.gov/

The FDA gives permission to manufacturers (or distributors or importers) to market certain kinds of products before they can be sold in interstate commerce. The FDA publishes their proposed regulations in the Federal

Register, which is published daily, Monday through Friday. Copies of this can usually be found in local libraries, county courthouses, or federal buildings.

To search FDA records for their rules about herbal products, you need to look at the Code of Federal Regulations (CFR). These regulations are updated on April 1 of each year and are available for sale some four months later. They are available in public libraries and on the Internet. The parts covering regulations about herbal products are in the sections entitled Food Additives: Title 21, parts 170 -199.

FDA Small Business Representatives

These have been set up to help small businesses whose products are regulated by the FDA; to provide information to help clarify how FDA laws and regulations apply to specific circumstances and products; to suggest methods of meeting those requirements. I would suggest you do some research first on your own, and then contact them with very specific questions. If their phones are very busy (which these days they certainly are) they may take a week or two to get back to you. The phone message will ask you to leave a detailed question about a product you wish to make, and to also leave your address so they can send you the relevant regulations. If you can reach them directly on the phone, they seem quite helpful, but the representative I spoke with reflected some of the confusion surrounding herbal products. "If you say you are making something you call a tincture, we will assume it is a homeopathic product, and it will have to meet those standards and regulations, which are different from those concerning products put out under the DSHEA regulations." What herbalists commonly call herbal tinctures are apparently considered "fluid alcohol extracts" in the regulatory arena. Be patient. And remember that the FDA is trying to cover this world of herbal product frenzy with very few people—most of whom are concerned with things like product recalls. With only 9,000 agents employed, they can hardly be expected to be up on every little nuance of the herb market sector that may be of concern to you or me. Don't use unsafe herbs, then stay with your local town, city, county, and health department rules and regulations, or sometimes your state agriculture department (if you are selling at a farmers' market), and worry about the FDA when your product will be sold to other states.

FDA Small Business Representatives are located as follows:

FDA Northeast Region
Small Business Representative
850 Third Ave.
Brooklyn, NY 11232
718-965-5300, Ext 5528
Fax 718-965-5759

FDA Mid-Atlantic Region
Small Business Representative
900 U.S. Customhouse
2nd & Chestnut St.
Philadelphia, PA 19106
215-597-0537
Fax 215-597-6649

FDA Southeast Region
Small Business Representative
60 Eighth St. N.E.
Atlanta, GA 30309
404-347-4001, Ext. 5256
Fax 404-347-4349

FDA Southwest Region
Small Business Representative
7920 Elmbrook Dr., Ste. 102
Dallas, TX 75247-4982
214-655-8100, Ext. 128
Fax 214-655-8130

FDA Midwest Region
Small Business Representative
20 N. Michigan Ave., Rm. 5120
Chicago, IL 60602
312-353-9400, Ext. 23
Fax 312-886-1682

FDA Pacific Region
Small Business Representative
Oakland Federal Bldg.
1301 Clay St., Ste. 1180-N
Oakland, CA 94612-5217
510-637-3980
Fax 510-637-3977

Labeling Laws: For FDA labeling information, check out the following Internet site: http://vm.cfsan.fda.gov/~ams/fig-1.html

Legal Guidelines for Unlicensed Practitioners, by Dr. Lawrence Wilson. 61 page booklet offering legal hints and help to those working in complementary medicine.
Cost is $16.50 + s&h
1718 E. Valley Parkway #n
Escondido, CA 92027
619-743-1790

Good Manufacturing Practices

To find out the GMPs that refer now to your product, see your local county health department. To find the recent GMPs proposed by the FDA, consult the Federal Register in your library, entry for 2-6-97.

Other Resources on Regulations

Natural Medicine Law Newsletter
Muscatatuck Publishers, Inc.
PO Box 1444, Rockville, MD 20849
Expensive, detailed journal of legal issues surrounding natural medicine.

Organic Resources
Certified Organic Associations of B.C.
c/o B.C. Ministry of Ag, Fisheries & Food
Food Industry Branch
808 Douglas St., Victoria, BC V8W 277
604-387-7166. Fax 604-356-2949

MARKETING RESOURCES
Publications

Whole Foods Magazine
They put out a source directory once a year listing product makers and processors.

WFC Inc.
3000 Hadley Rd.
So. Plainfield, NJ 07080-1117

Richo Cech: *Finding Your Niche: Making a Living With Medicinal Plants.* 1995. Available From Horizon Herbs, PO Box 69, Williams, OR 97544. 12 pp.

Small Directory of Flower & Herb Buyers. Available from Prairie Oak Seed, PO Box 382, Maryville, MO 64468.

Market Report in *HerbalGram.* Usually several pages of details on current herb market world wide. (see media listing)

Check classified ads in both *Herb Growing and Marketing Network* and *Business of Herbs* newsletters. See their listings on page 278.

See the listings in Resources for Product People. Several bulk herb suppliers are also seeking herbs.

Medicinal Herb Consultants
The following people and companies are active consultants with medicinal herbs, issues, and products.

Integrated Crop Management Inc.
Box 43004, Stn. Main
Okanagan Centre, BC V4B1Z6

Agricultural & Horticultural Consulting & Research
Craig Winters
6920 Roosevelt Way N.E. #250
Seattle, WA 98115
206-775-7644. Fax 206-776-3262
fshealth@aol.com

JR Labs
12/13 3871 No. Fraser Way
Burnaby, BC V5J 5G6
604-432-9311. Fax 604-432-7768
jrlabs@istar.ca

Biosciences Enterprise Centre
1721 Lower Water St.
Halifax, Nova Scotia B3J 1S5
902-420-0288. Fax 902-420-0688
jrlabs@ns.sympatico.ca

Andrea Gunner, Ag consultant & business planner. Armstrong, BC. 250-546-2712.

International Directory of Specialists in Herbs, Spices and Medicinal Plants. Lyle Craker, Dept. of Plant and Soil Sciences, University of Massachusetts, Amherst, MA 01003

The Sage Group
Consultants for Herbal Product Makers
1928 8th Ave., W.
Seattle, WA 98119
206-282-1789

North American Herb Professionals Mentioned in
Medicinal Herbs in the Garden, Field & Marketplace

Rather than present a long list of important books on Medicinal Herbs
(and believe me, it would be long), following is a list of well-known American and Canadian herb professionals who are mentioned in this book, or
whose schools or companies we recommend. They often speak and teach
at herbal conferences. Reading their books, or listening to them talk, is a
good way to further your own medicinal herb education. They will lead
you to the other important herbalists you'll want to read. Most medicinal
herb people are remarkably open and supportive, both to each other and
to newcomers.

Branka Barl	Paul Bergener
Peggy Brevoort	Mark Blumenthal
Chanchal Cabrera	Richo Cech
Amanda McQuade Crawford	Ryan Drum
Jim Duke	Steven Foster
Daniel Gagnon	Rosemary Gladstar
James Green	Christopher Hobbs
David Hoffman	Marlin Huffman
Feather Jones	Kathi Keville
Rob McCaleb	Alison McCutcheon
Michael Moore	Jeanne Rose
Ed Smith	Deb Soulé
Elaine Stevens	Michael Tierra
Varro Tyler	Roy Upton
Susan Weed	

How to Contact Us
Lee Sturdivant
PO Box 642P
Friday Harbor, WA 98250
360-378-2648
Toll free book orders: 1-800-770-9070
E-mail: naturals@bootstraps.com
Or visit the Bootstrap Guide Web Site: http://www.bootstraps.com

Tim Blakley
33560 Beech Grove Rd
Rutland, OH 45775
E-mail: tim.blakley@frontierherb.com

Please drop a line if any of these resources come up short for you.

Herb Company Surveys

Following are the companies who responded to our random survey about their needs for new medicinal herb growers. Be sure to also see the Recommended Bulk Herb Suppliers in the Resources section for a few other companies that may well be interested in purchasing what you grow.

Medicinal Tincture & Teamaker Survey

Name of your company: ABCO Laboratories Inc.
Address: 2377 Stanwell Dr., Concord, CA 94520
Telephone: 510-676-1060   *Fax#:* 510-603-7788
email: kbabco@aol.com
Web Site URL:
Your name: David S. Baron

Do you use organically grown herbs in your tinctures? Yes
Please describe or name your present suppliers:
As your needs increase, will you be interested in hearing from other growers? Yes
What specific plants will probably be of most interest to you? All
How small a beginning quantity would you be willing to deal with? One pound
Do you deal primarily with fresh or dried herbs? Both
Do you have special herb crop needs that you wish experienced market gardeners would learn to grow? No
Do you offer written grower guidelines? No
If interested in hearing from other growers, how would you wish to be contacted?: By mail, with a sample.
What person in your company should be contacted? Kristin Bradley, mgr. purchasing/inventory
Do you have any comments you would like to make to those considering growing herbs for your company?

Medicinal Tincture & Teamaker Survey

Name of your company: Alaskan Phytomedicinals
Address: 2986 Gold Hill Rd., Fairbanks, AK 99709-2319
Telephone: 907-479-0992   *Fax#:* 907-479-0992
email: phyto@mosquitonet.com
Web Site URL: www.seedman.com
Your name: Anne-Line J Rochet

Do you use organically grown herbs in your tinctures?
No. see below.

Please describe or name your present suppliers: We have exclusively
harvested and used our own wildcrafted herbs. We insist on 100%
control of the source of our botanicals. We consciously harvest the
best in the Alaskan wilderness.

*As your needs increase, will you be interested in hearing from other
growers?* Recently, I have been looking for an organic source of
roots of plants which do not grow wild in Alaska. Since we insist on
using fresh herbs we have thus excluded buying botanicals other
than roots, due to the shipping factor to Alaska. Leaves or flowers
would reach us wilted, and thus not fresh.

What specific plants will probably be of most interest to you?
I have been looking for organically grown roots of ginseng,
goldenseal and echinacea. I have tried several growers found in the
Herbal Green Pages Directory, but so far have had no response.

How small a beginning quantity would you be willing to deal with?
Ten pounds

Do you deal primarily with fresh or dried herbs? Fresh

*Do you have special herb crop needs that you wish experienced market
gardeners would learn to grow?* Stevia

Do you offer written grower guidelines? No

*If interested in hearing from other growers, how would you wish to be
contacted?* Difficult to get me 'live' on the phone. Mail, Fax or
email might be best.

What person in your company should be contacted? I am the main
decision maker.

*Do you have any comments you would like to make to those considering
growing herbs for your company?* As long as it is organically grown
and harvested at peak of potency (right season/year/time of day).
I have no further requests for now.

Medicinal Tincture & Teamaker Survey

Name of your company: Ancient Mother Herbal Pharmacy
Address: Rt. 1, Box 90, Windom, TX 75492
Telephone: 903-623-4744   *Fax#:* same
email:
Web Site URL:
Your name: Virginia Baker

Do you use organically grown herbs in your tinctures? Yes
Please describe or name your present suppliers: San Francisco Herb Co.,
Trinity Herb Co., and we grow and wildcraft for ourselves.
As your needs increase, will you be interested in hearing from other growers? Yes
What specific plants will probably be of most interest to you? We are
interested in all herbs. We currently stock over 150 herbs used in our
products.
How small a beginning quantity would you be willing to deal with?
One pound.
Do you deal primarily with fresh or dried herbs? Use both but as many
fresh as possible.
*Do you have special herb crop needs that you wish experienced market
gardeners would learn to grow?* Southern Prickly Ash (Xanthoxylum
clava-herculis).
Do you offer written grower guidelines? Not currently
*If interested in hearing from other growers, how would you wish to be
contacted?* Phone or mail is fine. I like to have a catalog or price list
available for reference as I'm looking at re-ordering.
What person in your company should be contacted? Virginia Baker;
William Trezise
*Do you have any comments you would like to make to those considering
growing herbs for your company?* It's very important to us, and anyone
using herbs for medicine, to be absolutely certain of the botanical
identity of the plant matter. We have had occasion to question items
we received and decided to return them to our supplier—due to an
obvious change of appearance for an herb that we work with quite
often. We are a small business and aren't able to carry as large an
inventory as we would like to, so it's even more important to us to
depend on accuracy concerning our products.

Medicinal Tincture & Teamaker Survey

Name of your company: Blessed Herbs
Address: 109 Barre Plains Rd., Oakham, MA 01068
Telephone: 508-882-3839   *Fax#:* 508-882-3755
email: michael@blessedherbs.com
Web Site URL: www.blessedherbs.com
Your name: Michael Volchok

Do you use organically grown herbs in your tinctures? Yes
Please describe or name your present suppliers: Many
As your needs increase, will you be interested in hearing from other growers? Yes
What specific plants will probably be of most interest to you? Calendula
How small a beginning quantity would you be willing to deal with? Ten pounds.
Do you deal primarily with fresh or dried herbs? 50/50
Do you have special herb crop needs that you wish experienced market gardeners would learn to grow? Calendula
Do you offer written grower guidelines? No
If interested in hearing from other growers, how would you wish to be contacted? Mail
What person in your company should be contacted? Michael
Do you have any comments you would like to make to those considering growing herbs for your company? Only call if you have something ready to sell. I am sorry, but 99% of callers have resulted in zero happening.

Medicinal Tincture & Teamaker Survey

Name of your company: Celestial Seasonings, Inc.
Address: 4600 Sleepytime Dr., Boulder, CO 80301
Telephone: 303-530-53   *Fax#:* 303-581-1209
email: kwright@ctea.com
Web Site URL: www.ctea.com
Your name: Kay Wright

Do you use organically grown herbs in your tinctures? Not certified.
Please describe or name your present suppliers: Bulk herb and herbal
extract suppliers—both domestic and international.
*As your needs increase, will you be interested in hearing from other
growers?* Yes
What specific plants will probably be of most interest to you? List
follows
How small a beginning quantity would you be willing to deal with?
500 pounds
Do you deal primarily with fresh or dried herbs? Dried
*Do you have special herb crop needs that you wish experienced market
gardeners would learn to grow?* No
Do you offer written grower guidelines? Yes
*If interested in hearing from other growers, how would you wish to be
contacted?* Fax with company information and product list.
What person in your company should be contacted? Kay Wright
*Do you have any comments you would like to make to those considering
growing herbs for your company?* Celestial Seasonings has established
the following minimum guidelines and requirements for those of
you interested in growing herbs as a livelihood.

1. Purchase of any herb by Celestial Seasonings depends upon
   sample approval by both the Purchasing and Quality Control
   departments. All samples must be a minimum of 500 grams to
   accommodate our complete testing procedures.
2. The grower should have adequate acreage to produce our
   minimum requirements. For the majority of our herbs this
   would be 2000 pounds. If you expect smaller yields we suggest
   that you sell your herbs locally or regionally.
3. The product must be clean, dried, and completely free of
   chemical residues or any extraneous material.
4. The product must be processed and packaged according to
   Celestial Seasonings' specifications (whole leaf and packed in
   bags weighing 50 pounds each, for most products.)

5. To supply Celestial Seasonings, competitive pricing is required. The pricing of agricultural commodities may fluctuate widely in the botanical market.

If you can meet these guidelines, Celestial Seasonings will try to provide information regarding harvesting and drying. We suggest contacting your County Extension Agent for local growing information.

Celestial Seasonings Botanical List

INGREDIENT	LATIN	PLANT PART
Agave Tequilana	*Agave tequilana*	leaves
Alfalfa	*Medicago sativa*	leaves
Allspice	*Pimenta dioica*	berry
Angelica Root	*Angelica archangelica*	root
Anise Seed	*Pimpinella anisum*	seed
Barley	*Hordeum vulgare*	grain
Black pepper	*Piper nigrum*	seeds
Blackberry Chinese	*Rubus suavissimus*	leaves
Blackberry	*Rubus fruticosus*	leaves
Calendula	*Calendula officinalis*	flower
Caramel Malt	*Hordeum vulgare*	grain
Cardamom	*Elettaria cardamomum*	seed
Carob	*Ceratonia siliqua*	fruit
Cassia	*Cinnamomum cassia*	bark
Catnip	*Nepeta cataria*	leaves
Cayenne Pepper	*Capsicum annuum*	seed/pod
Chamomile	*Matricaria chamomilla*	flower
Chamomile Pollen	*Matricaria chamomilla*	pollen
Chicory	*Cichorium intybus*	root
Cloves	*Syzygium aromaticum*	bud
Coriander	*Coriandrum sativum*	seed
Crystal Malt	*Hordeum vulgare*	grain
Dandelion Root	*Taraxacum officinale*	root
Echinacea	*Echinacea angustifolia & purpurea*	leaf/stem & root
Eucalyptus	*Eucalyptus globulus*	leaves
Fennel	*Foeniculum vulgare*	seed
Ginger	*Zingiber officinale*	root
Ginkgo	*Ginkgo biloba*	leaves
Ginseng Eleuthero	*Eleutherococcus senticosus*	root

Celestial Seasonings Botanical List

INGREDIENT	LATIN	PLANT PART
Ginseng Panax	*Panax ginseng*	root
Goldenseal	*Hydrastis canadensis*	leaf/stem
Goldenseal Root	*Hydrastis canadensis*	root
Gotu Kola	*Centelia asiatica*	leaves
Green Tea	*Camellia sinesis*	leaves
Hawthorn	*Crataegus spp*	berry
Hibiscus	*Hibiscus sabdariffa*	calyx
Hops	*Humulus lupulus*	cone
Kola Nut	*Cola acuminata*	nut
Lavender	*Lavandula angustifolia*	flower
Lemon Grass	*Cymbopogon citratus*	leaf
Lemon Peel	*Citrus limon*	fruit
Lemon Verbena	*Lippia citrodora*	leaves
Licorice Root	*Glycyrrhiza glabra*	root
Lo Han Kuo	*Cucurbitaceae ficifolia*	fruit
Lovage	*Levisticum officinale*	root
Milk Thistle	*Silybum marianum*	seed
Nutmeg	*Myristica fragans*	seed
Orange Blossoms	*Citrus sinesis*	flower
Orange Peel	*Citrus sinesis*	fruit
Passion Flower	*Passiflora incarnata*	leaf/pod
Peppermint	*Mentha piperita*	leaves
Quinoa	*Chenopodium*	chaff
Raspberry Pellets	*Rubus idaeus*	leaves
Red Clover	*Trifolium prantense*	leaf/stem
Rooibus	*Aspalathus lineans*	stem/neels
Rosebuds	*Rosa spp*	flower
Rosehips	*Rosa Canina*	fruit
Rosehip Shells	*Rosa canina*	fruit
Sarsaparilla Root	*Smila anstolochiaefolia*	root
Slippery Elm	*Ulmus fulva*	bark
Spearmint	*Mentha spicata*	leaves
Star Anise	*Illicium verum*	fruit
Tilia	*Ternstroemia*	fruit/bud
Wild Cherry Bark	*Prunus serotonia*	bark
Wintergreen	*Gaultheria procumbens*	leaves

Medicinal Tincture & Teamaker Survey

Name of your company: Devonshire Apothecary
Address: 2105 Ashby Ave., Austin, TX 78704
Telephone: 512-444-5039   *Fax#:* 512-443-8176
email:
Web Site URL:
Your name: Nancy Levy

Do you use organically grown herbs in your tinctures? Yes
Please describe or name your present suppliers: Pacific Botanicals,
Blessed Herbs, Frontier Herbs. We pick and grow a few ourselves.
Also purchase direct from other growers.
*As your needs increase, will you be interested in hearing from other
growers?* Yes
What specific plants will probably be of most interest to you?
Echinacea, arnica, valerian root
How small a beginning quantity would you be willing to deal with?
20 to 40 pounds of fresh herbs
Do you deal primarily with fresh or dried herbs? Both
*Do you have special herb crop needs that you wish experienced market
gardeners would learn to grow?*
Do you offer written grower guidelines? No
*If interested in hearing from other growers, how would you wish to be
contacted?* Phone first to see if I need what you have; mail, with a
sample, if it's something I use and your price is competitive.
What person in your company should be contacted? Nancy Levy
*Do you have any comments you would like to make to those considering
growing herbs for your company?* Don't tie up your whole crop with
big companies. Remember some of us are small, too. Be willing to
work with us. Don't compete with your customers. If you want me
to buy your herbs, don't be making my product. That's why we
don't buy from several suppliers.

Medicinal Tincture & Teamaker Survey

Name of your company: Dragon River Herbals
Address: PO Box 28, El Rito, NM 87530
Telephone: 505-581-4441   *Fax#:* 505-581-9149
email:
Web Site URL:
Your name: Patty Shure

Do you use organically grown herbs in your tinctures? Yes
Please describe or name your present suppliers:
As your needs increase, will you be interested in hearing from other growers? Yes
What specific plants will probably be of most interest to you? Echinacea angustifolia, arnica, goldenseal, etc.
How small a beginning quantity would you be willing to deal with? 2-5 pounds.
Do you deal primarily with fresh or dried herbs? Both
Do you have special herb crop needs that you wish experienced market gardeners would learn to grow?
Do you offer written grower guidelines?
If interested in hearing from other growers, how would you wish to be contacted? Phone or mail. I'd love to receive a growing list by mail.
What person in your company should be contacted?: Patty Shure.
Do you have any comments you would like to make to those considering growing herbs for your company? We are very small and particular about our herbs, but also easy to work with.

Medicinal Tincture & Teamaker Survey

Name of your company: East Earth Herb
Address: 4091 W 11th Ave., Eugene OR 97402
Telephone: 541-687-0155   *Fax#:* 541-485-7347
email: david@eastearth.com
Web Site URL:
Your name: David Doty

Do you use organically grown herbs in your tinctures? Rarely
Please describe or name your present suppliers: Confidential global network of growers and distributors
As your needs increase, will you be interested in hearing from other growers? yes
What specific plants will probably be of most interest to you? gold-enseal, echinacea angustifolia, black cohosh
How small a beginning quantity would you be willing to deal with? 1,000 pounds
Do you deal primarily with fresh or dried herbs? Dried
Do you have special herb crop needs that you wish experienced market gardeners would learn to grow? As above.
Do you offer written grower guidelines? Yes
If interested in hearing from other growers, how would you wish to be contacted? Mail. I have a questionnaire.
What person in your company should be contacted? David Doty
Do you have any comments you would like to make to those considering growing herbs for your company? See below.

Contract Grower Questionnaire from East Earth Herb, Inc.

Grower Name _____

Firm Name _____

Address _____

Phone, Fax etc._____

1. Current acreage owned:

2. Current acreage leased:

3. Crops grown this year and acreage of each:

4. What other crops do you have experience at growing for sale:

5. What other crops are grown in your area:

6. What crops are being grown on immediately neighboring land:

7. Do you have irrigation? If so, what type?

8. Climatic conditions, annual rainfall, average temps, low temps, high temps, special considerations (hail, monsoon, etc.):

9. What are the major insect pest problems:

10. What are the major weed problems:

11. What are the major fungal, or bacteriological problems:

12. What philosophy do you use to control your problems:

13. What philosophy do you use for nutrition:

Medicinal Tincture & Teamaker Survey

Name of your company: Eclectic Institute, Inc.
Address: 14385 SE Lusted Rd., Sandy, OR 97055
Telephone: 503-668-4120   *Fax#:* 503-668-3227
email:
Web Site URL:
Your name: Ed Alstat

Do you use organically grown herbs in your tinctures? Of course
Please describe or name your present suppliers: We grow our own, as
well as use Trout Lake Farm, Pacific Botanicals.
*As your needs increase, will you be interested in hearing from other
growers?* I've been preaching this for ten years.
What specific plants will probably be of most interest to you? St. John's
wort, echinacea angustifolia, milk thistle, ginkgo, feverfew
How small a beginning quantity would you be willing to deal with?
25 pounds.
Do you deal primarily with fresh or dried herbs? Fresh
*Do you have special herb crop needs that you wish experienced market
gardeners would learn to grow?*
Do you offer written grower guidelines? Yes
*If interested in hearing from other growers, how would you wish to be
contacted?* Mail only.
What person in your company should be contacted? Ed Alstat
*Do you have any comments you would like to make to those considering
growing herbs for your company?*

Medicinal Tincture & Teamaker Survey

Name of your company: Essence of Life Ministries & Herbal Products
Address: Rt. 1, Box 172, Little Hocking, OH 45742
Telephone: 614-989-2300   *Fax#:*
email:
Web Site URL:
Your name: Michael Minear, ND; Debby Minear, MH

Do you use organically grown herbs in your tinctures? No.
Please describe or name your present suppliers: Local family; wildcrafters; Blessed Herbs; Frontier.
As your needs increase, will you be interested in hearing from other growers? Yes
What specific plants will probably be of most interest to you? We work with over 100 varieties.
How small a beginning quantity would you be willing to deal with? ½ to one pound.
Do you deal primarily with fresh or dried herbs? Both
Do you have special herb crop needs that you wish experienced market gardeners would learn to grow?
Do you offer written grower guidelines? No.
If interested in hearing from other growers, how would you wish to be contacted? Mail with a sample.
What person in your company should be contacted? Debby Minear.
Do you have any comments you would like to make to those considering growing herbs for your company?

Medicinal Tincture & Teamaker Survey

Name of your company: Frontier Natural Products Co-op
Address: 3021 78th St. Norway, Iowa 52318
Telephone: 319-227-7996   *Fax#:* 319-227-7966
email: barb.letchworth@frontierherb.com
Web Site URL: www.frontierherb.com
Your name: Barb Letchworth

Do you use organically grown herbs in your tinctures? Most
Please describe or name your present suppliers: For fresh herbs, I deal
directly with growers
*As your needs increase, will you be interested in hearing from other
growers?* Yes!!
What specific plants will probably be of most interest to you? Certified
Organic: Ginkgo leaves, donquai root, black cohosh root, astraga-
lus root, eyebright herb
How small a beginning quantity would you be willing to deal with?
100 pounds for dry; 50-100 pounds for fresh
Do you deal primarily with fresh or dried herbs? Dried
*Do you have special herb crop needs that you wish experienced market
gardeners would learn to grow?* Lemon balm leaf, more valerian
root, dandelion leaf & root, in addition to the list above.
Do you offer written grower guidelines? Not yet, but Tim Blakley
will be working on this, too.
*If interested in hearing from other growers, how would you wish to be
contacted?* Fax, phone, e-mail. If already a grower, with sample.
What person in your company should be contacted? Barb Letchworth
*Do you have any comments you would like to make to those considering
growing herbs for your company?* Frontier quality standards are very
high and we prefer to work closely with growers on our requirements. This can include a visit to Frontier, meeting with quality
control, seeing what the herb should look like when we receive it.

Medicinal Tincture & Teamaker Survey

Name of your company: Harvest Moon / Flower Power Teas
Address: PO Box 2877, Santa Cruz, CA 95063
Telephone: 408-425-3310   *Fax#:*
email:
Web Site URL:
Your name: Julie Rothman

Do you use organically grown herbs in your tinctures? Yes
Please describe or name your present suppliers: Pacific Botanicals,
local growers, Oregon's Wild Harvest
*As your needs increase, will you be interested in hearing from other
growers?* Yes
What specific plants will probably be of most interest to you? Gotu
Kola, organic goldenseal
How small a beginning quantity would you be willing to deal with?
Do you deal primarily with fresh or dried herbs? Fresh
*Do you have special herb crop needs that you wish experienced market
gardeners would learn to grow?*
Do you offer written grower guidelines? No
*If interested in hearing from other growers, how would you wish to be
contacted?* Mail or call the Herb Room at 408-429-8108. Samples
would be great.
What person in your company should be contacted? Julie Rothman
*Do you have any comments you would like to make to those considering
growing herbs for your company?* I own a tea company and would be
interested in organically grown dried herbs for my teas, along with
fresh organic herbs for the tincture business: Harvest Moon, that is
owned by the Herb Room, where I work part time.

Medicinal Tincture & Teamaker Survey

Name of your company: Hawk Canyon Herb Farm
Address: 2280 Grass Valley Hwy. #136, Auburn, CA 95603
Telephone: 916-887-0626   *Fax#:*
email:
Web Site URL:
Your name: Kendra Douglass

I am no longer an herb grower, but would like to say that the hardest part of starting a business growing herbs for medicinal use is hooking up with someone who will buy a small quantity of herbs: ten to twenty pounds of echinacea root, for example. The second hardest thing is knowing how to ship the product so fresh root gets there without spoilage.

I only got as far as selling at the local Farmers' Market. It wasn't financially feasible to continue.

Medicinal Tincture & Teamaker Survey

Name of your company: Health 4 All Products Ltd.
Address: 545 Welham Rd., Barrie, ON LYN 8Z7
Telephone: 705-733-2117   *Fax#:* 705-733-2391
email:
Web Site URL:
Your name: Kathy Vessair

Do you use organically grown herbs in your teas? Yes
Please describe or name your present suppliers: Farmers, bulk suppliers, importers.
As your needs increase, will you be interested in hearing from other growers? yes
What specific plants will probably be of most interest to you?
echinaceas, golden seal, St. John's wort, yarrow, etc.
How small a beginning quantity would you be willing to deal with?
Do you deal primarily with fresh or dried herbs?
Do you have special herb crop needs that you wish experienced market gardeners would learn to grow?
Do you offer written grower guidelines? attached
If interested in hearing from other growers, how would you wish to be contacted? Either phone or Fax. See Buyers Wish List.
What person in your company should be contacted? Kathy Vessair
Do you have any comments you would like to make to those considering growing herbs for your company?

Buyers Wish List from Health 4 All Products

One of the requirements being placed upon the wholesaler is a stringent and detailed paper trail. In addition to lot specific Certificates of Analysis, this paper trail must document the crop from its conceptual stages to its final delivery to us, the Purchaser.
We will be required to keep the following information for each product lot purchased.

- What crops were grown on the land prior to the lot being offered for sale.
- If the land is certified organic, or in the process of becoming so. (If certified, a copy of the certificate will be required with the other documentation.)

Buyers Wish List from Health 4 All Products *(Continued)*

- What sprays (insecticides, fertilizers, etc.) were used on this land prior to and during the production of the lot being offered for sale.
- Where the seed for the lot being offered for sale was purchased.
- What type of machinery was used to plant the product, and how and when it was planted.
- How the product was grown, and what it was grown beside.
- Any machinery used in the weeding and harvesting of the product.
- What geographical location the product was grown in.
- How the product was dried. (Specific procedures including times and temperature, as well as machinery used.)
- If the product was cut, what machinery was used, and the procedure used to process it.
- A sample of the product being offered is appreciated prior to the purchase of the product.
- What the product is packed in. (Specific packaging materials.)
- If any other agencies assisted in the production of this product, and if so, who. (Example: Agriculture Canada or Agriculture Ontario.)
- A detailed Certificate of Analysis which includes microbiological and chemical analysis that is lot specific to the crop.
- As the Purchaser, we would also like to keep in contact with you, the Farmer, during the growing process. In this way, both of us may have our questions and/or concerns addressed.
- To aid in production scheduling, we would like to be informed as soon as possible of any anticipated delays in availability dates, or adjustments in the anticipated harvested yield.

By keeping detailed records of your crops and supplying complete certificates, which are lot specific, helps to aid in the marketability of your product. If we can easily obtain the information requested, it saves us time and money and makes your crop that much more attractive. Happy Growing!

Medicinal Tincture & Teamaker Survey

Name of your company: Herb Pharm
Address: PO Box 116, Williams, OR 97544
Telephone: 541-846-6162   *Fax#:*
email: *Web Site URL:*
Your name: Richard A. Cech

Do you use organically grown herbs in your tinctures? Yes
Please describe or name your present suppliers: Confidential
As your needs increase, will you be interested in hearing from other growers? No, I will contact or increase orders to existing vendors. We cannot accept new growers at this time.
What specific plants will probably be of most interest to you? Echinacea, valerian in 500 lb. lots.
How small a beginning quantity would you be willing to deal with?
Do you deal primarily with fresh or dried herbs? Both
Do you have special herb crop needs that you wish experienced market gardeners would learn to grow? Ginseng, goldenseal, black cohosh, wild yam, collinsonia, bloodroot, gentian, blue cohosh—all in 100 lb lots.
Do you offer written grower guidelines? No.
If interested in hearing from other growers, how would you wish to be contacted? We have too many people contacting us. If you have any of these organically grown plants in 100 lb lots, please write ONLY. We really do not wish to be listed as buyers at this time.
What person in your company should be contacted?
Do you have any comments you would like to make to those considering growing herbs for your company?

Medicinal Tincture & Teamaker Survey

Name of your company: Herb Technology
Address: 1305 NE 45th, Ste # 205, Seattle, WA 98105
Telephone: 206-547-2007   *Fax#:* 206-547-4240
email:
Web Site URL:
Your name: K. P. Khalja

Do you use organically grown herbs in your tinctures? Emphatically yes
Please describe or name your present suppliers: World wide procurement and brokering in North America, Europe, and Asia. $20 million per annum company.
As your needs increase, will you be interested in hearing from other growers? Absolutely. We are in process of going 100% organic; especially in Europe.
What specific plants will probably be of most interest to you? Full spectrum of culinary and medicinal herbs
How small a beginning quantity would you be willing to deal with? One pound
Do you deal primarily with fresh or dried herbs? Dried
Do you have special herb crop needs that you wish experienced market gardeners would learn to grow?
Do you offer written grower guidelines? Yes, call procurement: Karam Singh @ 541-461-2160
If interested in hearing from other growers, how would you wish to be contacted? Phone as above
What person in your company should be contacted? Karam Singh 541-461-2160
Do you have any comments you would like to make to those considering growing herbs for your company?

Medicinal Tincture & Teamaker Survey

Name of your company: Herbalist & Alchemist, Inc.
Address: PO Box 553, Broadway, NJ 08808
Telephone: 908-689-9020   *Fax#:* 908-689-9071
email:
Web Site URL:
Your name: Betzy Bancroft

Do you use organically grown herbs in your tinctures? Yes
Please describe or name your present suppliers: Some herb farms and established gatherers. (Pacific Botanicals, Ryan Drum); some local friends, farmers. Trying to do business with primary sources—not brokers.
As your needs increase, will you be interested in hearing from other growers? Yes
What specific plants will probably be of most interest to you? Eyebright (*Euphrasia canadensis*), Sundew (*drosera*), Helonias. Other swamp things, cultivated scarce species.
How small a beginning quantity would you be willing to deal with? Five pounds
Do you deal primarily with fresh or dried herbs? Both
Do you have special herb crop needs that you wish experienced market gardeners would learn to grow? Eyebright, goldenseal, etc.
Do you offer written grower guidelines? Yes. We tell what part, harvested when and how etc. We also have growers and a horticulturist on staff here in lab and office.
If interested in hearing from other growers, how would you wish to be contacted? Initially phone is nice, but backed up with clear list of available species, specs and pricing. Samples are nice, too.
What person in your company should be contacted? Betzy Bancroft or David Winston
Do you have any comments you would like to make to those considering growing herbs for your company? Reliability is a crucial issue. Straight and honest info on availability, price, quality, etc; return phone calls promptly, pack fresh shipments properly; have shipping guidelines worked out in advance; clean plants, etc.
Here's the story from the purchaser's point of view. I have worked with established suppliers like Pacific and Island herbs for 10 years and have tried many smaller and newer suppliers also.

Herbalist & Alchemist, Inc. *(Continued)*

#1. Be honest about what we can get from you. (I have ordered herbs that the gatherer never bothered to pick.) If you will not be able to supply the plant, let the purchaser know as soon as possible to make other arrangements—well before the plant is out of season. This includes returning purchaser's calls when checking up.

#2. As a purchaser, I try to be clear about what part, when harvested, etc. In return, we expect what we ask for, gathered carefully. Herbs should be clean, not contaminated with stuff, other plants, dead leaves, etc.

#3. Shipping fresh material is often a problem. Learn how to pack fresh herbs so they stay vibrant and fresh. Work out how to ship ahead of time and let purchaser know when to expect shipment. Then pack herbs as soon as possible after harvest and send agreed-upon way. Pack in brown or plain paper, wrapped ice packs layered between bags. Watch out for oversize boxes!

Communication and reliability are crucial.

Quality of herbs is crucial.

Co-ordinate shipping w/purchaser; don't ship airs before weekend or holidays, etc.

Medicinal Tincture & Teamaker Survey

Name of your company: Herbs Etc. Inc
Address: 1340 Rufina Circle, Santa Fe, NM 87505
Telephone: 505-471-6488   *Fax#:* 505-471-0941
email: botandan@aol.com
Web Site URL:
Your name: Daniel Gagnon, President & medical herbalist.

Do you use organically grown herbs in your tinctures? Yes. Many
Please describe or name your present suppliers: Pacific Botanicals,
Trout Lake Farm, Windy Pines
*As your needs increase, will you be interested in hearing from other
growers?* Yes. We are especially looking for third party certified
organic farmers and medicinal plant growers.
What specific plants will probably be of most interest to you? Yerba
Mansa, Goldenseal, Ginkgo, Jack in the Pulpit, Passion Flower.
How small a beginning quantity would you be willing to deal with?
25 pounds if fresh, 10 pounds if dry.
Do you deal primarily with fresh or dried herbs? Both, about equally
*Do you have special herb crop needs that you wish experienced market
gardeners would learn to grow?* We would love to get the above
herbs to be certified organically grown.
Do you offer written grower guidelines? Yes
*If interested in hearing from other growers, how would you wish to be
contacted?* Please contact us by mail with samples, if appropriate.
Include a list of herbs you are growing or specific herbs you would
like to grow (top 10 list).
What person in your company should be contacted? Jamie Reagan,
Herb Buyer.
*Do you have any comments you would like to make to those considering
growing herbs for your company?* We love it when serious homework
has been done prior to contacting us. Growing a medicinal crop of
some kind prior to contacting us is a definite plus because we see
that you understand the market. We are willing to work with you as
you grow with us.

Medicinal Tincture & Teamaker Survey

Name of your company: Herbs For Kids
Address: 151 Evergreen Dr., Bozeman, MT 59715
Telephone: 406-587-0180   *Fax#:* 406-587-0111
email:
Web Site URL:
Your name: Rick Cooper

Do you use organically grown herbs in your tinctures? Yes
Please describe or name your present suppliers: Proprietary info
As your needs increase, will you be interested in hearing from other growers? Yes
What specific plants will probably be of most interest to you? Astragalus membranaceus, echinacea purpurea root and flower, Oregon grape root.
How small a beginning quantity would you be willing to deal with? Depends on herb; 50 to 100 pounds of some; 1,000 pounds of others.
Do you deal primarily with fresh or dried herbs? Dried
Do you have special herb crop needs that you wish experienced market gardeners would learn to grow? Astragalus
Do you offer written grower guidelines? No, but we do require organic certification proof from growers.
If interested in hearing from other growers, how would you wish to be contacted? Mail, with sample.
What person in your company should be contacted? Jeanne Harper
Do you have any comments you would like to make to those considering growing herbs for your company? Good luck!

Medicinal Tincture & Teamaker Survey

Name of your company: Motherlove Herbal Company
Address: PO Box 101, Laporte, CO 80535
Telephone: 970-493-2892   *Fax#:* 970-224-4844
email: mother@motherlove.com
Web Site URL: www.motherlove.com
Your name: Kathryn Cox

Do you use organically grown herbs in your tinctures? Yes
Please describe or name your present suppliers: Shortgrass in
Longmont, CO, Pacific Botanicals in Grants Pass, OR.
*As your needs increase, will you be interested in hearing from other
growers?* Yes
What specific plants will probably be of most interest to you? Fresh
blessed thistle, nettles, dandelion, raspberry, yellow dock, red
clover blossoms, horsetail, St. John's wort, motherwort, cleavers,
oats, skullcap.
How small a beginning quantity would you be willing to deal with?
10 pounds.
Do you deal primarily with fresh or dried herbs? Fresh
*Do you have special herb crop needs that you wish experienced market
gardeners would learn to grow?* Not right now
Do you offer written grower guidelines? No
*If interested in hearing from other growers, how would you wish to be
contacted?* By phone or mail first, then I would call and request
samples of herbs I'd be interested in quantity.
What person in your company should be contacted? Kathryn Cox
*Do you have any comments you would like to make to those considering
growing herbs for your company?* Most of the herbs I use are grown
in this area (do well in the Rocky Mtn. environment.) Shortgrass
can deliver right to my door within hours of picking, eliminating
shipping costs and time before processing. So I would rely mostly
on growers closer to my area. I do get certified organic dried herbs
from growers further away for our teas. We personally wildcraft
some of our herbs, especially ones I've found hard to buy, such as
fresh mullein flower (not stalk), malva neglecta (common garden
mallow) and rose petals.

Medicinal Tincture & Teamaker Survey

Name of your company: Nature's Meadow™
Address: PO Box 510, Gainesville, MO 65655
Telephone: 417-679-2300   *Fax#:* 417-679-3760
email:
Web Site URL:
Your name: Mary Spencer

Do you use organically grown herbs in your tinctures? Yes
Please describe or name your present suppliers: San Francisco Herbs,
Frontier Herbs. (Almost all of our herbs are wildcrafted.)
*As your needs increase, will you be interested in hearing from other
growers?* Yes
What specific plants will probably be of most interest to you? Chaparral
How small a beginning quantity would you be willing to deal with?
25 pounds
Do you deal primarily with fresh or dried herbs? Fresh
*Do you have special herb crop needs that you wish experienced market
gardeners would learn to grow?*
Do you offer written grower guidelines?
*If interested in hearing from other growers, how would you wish to be
contacted?* Mail
What person in your company should be contacted? Michael or Mary
*Do you have any comments you would like to make to those considering
growing herbs for your company?* We test every herb for toxins and
chemicals, and will return them if they are not pure and clean.

Medicinal Tincture & Teamaker Survey

Name of your company: Terra Firma Botanials, Inc.
Address: PO Box 5680, Eugene OR 97405
Telephone: 541-485-7726   *Fax#:* 541-485-8600
email: terrafirm@continet.com
Web Site URL:
Your name: River Kennedy

Do you use organically grown herbs in your tinctures? Yes
Please describe or name your present suppliers: Pacific Botanicals,
Oregon's Wild Harvest
*As your needs increase, will you be interested in hearing from other
growers?* Yes
What specific plants will probably be of most interest to you? Fresh
pleursy root, cayenne, fresh spilanthes and others.
How small a beginning quantity would you be willing to deal with?
Do you deal primarily with fresh or dried herbs? Fresh
*Do you have special herb crop needs that you wish experienced market
gardeners would learn to grow?* No
Do you offer written grower guidelines? No
*If interested in hearing from other growers, how would you wish to be
contacted?* Mail
What person in your company should be contacted? River Kennedy
*Do you have any comments you would like to make to those considering
growing herbs for your company?* Certified organically grown is
essential

Medicinal Tincture & Teamaker Survey

Name of your company: Unitea Herbs
Address: 1705 14th St., Ste. 318, Boulder, CO 80302
Telephone: 303-443-1248   *Fax#:* 303-442-1316
email:
Web Site URL: www.indra.com/~brigitte
Your name: Rob Wilcox

Do you use organically grown herbs in your teas? Yes
Please describe or name your present suppliers: Trout Lake Farms,
Pacific Botanicals
*As your needs increase, will you be interested in hearing from other
growers?* yes
What specific plants will probably be of most interest to you? Many
"weeds," those which are not currently available from Trout Lake
or Pacific. Can contact us for complete list.
How small a beginning quantity would you be willing to deal with?
25 to 50 lbs.
Do you deal primarily with fresh or dried herbs? Dried, exclusively.
*Do you have special herb crop needs that you wish experienced market
gardeners would learn to grow?* Yellow dock, chamomile, thyme,
rosemary, Chinese herbs, etc.
Do you offer written grower guidelines? Amounts used per year and
form of cut needed.
*If interested in hearing from other growers, how would you wish to be
contacted?* Either phone or mail is fine; we would definitely need to
see a sample and third party organic certification.
What person in your company should be contacted? Rob Wilcox
*Do you have any comments you would like to make to those considering
growing herbs for your company?* That we do require 3rd party
organic certification, and that the herbs must be dried and milled
to our specifications.

Medicinal Tincture & Teamaker Survey

Name of your company: Wilderness Herbs
Address: PO Box 518, Ishpeming, MI 49849
Telephone: *Fax#:*
email:
Web Site URL:
Your name: Victoria Jungwirth

Do you use organically grown herbs in your tinctures? Yes
Please describe or name your present suppliers: Ameriherb, Inc., Wild
Botanicals, Wild Weeds
*As your needs increase, will you be interested in hearing from other
growers?* Yes, but I expect our needs to remain small.
What specific plants will probably be of most interest to you?
Echinacea, ginseng, and goldenseal.
How small a beginning quantity would you be willing to deal with?
Five pounds.
Do you deal primarily with fresh or dried herbs? Fresh
*Do you have special herb crop needs that you wish experienced market
gardeners would learn to grow?*
Do you offer written grower guidelines? No.
*If interested in hearing from other growers, how would you wish to be
contacted?* Mail
What person in your company should be contacted? Victoria
Jungwirth
*Do you have any comments you would like to make to those considering
growing herbs for your company?* We primarily wildcraft our herbs
and our need for organically grown herbs is small.

Medicinal Tincture & Teamaker Survey

Name of your company: Wise Woman Herbals, Inc.
Address: PO Box 279, Creswell, OR 97426
Telephone: 541-895-5152   *Fax#:* 541-895-5174
email: wwh@rio.com
Web Site URL:
Your name: Sharol Tilgner, N.D.

Do you use organically grown herbs in your products? Yes
Please describe or name your present suppliers: Many suppliers.
A huge amount of both organic growers and wildcrafters.
As your needs increase, will you be interested in hearing from other growers? Yes. We also grow our own herbs now due to a lack of quality on the market.
What specific plants will probably be of most interest to you? Those we can't grow in the Pacific Northwest.
How small a beginning quantity would you be willing to deal with? 10 lbs. We buy up to 1000 lbs of a kind.
Do you deal primarily with fresh or dried herbs? Both
Do you have special herb crop needs that you wish experienced market gardeners would learn to grow?
Do you offer written grower guidelines? Yes
If interested in hearing from other growers, how would you wish to be contacted? By mail. Need info on who growers are; copy of organic certification; list of fresh and dry products and prices.
What person in your company should be contacted? Vincent.
Do you have any comments you would like to make to those considering growing herbs for your company? Quality is #1 concern. Price is #2 concern.

Index

Plant Index

Bootstrap $\int$ *Guides* Order Form

QTY	TITLE	PRICE	TOTAL
	FLOWERS FOR SALE: *Growing and Marketing Cut Flowers,* *Backyard to Small Acreage* 225 pages	$14.95	
	HERBS FOR SALE: *Growing and Marketing Herbs, Herbal Products* *and Herbal Know-How* 250 pages	$14.95	
	PROFITS FROM YOUR BACKYARD *HERB GARDEN* *A First Steps Guide* 120 pages	$10.95	
	MEDICINAL HERBS: *In the Garden,* *Field & Marketplace* 336 pages	$24.95	
	Subtotal		
	Postage and Handling (Add $2.00 for one book, 50¢ for each additional book.)		
	Sales tax (WA residents only, add 7%)		
	Total Enclosed		

I understand that I may return any books for a full refund if not satisfied.

Your Name _____

Address _____

City_____

State / Zip _____

Daytime Phone _____

Enclosed is my check payable to San Juan Naturals , or
Please charge my _____ MasterCard _____ Visa

Account No. _____

Exp. Date _____ Signature _____

Mail or Fax to: SAN JUAN NATURALS
PO Box 642P Friday Harbor, WA 98250
Toll Free Order Phone: 1-800-770-9070
Fax: 206-378-2548
E-mail: naturals@bootstraps.com
Web site: www.bootstraps.com

IF THIS IS A LIBRARY BOOK,
PLEASE PHOTOCOPY
THIS PAGE.
THANK YOU
FOR YOUR ORDER!